DATE DUE

JUL 01 1992		
Jul 11·8·92		

DEMCO 38-297

Obstetrics:
Psychological
and Psychiatric
Syndromes

CURRENT TOPICS IN OBSTETRICS AND GYNECOLOGY

Series Editor

Morton A. Stenchever, MD

Professor and Chairman
Department of Obstetrics and Gynecology
University of Washington
School of Medicine
Seattle, Washington

Controversies in Reproductive Endocrinology and Infertility

Michael R. Soules, MD

Caring for the Older Woman

Morton A. Stenchever, MD and George A. Aagaard, MD

Caring for the Exercising Woman

Ralph W. Hale, MD

Gynecologic Oncology: Treatment Rationale and Techniques

Benjamin E. Greer, MD and Jonathan S. Berek, MD

Obstetrics: Psychological and Psychiatric Syndromes

John Patrick O'Grady, MD

Obstetrics: Psychological and Psychiatric Syndromes

Editor
John Patrick O'Grady, MD

Associate Professor
Department of Obstetrics and Gynecology
Tufts University School of Medicine

Chief, Division of Maternal-Fetal Medicine
Baystate Medical Center
Springfield, Massachusetts

Associate Editor
Miriam Rosenthal, MD

Associate Professor
Department of Psychiatry and Reproductive Biology
Case Western Reserve University School of Medicine
University MacDonald Womens Hospital
Cleveland, Ohio

Elsevier
New York • Amsterdam • London • Tokyo

Elsevier Science Publishing Co., Inc.
655 Avenue of the Americas, New York, New York 10010

Sole distributors outside the United States and Canada:
Elsevier Science Publishers B.V.
P.O. Box 211, 1000 AE Amsterdam, The Netherlands

Library of Congress Cataloging-in-Publication Data

Obstetrics: psychological and psychiatric syndromes/ editor,
    John Patrick O'Grady; associate editor, Miriam Rosenthal.
       p. cm. — (Current topics in Obstetrics and gynecology)
    Includes index.
    ISBN 0-444-01620-1 (hardcover : alk. paper)
    1. Mental illness in pregnancy. 2. Pregnancy—Psychological aspects.
I. O'Grady, John Patrick, 1945- . II. Rosenthal, M.B. (Miriam B.) III. Series.
    [DNLM: 1. Mental Disorders —pregnancy. 2. Pregnancy—psychology.
3. Pregnancy Complications—psychology. WQ 240 0138]
RG588.027 1992
618.3'001'9—dc20   91-34475
                                              CIP

Current printing (last digit):
10 9 8 7 6 5 4 3 2 1

Manufactured in the United States of America

To Caitlin, Cristin, and Sean
  who never stop teaching me new things

To Justin, Alison, and Conner
  the brightness of the future

Contents

Foreword

For many years physicians practicing obstetrics and gynecology have been well-trained and well-versed in the diagnosis and management of the pathophysiologic conditions that affect the patients they serve. Training programs, postgraduate courses, and other CME activities have been heavily weighted with up-to-date information that relates to these entities. On the other hand, psychological and psychosocial problems have tended to be dealt with only superficially in residency, fellowship, and CME programs. Although women in their reproductive years often suffer from depression, anxiety reactions, personality disorders, psychoses, and other emotional disorders, physicians caring for their reproductive needs often are not trained to identify or manage the problems that occur when pregnancy is superimposed on these conditions. Also, women who are pregnant must often face losses, not only of the pregnancy but in other aspects of their lives as well. Their obstetricians, however, are rarely trained to identify and deal with the grief that will always accompany these losses.

This book deals with the psychological and psychosocial problems that occur during pregnancy. John Patrick O'Grady, the volume editor, is a perinatologist with a long-term interest in the psychiatric aspects of obstetrics. Miriam Rosenthal is a psychiatrist who has devoted her career to studying the psychiatric problems of patients with medical and reproductive illness. The chapter authors span the spectrum of obstetricians, psychiatrists, and other mental health workers with a specific interest in the emotional problems that women face. This book should be of great value in helping obstetricians and other physicians who care for pregnant women to identify psychiatric, psychosocial, and other emotional problems in their patients and to deal with them effectively. It should also be of particular value to individuals training in obstetrics and gynecology and other specialties that relate to women in their reproductive years.

Morton A. Stenchever, MD

Preface

Whoever thinks a faultless piece to see
Thinks what ne'er was, nor is, nor e'er shall be
An Essay on Criticism
Alexander Pope
1688–1744

Practitioners of obstetrics, midwifery, and family medicine are repeatedly drilled to recognize abnormalities in the physiology of pregnant women. Also, a great deal of effort in modern obstetric training is expended in reviewing various techniques of operative obstetrics and in the interpretation of electronic fetal monitoring strips and ultrasonic scans. Despite this emphasis in their training on technical competence in operative obstetrics and understanding of the physiology of medical disorders, these same clinicians are, in general, much less knowledgeable concerning the psychological disturbances that may develop during gestation. Further, little is found in many standard textbooks of obstetrics concerning the management of uncommon obstetric and psychological disorders such as pseudocyesis, postpartum psychosis, or denial of pregnancy/infanticide. Often the clinician is bewildered or overcome by the complexity and the intensity of the psychological reactions observed in these and other conditions. In the management of the much more common problems of postpartum depression, illicit drug use, and maternal reactions to induced or spontaneous abortion, similar difficulties of limited training and inadequate reference sources exist. All too commonly, formal obstetric education in the handling of such conditions is either incomplete or nonexistent, reflecting the uncertainty or inexperience of even senior clinicians in such disorders.

The obstetric attendant is not alone in these difficulties. Many psychiatrists or psychologists attempting to treat pregnant women are similarly bothered by uncertainties concerning which drug therapies are safe, the effects of the physiology of pregnancy on treatment, and, inevitably, medicolegal considerations if the outcome of treatment is not good.

In dealing with pregnancy, the clinician faces dilemmas not encountered in other types of medical practice. The interests of the fetus, mother, family, and society commonly do not coincide and may be entirely at odds. This is especially true when maternal behavior is recognized to be dangerous to the fetus—for example, in instances of maternal drug addiction. Even basic physiology is a problem. The metabolism of any drugs administered recreationally or therapeutically is altered by the physiology of pregnancy. The effects of drugs on the fetus are not entirely predictable and may vary considerably depending upon the trimester when they are administered. Finally, maternal physiology rapidly alters postpartum, and drug distribution, especially into breast milk in nursing mothers, is a persisting concern. Despite these difficulties and many others, management decisions must be made. The classic resort to masterful inaction and determined optimism when it is unclear how to proceed is simply not acceptable.

This book evolved from a series of lectures originally prepared by the associate editor for obstetrical residents and medical students at Case Western Reserve University. The original intention was to provide direction on the management of depressed and psychotic postpartum patients. From that beginning, the original idea has grown into a full text.

This book is divided into four sections. The introductory chapter reviews the demography of clinical obstetrics with special attention to recent changes in the obstetric population and the experience of childbirth. The second section serves as a general clinical introduction, reviewing patient interviewing skills and the legal and ethical issues that underlie medical practice. An attempt is made in this section to outline the major current problems in these fields. The central bulk of the text discusses the psychophysiology of normal gestation and the psychopathology of a number of selected conditions. The aim here is to pay special attention to the recognition of problems and to suggest practical clinical management. In the concluding section various methods of treatment are critically reviewed.

One of the most difficult tasks for an editor is that of selection. In the preparation of this book selection was a particular problem. The topics included reflect the clinical experience of the editors as well as their opinion of the major issues that practitioners are likely to encounter. This book is not intended as an encyclopedic review but as a tool to assist obstetrical clinicians in everyday practice.

Managing the health care of pregnant women is both a privilege and a responsibility. Insofar as this monograph assists clinicians in identifying, understanding, and treating selected psychophysiologic disturbances occurring during gestation, the expectations of the authors will be amply fulfilled.

John Patrick O'Grady, MD

Contributors

Zev S. Ashenburg, PhD
Assistant Professor of Psychology, Department of Neurology,
Associate Director, Case Western Reserve University School of Medicine, Pain Center,
University Hospitals of Cleveland, 2074 Abington Road, Cleveland, Ohio 44106

Lucy A. Bayer-Zwirello, MD
Assistant Professor, Department of Obstetrics and Gynecology,
Tufts University School of Medicine,
Baystate Medical Center, 759 Chestnut Street, Springfield, Massachusetts 01199

Max Chorowski, MD
Assistant Clinical Professor, Department of Obstetrics and Gynecology,
Clinical Instructor, Department of Psychiatry
Tufts University School of Medicine,
Baystate Medical Center, The Counseling and Gynecology Group,
760 Chestnut Street, Springfield, Massachusetts 01107

Lewis Cohen, MD
Assistant Professor, Department of Psychiatry,
Tufts University School of Medicine, Baystate Medical Center,
759 Chestnut Street, Springfield, Massachusetts 01199

M. Gayle Doucette, MSSA
Director of Social Work,
University MacDonald Womens Hospital,
2074 Abington Road, Cleveland, Ohio 44106

Shelley Falkin, PhD
Assistant Professor, Department of Psychiatry and Behavioral Medicine,
University of Illinois College of Medicine, 7725 N. Knoxville, Peoria, Illinois 61614

Timothy K. Fitzpatrick, MD
Clinical Instructor, Department of Obstetrics and Gynecology,
Tufts University School of Medicine, Baystate Medical Center,
299 Carew Street, Springfield, Massachusetts 01104

Martin L. Gimovsky, MD
Associate Professor, Department of Obstetrics and Gynecology,
Tufts University School of Medicine,
Associate Chairman, Department of Obstetrics and Gynecology,
Baystate Medical Center, 759 Chestnut Street, Springfield, Massachusetts 01199

Paul A. Greve, Jr., JD
Vice President/General Counsel, Legal Affairs Office,
St. Luke's Hospital, 11311 Shaker Blvd., Cleveland, Ohio 44104

Camille Kanaan, MD
Assistant Professor, Department of Obstetrics and Gynecology,
Tufts University School of Medicine, Baystate Medical Center,
759 Chestnut Street, Springfield, Massachusetts 01199

Paul Kirk, MD
Professor and Chairman, Department of Obstetrics and Gynecology,
Oregon Health Sciences University, 3181 SW Sam Jackson Park Road,
Portland, Oregon 97201-3098

Mary B. Mahowald, PhD
Professor and Senior Scholar, Department of Obstetrics and Gynecology,
Center for Clinical Medical Ethics,
University of Chicago, The Chicago Lying-in-Hospital,
5841 S. Maryland Avenue, Chicago, Illinois 60637-1463

Therese M. Madden-Fitzsimons, MB
Staff Psychiatrist, Consultation-Liaison Division and Lecturer,
Department of Psychiatry, Mount Sinai Hospital, Toronto, Ontario, Canada M5G 1X5

William H. Miller, MD
Assistant Professor, Department of Psychiatry,
Director: Inpatient Psychiatry Service,
University of Kentucky College of Medicine, Chandler Medical Center,
Annex 2, Room 206, Lexington, Kentucky 40536-0080

John Patrick O'Grady, MD
Associate Professor, Department of Obstetrics and Gynecology,
Tufts University School of Medicine,
Chief: Division of Maternal-Fetal Medicine,
Baystate Medical Center, 759 Chestnut Street, Springfield, Massachusetts 01199

Miriam Rosenthal, MD
Associate Professor, Department of Psychiatry and Reproductive Biology,
Case Western Reserve University School of Medicine,
University MacDonald Womens Hospital, 2074 Abington Road, Cleveland, Ohio 44106

Patricia L. Schwiebert, RN
Director: Perinatal Loss,
2116 NE 18th Avenue, Portland, Oregon 97212

Dennis H. Smith, MD
Professor, Department of Reproductive Biology,
Associate Professor, Department of Psychiatry,
Case Western Reserve University School of Medicine,
Medical Director Obstetrics and Gynecology Out-Patient Department,
Metro Health Medical Center, 3395 Scranton Road, Cleveland, Ohio 44109

Leon Speroff, MD
Professor, Department of Obstetrics and Gynecology,
Oregon Health Sciences University, 3181 SW Sam Jackson Park Road,
Portland, Oregon 97201-3098

Halina P. Wiczyk, MD
Assistant Professor, Department of Obstetrics and Gynecology,
Tufts University School of Medicine,
Chief: Division of Reproductive Endocrinology,
Baystate Medical Center, 759 Chestnut Street, Springfield, Massachusetts 01199

Obstetrics: Psychological and Psychiatric Syndromes

PART I

Perspectives

Chapter 1

The New Obstetrics

John P. O'Grady, MD, and Camille Kanaan, MD

> Obstetrics is not one of the exact sciences, and in our penury of truth we ought
> to be accurate in our statements, generous in our doubts, tolerant in our
> convictions . . .
> —*James Young Simpson (1875)*

The practice of obstetrics in the last quarter of the 20th century has been re-modeled by rapid technological advances as well as by changing social norms and cultural trends. Today, more so than in the past, the obstetrician is faced with new challenges and stresses in caring for women from different ethnic, social, and economic backgrounds in a sensitive and nonjudgmental way.[1] While technology has made many aspects of childbirth safer, it has resulted in a process that is more intricate and less natural. This in turn has raised the concern of many pregnant women and care providers that the patient-physician relationship has turned into an interaction between actors performing in a play involving simply physiologic if not pathologic processes.[2,3]

The sociology of human reproduction is rapidly changing. The influence of these changes on obstetrical practice is profound. The population is aging and the baby boom cohort has now reached its middle 30s and early 40s. Within this cohort is an increasing number of women who postponed reproduction until later in life. At the other end of the spectrum, there is an epidemic of adolescent pregnancies with serious medical and social consequences. In addition, both work patterns and family life have changed from traditional models.[4] The proportion of single men and women is increasing as over one million divorces occur annually. Over half of the women with children under 3 years of age are in the work force. Many are single or divorced and live far from the usual extended family. Changes in social arrangements, sexual practices, and technological advances are creating situations unthought of in previous years. These are not only difficult to understand and discuss with patients but they also raise legal and ethical issues when the interests of the mother and the fetus are in conflict.

While the health of the mother used to be the primary concern and focus of attention of the obstetrician, new technology such as visualization of the fetus by ultrasound and the possibility of in utero surgery has brought about a new emphasis on the fetus as a patient. Knowledge about the effects of drugs, alcohol, diet, and exercise is accumulating and the field of fetal physiology is expanding. Early detection of fetal anomalies commonly generates dilemmas and controversies in the management of the pregnancy. Although abortion is frequently an option, the emotional overtones of such a procedure cannot be overlooked. About 1.3 million abortions are performed yearly in the United States[5] and major societal conflicts concerning terminations continue to color the political process and echo through the media and the courts.

Other social changes such as the rise of the women's movement, the creation of self-help groups, the education and participation of the "consumer," and heightening of the medicolegal climate are all part of the practice of obstetrics in the 1990s. It is a paradox that precisely at the time when science permits better understanding of our patients' problems, when communication is easier, and when therapy is more effective, there is more interference limiting our achievement of these same goals.

This introductory chapter briefly reviews the major trends facing obstetrics, and emphasizes the importance of education and flexibility as virtues necessary for the continued survival of the obstetrician in the future.

Current Problems

Prenatal Care

The number of births in the United States is about 3.8 million, reflecting a fertility rate of 65.7/1000 women.[6] While the overall fertility rate has been constant since 1975, its demographic characteristics are changing. The number of births to unmarried mothers and to older women is rising steadily. A particularly disturbing national trend is the decline in the percentage of pregnant women receiving adequate prenatal care.[7,8]

In 1987, 24% of women received no prenatal care in the first trimester.[6] Demographic characteristics closely linked to insufficient prenatal care include teenagers; blacks, Hispanics, or Native Americans; unmarried women; recent immigrants to the United States; and those of limited education at the poverty level.[7-9] These conditions contribute heavily to the infant mortality rate of 10.1 per 1000 live births.[5] As a result, in 1987, the United States ranked 19th among the industrialized countries of the world for infant mortality. This high death rate is related to low birth weight and prematurity, both of which correlate with poor nutrition, medical complications, and substance abuse. Prenatal care programs play an important role in the reduction of infant mortality. Accessibility to prenatal care is frequently impeded by the inability to pay, shortage of clinics, unavailability of physicians, restrictions on nurse midwives, and fear and suspicion of clinics and their personnel.[7] Pregnant women may also face difficulties of transportation or child care, and in coping with long waiting times or limited clinic hours. Those women who use illicit drugs may fear being arrested or having their babies taken away. For these reasons, universal delivery of prenatal care presents serious challenges for practitioners and health care planners. An obvious response is to argue that financial barriers to medical care should be reduced. Unfortunately, under the current political and economic conditions, it is difficult to foresee much improvement as the trend has been a declining level of support from state and federal sources. Lobbying the legislature and taking action within professional societies are necessary; however, practitioners should also consider the means by which their communities can help them deliver better prenatal care. Educational programs for women need to emphasize that prenatal care is not only cost-effective but also capable of reducing maternal and neonatal complications. Community support systems can assist and encourage women to adhere to prenatal programs. Finally, more research is needed in the field of prenatal care to address the following issues[10]: (1) understanding more about intrauterine growth retardation and premature onset of labor, so that preventive measures can be developed; (2) understanding what factors make some programs more successful in drawing women into prenatal care clinics; (3) understanding what psychological and educational factors keep women away from clinics; (4) developing cost-effective ways for workers to visit homes and neighborhoods to reach out to pregnant women; (5) changing lifestyles harmful to fetuses, with treatment facilities available to pregnant women with drug and alcohol problems; and (6) learning the kind of educational programs that are most effective.

Prematurity

While the picture of current prenatal care appears bleak and infant mortality rates remain high, the successful application of new medical technology to the care of very-low- birth-weight infants (1000 g or less) is a success story, but it has proven to be a mixed blessing for obstetrical practitioners. While the statistics vary among institutions, currently, the bitter edge of viability falls at approximately 24 weeks gestation and 600 g birth weight but it may be even lower in some clinical services.[11] Clinicians may look at these numbers as "cutoff" values for viability, but the message that needs to be conveyed along with the statistics is that only 10% or less of infants below this gestational age and birth weight survive. When fetal age and weight exceed these limits, survival rapidly rises to 40% or more. Viability may not be the only acceptable outcome for parents. Although approximately 70% of the eventual survivors are normal, the remainder will suffer from long-term sequelae of varying severity. The problem for the clinician is to decide, along with the patient, whether and when to intervene for fetal indications.

It is easy to suggest that such problems are the province of the hospital ethics committee. In truth, there are times when such evaluations can be leisurely performed and balanced judgments reached. The participation of the neonatologist, frequently with an optimistic outlook, is invaluable. Yet in many circumstances clinicians are forced to make decisions about interventions, almost instantaneously, in the face of acute obstetrical catastrophes related to fetal distress, abruptio placentae or advanced premature labor. This difficulty is often compounded by the inability to convey all appropriate information to a distraught patient in crisis or in severe pain. There are no easy answers to such dilemmas. Rather than correct responses, there are reasonable alternatives and these must be presented in the context of standards of care and success rates for the particular institution. The appropriateness of performing a cesarean delivery when fetal survival rates are known to be poor is at best problematic. No rigid rules can be established. Clinicians should be unequivocally clear about their data, yet flexible enough to allow participation of the woman and her family in the decision making.

The Older Pregnant Woman

Among the most striking trends in childbearing in recent years is the increase in birthrate among older women.[8,12–15] Part of this increase is accounted for by the aging of the baby boom generation, which now tends to outnumber the cohorts coming before and after it. However, this is not the only explanation for the observed increase in the number of women becoming pregnant in their fourth and even fifth decades. Several important socioeconomic changes have also been implicated.[14] Increased numbers of divorces and remarriages bring about a desire for additional children. Many women defer childbearing while developing their careers. Infertility treatments are more successful, allowing some women with long-standing infertility to conceive. Whether age by itself represents a greater risk for a pregnant woman in her late 30s or in her 40s is controversial.[12,13]

Risk estimates appear to be related to specific characteristics of the group studied and the availability of adequate care. The greater the proportion of middle-class "postponers" with access to good prenatal care in the population studied, the better the overall outcome.[12,15] In contrast, a high rate of complications is incurred by women with advanced multiparity who are ending their reproductive careers, or with involuntary infertility, and by those living at or below the poverty level.[13] Occasionally, some obstetric complications are brought about in this group of older mothers by excessive zeal and intervention due to practitioner anxiety or the misconceived belief of increased risk.[13] However, with the use of ultrasonic surveillance, prenatal diagnosis, fetal monitoring, and early intervention for medical complications such as gestational diabetes, pregnancy risks for older mothers and their babies are reduced to acceptable levels.

New Reproductive Technologies

Infertility is increasingly common, with at least 3.5 million infertile couples in the United States. This increase, due to the spread of sexually transmitted diseases, environmental toxins, and delayed childbearing, has fueled the demand for infertility services. As a result, the greatest developments of the 1980s in the field of reproduction were brought about by the rapid expansion of new technologies including in vitro fertilization, gamete intrafallopian transfer, and artificial insemination. Previously available diagnostic and therapeutic modalities such as ultrasound, laparoscopic surgery or pelviscopy, sperm banking, and the administration of gonadotropins and their analogues have all been refined.[16] This wave of developments is flooding the legal and ethical systems with problems hitherto unheard of (see Chapter 16). The frantic attempts of couples to conceive at great personal difficulty, some risk, and often considerable expense are commonly observed in infertility practice. While about half of all infertile couples will eventually conceive with assistance, many if not most couples experience a roller coaster of elation alternating with depression associated with the various attempts and failures. Conception becomes an obsession driving personal lives, commanding sexual function, and destabilizing family finance.[16,17] For couples unable to conceive despite technical assistance, private adoption and surrogate parenthood provide controversial and expensive options. Despite the fact that the legal underpinnings of these options are still unsettled, at least 500 children have been born in recent years in formally arranged surrogacy contracts. In a few instances, legal actions by the contracting couple or the surrogate mother have been initiated, raising serious and unresolved questions about the meaning of motherhood, the ethics of contractual relationships for surrogacy, and the psychological implications for the surrogate as well as the newborn.

Most recent technologies involving embryo freezing and embryo biopsy with preimplantation determination of genetic makeup are only a few examples of the increasing complexity of this field. They also emphasize how far our thinking about such issues has lagged behind our technical capabilities.

These new technologies continue to raise controversies relative to their virtual restriction to the affluent class of society, who can afford the tremendous expense incurred in these programs. Whether insurance companies should cover these expenses remains unsettled. Alternate means of obtaining normal children through adoption are constantly shrinking due to the widespread use of birth control, the availability of abortions, and the reluctance of women with unplanned or unwanted pregnancies to give up their babies.

Substance Abuse

It is no secret that abuse of various illicit and prescription drugs as well as the excessive use of alcohol and cigarettes presents serious and increasing problems for society.[18–20] At least 8 million women of childbearing age are chemically dependent and about 10% to 15% of pregnant women use illicit drugs and/or alcohol.[18] Though substance abuse afflicts both low and high socioeconomic classes, poorer women and those of minority groups are most likely to be identified. The medical complications and psychological implications of this behavior will be addressed later, but suffice to say that the dilemma facing the clinician is considerable (see Chapter 11). Screening programs can be justified only if treatment and rehabilitation are integral parts of them. The identification of these patients frequently elicits anger on the part of the obstetrician, who feels that the woman is deliberately harming her baby. Though punitive legal implications of substance abuse in pregnant women have surfaced in several states,[21] for the clinician, maternal addiction is best considered as a complex medical and social disorder.

Ethical Dilemmas

Ethical issues have always been an integral part of obstetrical and gynecological practice.[1] Recent technological advances, as mentioned previously, are bringing some of these issues to the forefront. Forced cesarean sections, attempts at preventive detention of pregnant drug abusers, the disposition of frozen embryos from in vitro fertilization programs, and treatment of the acquired immunodeficiency syndrome in pregnancy are all examples of new problems with important ethical implications. Hospital ethics committees and legal departments are not only of great assistance but are a necessity in addressing these dilemmas. The input of the bioethicist in conferences and clinical rounds is helpful in keeping an ethical focus on the teaching and practice of obstetrics.

Conclusions

The stress on the modern obstetrician is considerable. The practitioner is asked not only to be sensitive to women's sexual and psychological needs, but also to have up-to-date technical and academic competence in the various settings of the office, labor and delivery room, operating room, and intensive care unit.[22] Further, the obstetrician is expected to counsel, educate, and cure patients in a way that keeps his practice cost effective and free from errors. It is little wonder that mere mortals encounter some difficulty with these complex and conflicting requirements.

As the world in which we practice changes, as members of the medical profession, so must we. In reviewing the trends of modern practice, the themes of increasing complexity and social reorganization—and at times disintegration—are particularly prominent. Communication and sensitivity are central to the rapidly changing needs of our patient population. Our challenge is to remain flexible and be able to face or adapt to these rapid social changes.

References

1. Park RC: Old bedfellows: Ethics and obstetrics and gynecology. *Obstet Gynecol* 1989;83:1–3.
2. Leavitt JW: *Brought to Bed: Childbearing in America, 1750–1950*. New York, Oxford University Press, 1986.
3. Leavitt JW: The medicalization of childbirth in the twentieth century. *Trans Stud Coll Physicians Phila* 1989;4:299–319.
4. American Psychiatric Association Task Force in Changing Family Patterns: *Task Force Report 25, Changing Family Patterns in the United States*. Washington, DC, American Psychiatric Association Press, 1986.
5. Mass Medical Society/Centers for Disease Control, U.S. Department of Health and Human Services: *MMWR* 1990;39:829–841.
6. U.S. Department of Health and Human Services; Public Health Service: *Health United States 1989 and Prevention Profile*. Washington, DC, U.S. Government Printing Office, 1990.
7. Brown SS (ed.): *Prenatal Care: Reaching Mothers, Reaching Infants*. Washington, DC, National Academy Press, 1988.
8. Massachusetts Department of Public Health: *Advance Data: Births 1987*. Boston, Department of Public Health, 1988.
9. Massachusetts Task Force on Infant Mortality: *Unfinished Business; Poverty, Race and Infant Survival in Massachusetts*. Boston, Department of Public Health, 1990.
10. Klerman LV: Prenatal care, in Wyinelenberg S (ed.): *Science and Babies: Private Decisions, Public Dilemmas*. Washington, DC, National Academy Press, 1990, pp. 96–125.
11. Hack M, Fanaroff AA: Outcomes of extremely-low-birth-weight infants between 1982 and 1988. *N Engl J Med* 1989;321:1642–1647.
12. Resnik R: The "elderly primigravida" in 1990. *N Engl J Med* 1990;322:693–694. Editorial.

13. Mansfield PK, McCool W: Toward a better understanding of the "advanced maternal age" factor. *Health Care Women Int* 1989;10:395-415.

14. Touleman L: Historical overview of fertility and age. *Maturitas* 1988;suppl:5-14.

15. Berkowitz GS, Skovron ML, Lapinski RH, Berkowitz RL: Delayed childbearing and the outcome of pregnancy. *N Engl J Med* 1990;322:659–664.

16. Holbrook SM: Adoption, infertility, and the new reproductive technologies: Problems and prospects for social work and welfare policy. *Social Work* 1990;35:333–337.

17. Valentine DD: Psychological impact of infertility: Identifying issues and medications. *Soc Work Health Care* 1986;11:61–69.

18. Chasnoff IJ: Drugs and women: Establishing a standard of care. *Ann NY Acad Sci* 1989;562:208–210.

19. Chasnoff IJ, Landress JH, Barrett ME: The prevalence of illicit drug or alcohol use during pregnancy and discrepancies in mandatory reporting in Pinellas County, Florida. *N Engl J Med* 1990;17:1202–1206.

20. Kilata GB: Behavioral teratology: Birth defects of the mind. *Science* 1978;202:732–734.

21. The American College of Obstetricians and Gynecologists: Substance abuse and pregnancy: State lawmakers respond with punitive and public health measures. *Legisletter* 1990;g(3).

22. Bradley DF, King JF, Effen SB: Psychology in obstetrics: Extinct or extant? *J Psychosom Obstet Gynecol* 1987;6:49–57.

Chapter 2

Law and the Practitioner

Paul A. Greve, Jr., JD and Martin L. Gimovsky, MD

The first thing we do, let's kill all the lawyers.
—*Henry VI, Part 2, IV, ii, 73*
William Shakespeare (1564–1616)

Legal Issues in Obstetric Practice

The law is a set of processes for the resolution of social issues. Clinicians in obstetrics and gynecology are acutely aware of the legal risks inherent in practicing medicine. Most physicians have difficulty accepting the fact that social conflicts involve competing values. Our society values individual liberty and autonomy in concert with a commitment to compassion, fairness, and equality. Thus, in general, law as applied to medical practice attempts to promote quality medicine, at a reasonable cost. How successful the current system is in this regard is at best controversial.

The American College of Obstetricians and Gynecologists reported in a 1985 survey of its members that fully 71% had experienced medical liability claims.[1] Rapidly rising costs for insurance and national discussion of alternatives to the traditional legal remedies for alleged malpractice are signs of the strains produced by this legal crisis. There are a number of reasons for this large and increasing burden of legal entanglements: consumerism, the increasingly litigious nature of American society, new applications of technology (eg, "assisted reproduction"), a greater potential of alienation of practitioners from patients, unrealistic expectations for immediate and ultimate results, and, in many jurisdictions, legal decisions or legislative actions widening the possibilities for suit.

Obstetric health care for women is a high-risk undertaking. Such practice inevitably includes medical and surgical care for two patients, the parturient and her fetus. Obstetrician- gynecologists also are at risk as they frequently perform surgery and are responsible for 5 of the 10 most common operative procedures performed in the United States: dilatation and curettage, hysterectomy, tubal ligation, oophorectomy, and cesarean delivery.[2]

In our increasingly complex medical care system even good practice cannot produce an invariably excellent result. Thus, patient expectations, partially fueled by prior extravagant claims by the medical profession, commonly exceed clinical performance. Ultimately, both practitioners and their patients practice an active form of denial concerning both predictable and unpredictable suboptimal or even disastrous outcomes. In such circumstances, dissatisfaction and legal entanglements are inevitable. Indeed, the medical profession may sometimes lose sight of how difficult is the plight of the patient who truly deserves compassion and compensation.[3]

Obstetrics: Areas of Major Concern

In considering obstetric legal liability it is helpful both to review general areas in which difficult situations can result in legal claims and to analyze claims information from a major insurance carrier critically. The St. Paul Fire and Marine Insurance Company underwrites approximately 20% of the liability insurance for hospitals and medical professionals in the United States. In reviewing the company's claims statistics, obstetric claims for improper birth-related treatment are the major problem (Table 2.1). In obstetric practice, legal claims commonly arise from cesarean delivery or its timing, surgical complications, traumatic birth injury, or failure to diagnose fetal distress properly. The single leading allegation for claims severity is pregnancy monitoring, specifically the failure to perform and interpret properly electronic fetal monitoring during "high-risk" pregnancy and labor.

Relative risks in practice are also related to complications of special and new technologies, as well as fertility control issues. The following brief review outlines several important issues in each of these areas.

Injuries

In any surgical field, actual operative complications and related patient injuries are a potentially fertile source of litigation. Most obstetric surgical claims

Table 2.1 Summary of Claims Reported by St. Paul Insured Physicians and Surgeons: Top Ten Allegations Involving Obstetricians/Gynecologists 1983–1987*

	Number of Claims	Average Costs†
1. Improper Treatment—Birth-Related	1167	$ 99,719
2. Surgery—Postoperative Complications	550	$ 28,047
3. Failure to Diagnose—Pregnancy Problems	450	$ 78,324
4. Surgery—Inadvertent Act	280	$ 24,627
5. Failure to Diagnose—Cancer	176	$101,755
6. Surgery—Inappropriate Procedure	140	$ 27,883
7. Surgery—Delay/Complications	76	$ 29,473
8. Improper Treatment—Drug Side Effect	62	$ 23,240
9. Surgery—Sponge Left	61	$ 22,595
10. Surgery—Postoperative Death	51	$ 76,982

*As of December 31, 1988.
†Average cost includes the total value of the claim, including legal and other expenses, with no cap on individual claims.

From St. Paul Fire and Marine Insurance Company, with permission.

arise from maternal complications of cesarean delivery due to infection and surgical injuries. Severe maternal injuries may rarely occur from episiotomy extensions or breakdown resulting from difficult vaginal deliveries requiring subsequent, often painful surgery. Except in the unusual association with a process such as necrotizing fasciitis these injuries are not life-threatening. Ureteric and bladder injuries are also possible with instrumental delivery but are infrequent in this era.

By far the most difficult cases involve *allegations* of malpractice involving "bad babies" in which it is claimed that permanent neurological injuries result from tardy or improperly performed operative deliveries or mismanaged labors. The potential dollar value of such cases can be astronomical. These are particularly difficult cases to deal with as there is not a consensus in the field concerning the cause of the vast majority of neurological and developmental disorders. To compound the problem, often such deficits are not identified until months or years after an obstetric delivery and the relationship of the abnormality to the events of parturition may be tenuous at best.[4,5] The wide variety of available "expert opinion" compounds and may further obscure the issue. Ethical considerations play an important part in deciding between medical maloccurrence and malpractice.[6] The "causation" of an injury is frequently the most difficult part of a suit to prove. This is especially true in situations involving abnormal neurologic outcomes.

Other injuries may result from intrauterine device (IUD) related complications or problems related to the administration of oral contraceptives. Alleged failures to recommend genetic testing or counseling may be held to deprive families of their rights to procreative choice or treatment and are also a potential source of litigation.[7]

Injuries to the fetus or newborn may also occur. A discussion of injury litigation in obstetrics must consider the related concepts of *wrongful life* and *wrongful birth*. The claim in both of these proceedings is that physician negligence resulted in the birth of either a defective child with a potentially diagnosable abnormality or a normal but unwanted child. Although the central event, the birth of an undesired child, is the same in both proceedings, the causes of action differ.[8]

Wrongful life claims are legal proceedings brought in the name of a child born with a defect.[9,10] The claim is that this defect was either not discovered during gestation or improperly managed.[11] The argument by the plaintiff is that except for the negligence of the clinician the defect would have been observed and an abortion performed. Such claims commonly involve infants with readily diagnosable genetic or chromosomal disorders such as Tay-Sachs or Down's syndrome, or those born injured as a result of an undiagnosed maternal disease, such as rubella. The legal basis for such claims is the contention that the legal duty owed by the clinician to the unborn child is similar to that owed to the parents.

A bizarre twist to such proceedings is the possibility that when wrongful life is accepted as a cause of action against physicians, the doctrine could then potentially be expanded to permit children to sue their parents for allowing their birth! In California, a specific statute precludes the enactment of this unusual legal scenario.[8]

A *wrongful birth* action is a legal proceeding brought by the parents of a defective or unexpected child based on the argument that the physician breached his or her duty to the patient by inadequate prenatal or early pregnancy testing or counseling or by faulty performance of sterilization. In this instance, *the alleged damage is birth itself*, a maternal injury, and *not an injury to the infant*. Such suits imply that the obstetrician has a legal duty to prevent the delivery of a defective child by appropriately performing and interpreting screening tests.[12] Alternatively, wrongful birth may also be claimed in the instance of a failed tubal ligation, even when the resulting child is normal. Claims of this type have proved successful in a number of jurisdictions, and with the increasing sophistication of prenatal diagnosis procedures, further expansion of this legal concept is possible.[13] Some states have, however, enacted statutes that have survived judicial review, prohibiting suits brought for wrongful birth.[14]

In a successful wrongful birth lawsuit, courts differ on how to calculate money damages. Depending on the jurisdiction, parents might receive money damages for the pain and suffering of the pregnancy and birth of a normal, healthy infant as well as an award for the associated medical expenses. However, most courts have held that the benefits of raising a normal healthy child outweigh any burdens imposed on the parents. Some courts use this "benefit" rule to offset the mother's injuries by the benefits of the birth of the normal child.[15,16] However, in the instance of the birth of a child with defects, courts can award damages to cover expenses directly attributable to the treatment of such abnormalities.[17]

Special Technologies

Techniques for in vitro fertilization and other related procedures of assisted reproduction are new and likely areas for complex legal entanglements[8] (see Chapter 15). These procedures combine complex laboratory manipulations, interpretation of sophisticated endocrinologic tests, possibility of multiple births, surgical complications, and potential for fetal or neonatal compromise. Surrogacy programs are also under close legal scrutiny, especially as the ethical and legal underpinnings of such plans are unclarified. In general, surrogacy contracts for profit or gain are of questionable legality and have been prohibited by statute in Utah and several other states.[18,19]

Fertility Control

Abortion and sterilization are of medicolegal importance as both involve problems of consent and surgical interventions. There is also potential for operative complications. In sterilization, problems result from errors in tubal ligation with inadvertent ligation of the round ligaments or other adnexal structures instead of the fallopian tubes. Alternatively, spontaneous recannulation of the tubes after an appropriately performed operation can also lead to failure of the procedure with subsequent unwanted pregnancy and a possible claim of wrongful birth.

Another snare for the unwary surgeon are procedures performed when the patient has an early, undiagnosed pregnancy. In such cases, usually, but not always, the menstrual history is uncertain or irregular.

Other risks concern informed consent. Many institutions require the use of specialized forms, signed well in advance of the contemplated procedure.

So long as the provider adheres to the usual requirements of informed consent, the risk of liability in the consent process for voluntary sterilization is effectively removed. In general, states cannot restrict access to voluntary sterilization on grounds of motive, marital status, or spousal consent.[20,21] Many writers advocate the use of a special consent form for sterilization that sets forth in lay language such facts as the loss of reproductive capability, failure rates, and possible operative complications.

Federal Medicaid pays for sterilization only when a special consent form is signed 1 month *before* to the surgery, unless an emergency occurs. Even in an emergency, a sterilization cannot be performed unless at least 72 hours has passed since the consent was obtained. Failure to document preoperative counseling and complete the related paperwork for the federal government properly does not establish either civil or criminal liability but does prevent payment for the procedure.

The physician should explain the potential for pregnancy after any sterilizing procedure as well as the limited success rate for reversal. Although spousal consent is no longer legally required, it is prudent to involve the husband or significant other in such discussions. It is not permissible to seek consent for sterilization from a woman's husband or companion while she is under anesthesia, absent a true emergency.

In less than a life-threatening emergency, sterilization procedures should not be performed on individuals whose decision- making capacity is in question because of psychiatric illness where the consent of a court-appointed guardian empowered to provide consent for medical treatment is not available. The same is true for minor patients or patients who have been previously adjudicated to be legally incompetent.[22–24] The case law and legislation for each jurisdiction vary greatly. Physicians should not proceed to seek consent for sterilization in uncertain or complex cases without the advice of a knowledgeable attorney who specializes in health care law.

Social Mores

Contemporary U.S. society places the threat of litigation in the role of social adjudicator. The lottery system of awards and relatively easy availability of "experts" to expedite costly and meaningless "settlements" fuel the distrust and disintegrating relationship between physicians and patients.[25]

A unique and dual responsibility is faced by the obstetrician under those rare circumstances in which patient demands or behavior are dangerous to fetal well-being. The courts have on occasion overridden concerns of individual maternal autonomy to order medical intervention.[26] This subject is discussed in substantial detail later in this chapter.

Infanticide

Under common law and in the absence of a specific state statute defining feticide or abortion as illegal, an act resulting in the death of a fetus is not a crime.[27] However, *if a child is born alive* and death results from felonious action, this act is considered homicide or manslaughter. The crime of homicide or manslaughter occuring at the time of birth is usually termed *infanticide* (see Chapter 12). However, states vary as to nomenclature or classification and the legal description for such killings is not consistent in all jurisdictions.

The first element of proof essential to establishing criminal responsibility in cases of suspected infanticide is the existence of the infant independent of the mother. The second element of proof is establishing that the death of the child was caused by a criminal act of the accused.[28] Not surprisingly, the courts have wrestled with the concept of what is meant by "live birth." There is no uniformity of case law on this point. In the past, courts would generally define "live birth" as meaning that the fetus was completely expelled from the mother's body and showed clear indications of independent viability, such as respiration.[29] Some courts require expulsion of the body as well as "independent circulation." Still others have stated that the umbilical cord must be severed, although this view has been modified in some jurisdictions to the extent that a live birth can be established where the child is alive after expulsion even though the cord is still intact.[30]

Most states continue to hold the position that homicide can only happen to persons who have been born alive by the definition of live birth accepted in that jurisdiction. However, some states, such as California, have revised their penal codes to include a category for killing of a fetus.[30]

Practitioners may become involved in legal cases in which there is evidence of maternal neglect in the minutes or hours after birth that results in or contributes to the death of the infant. In many cases mothers have been prosecuted for homicide under these circumstances.[31] In reviewing such cases, the court must initially determine that there is sufficient evidence that maternal neglect immediately after delivery was the cause of death. Prosecutions have been successful on the basis of confessions by the mother or of testimony that the mother failed to attend to the child immediately after birth.[32] A mother's conduct can be excused from criminal responsibility if it can be proved that her mental and physical condition prevented her from exercising reasonable newborn care. As with any alleged crime, the mother's mental state at the time of the incident must be proved by the prosecution. Hospital staff who attend a woman who is accused of childhood murder can be subpoenaed to testify as to the mother's mental and physical condition at the time of her hospital admission. The medical record can be introduced into evidence. Thus, careful objective documentation of the actions and mental state of the mother and any others involved is necessary and will assist the court in determining whether criminal conduct has occurred. State child abuse laws in all jurisdictions require health care personnel to report deaths or injuries to newborns occurring under suspicious circumstances to law enforcement personnel and/or to the coroner's office.

Maternal and Fetal Rights

Recent advances in maternal-fetal medicine permit clinicians to diagnose and treat a number of fetal disorders. This raises the legal question to what extent the fetus is an individual distinct from the mother. Specifically, does the physician owe a legal duty to the fetus, distinct from his or her legal duty to the mother? If so, the physician's and hospital's legal duty to intervene through the courts is likely to be in conflict with maternal rights if her activities place the fetus in jeopardy. Does the stage of pregnancy affect the appropriateness of court intervention? How far should the hospital and physician go in forcing the mother to undergo treatment?

This discussion is currently spirited and the outcome uncertain. Both maternal rights advocates and fetal rights advocates cite specific laws and general legal concepts to support their respective positions (Table 2.2).

In addition to the arguments put forth by the advocacy groups, there are other ethical and legal considerations. Under both common and constitutional law the right of privacy empowers the mother to make decisions about her body. That is the foundation for the legal doctrine of informed consent. Under the right of privacy and the doctrine of informed consent, competent individuals have the right to refuse treatment. This right has often been used in cases involving competent adult patients with terminal illness or injury. The legal and ethical issue is whether a mother's right to refuse treatment is valid if the fetus is placed at risk by her actions.[26]

When parents fail to make health care decisions that are in the best interest of their children, the state can intervene through the juvenile courts' enforcement of abuse and neglect laws. The court attempts to decide whether the proposed treatment is in the best interests of the child. But should this same test be applied to the fetus and if so, when in gestational age? Fetal rights advocates, including many pediatricians and obstetricians, would answer yes to this question but differ on the "acceptable" gestational age for potential intervention.

Before 1990, the medical-legal literature on court-ordered obstetric intervention cited an 86% success rate (18 of 21 cases) for providers seeking court orders for treatment against the mother's wishes.[36] For example, one of the first decisions to uphold the fetal rights position was *Jefferson v Griffin Spalding County Hospital*.[37] In this case, the Supreme Court of Georgia denied a motion to stay an order compelling a woman who was 39 weeks pregnant with complete placenta previa to submit to a cesarean section and transfusions. The

Table 2.2 Conflicts: Maternal-Fetal Rights

Maternal Rights Position	Fetal Rights Position
Unless fetus born alive, feticide is not a crime.[33] Also, the law imposes no duty to rescue after a child is born; parents are not legally required to risk their lives to save a child's life	Fetus has had rights under common law, including property and inheritance rights
The right of privacy guarantees women a constitutional basis to be free of state interference and unwarranted bodily intrusions. Case law precedents protect privacy rights in regard to procreation and the family	Rejection of privacy arguments: if the woman has chosen to carry a child to term, neither she nor others may take actions that will endanger the fetus.[35,36] *Roe*[35] and *Griswold*[36] do not govern all aspects of procreation
Efforts of the state to regulate the mother while protecting the fetus involve potentially enormous intrusions into personal privacy and thus are unacceptable	If the state has the power to regulate and prohibit abortion, it can prohibit other acts harmful to the fetus; ie, state has an interest once child is viable[35]
	State has had a traditional interest in the welfare of children that can be extended to the fetus (abuse and neglect laws)

trial court balanced the rights of the mother (religious freedom) against the rights of the fetus (risk of exsanguination). The original court held that the unborn child was a human being and that the intrusion on the parents' right to refuse treatment was outweighed by the duty of the state to protect a living, unborn human being from meeting his or her death before being given the opportunity to live. As with many of the court cases that have upheld the fetal rights position, the court cited *Roe v Wade*,[35] among other cases, as precedent for its decision. The county welfare department was granted custody of the unborn child and the mother was ordered to submit to a sonogram and other related procedures to protect and promote fetal well-being, including a cesarean section.

The legal opinion in such settings is now more complex. In a case decided in 1990 that many commentators in bioethics and law have stated will be a landmark in the maternal-fetal rights debate, the District of Columbia's highest court held that a court- ordered cesarean delivery should not have been authorized.[38,39] Angela Carder was a 27-year-old pregnant patient with cancer who was 25 weeks pregnant. Admitted to George Washington University Hospital, both mother and infant died shortly after the court-ordered surgery. The District of Columbia Court of Appeals held that issues such as competency, informed consent, and substituted judgment were not adequately considered by the judge who authorized the cesarean section.

Among other findings the appellate court placed great emphasis on the patient's right of bodily integrity and informed consent.[39,40] The court stated that the law cannot compel individuals to submit to a significant bodily intrusion for the benefit of others. The appellate court rejected the argument that a mother has a legal duty to her fetus sufficient to compel forced treatment because "a fetus cannot have rights in this respect superior to those of a person who has already been born."[38] The court concluded, "It would be an extraordinary case indeed in which a court might ever be justified in overriding the patient's wishes and authorizing a major surgical procedure such as a cesarean section." The court did not discuss the circumstances under which the state's interests might prevail over the interests of a pregnant patient. In a subsequent civil suit by Angela Carder's survivors, the hospital paid her parents an undisclosed cash award and promised to enact policies protecting pregnant women's rights.

In a report adopted by the American Medical Association at its annual meeting in June 1990, the AMA Board of Trustees recommended adoption of the following statement[40]:

1. Judicial intervention is inappropriate when a woman has made an informed refusal of a medical treatment designed to benefit her fetus. If an exceptional circumstance could be found in which a medical treatment poses an insignificant or no health risk to the woman, entails a minimal invasion of her bodily integrity, and would clearly prevent substantial and irreversible harm to her fetus, it might be appropriate for a physician to seek judicial intervention. However, the fundamental principle against compelled medical procedures should control in all cases that do not present such exceptional circumstances.

2. The physician's duty is to provide appropriate information, such that the pregnant woman may make an informed and thoughtful decision, not to dictate the woman's decision.

3. A physician should not be liable for honoring a pregnant woman's informed refusal of medical treatment designed to benefit the fetus.

4. Criminal sanctions or civil liability for harmful behavior by the pregnant woman toward her fetus are inappropriate.

5. Pregnant substance abusers should be provided with rehabilitative treatment appropriate to their specific physiological and psychological needs.

6. To minimize the risk of legal action by a pregnant patient or an injured child or fetus, the physician should document medical recommendations made including the consequences of failure to comply with the physician's recommendations.

The report also draws the following three conclusions: (1) the physician's duty is to ensure that the pregnant woman makes an informed and thoughtful decision, not to dictate that decision; (2) physicians should not have a legal duty to seek court-ordered interventions; (3) seeking court orders is permissible only in exceptional circumstances.[40]

Termination of Pregnancy

The law of abortion is greatly influenced by constitutional law as set forth in U.S. Supreme Court decisions. Access to abortion in U.S. society is an important political issue, and the law of abortion will continue to be influenced by the dominance of either the liberal or conservative wing of the Supreme Court. Thus, the law on abortion in each state is likely to change in reaction to new legislation or case law determined by state or federal courts. For example, on July 3, 1989, the Supreme Court handed down the decision *Webster v Reproductive Health Services*.[41] This decision is generally regarded as a curtailment of the woman's right to terminate a pregnancy, as set forth in the landmark case of *Roe v Wade* decided in 1973. *Webster* indicated the court's recognition of a greater state interest in regulating abortions. In this complex, controversial, and changing field of law, it is essential for the clinician to obtain competent and current legal advice on abortion laws applicable in his or her jurisdiction. This section will provide a brief summary of significant constitutional law cases concerning abortion. Given the intensity of the rational debate on abortion and the trend toward reduced access to terminations, the 1990s will likely witness significant changes in American abortion law.

Roe v. Wade

Since the landmark case of *Roe v Wade*,[35] women have had a constitutionally protected right to an abortion during the first trimester of pregnancy. This right to terminate the pregnancy is based on the constitutional right to privacy. In the first trimester, a woman and her doctor are free to conclude, without state regulation, that it is appropriate to terminate the pregnancy. However, *Roe v Wade* established a trimester framework for consideration of the legality of state intervention. After the first trimester, the state was empowered to regulate abortion if the regulations reasonably related to preservation and protection of maternal health. The state may further proscribe abortion in the third trimester on the basis of fetal viability, except when necessary to preserve the life or health of the mother.

In sum, *Roe* held that the right to an abortion was a qualified right, to be balanced against two competing state interests: preservation of maternal health and acknowledgment of potential fetal viability. The court's trimester framework was an attempt to define the scope and limits of state regulations of these competing interests.

Webster v Reproductive Health Services

The *Webster* case[41] arose out of 1986 legislation enacted by the state of Missouri to revise existing abortion statutes. Although there were other issues discussed or dismissed by the court, the issue of viability testing remains the most controversial. The court seemingly rejected the trimester framework of *Roe*, without expressly doing so. It was not necessary to overturn *Roe* completely because the Missouri statute did not attempt to restrict abortion before viability. The court recognized the state's interest in protecting potential human life by requiring viability testing before pregnancy termination. The *Webster* decision had no immediate impact beyond Missouri, for no other state had an identical abortion statute. Its significance lies in its implications for state legislation concerning abortion. In effect, the *Webster* decision reversed *Roe* to the extent that it permits states to exercise a greater degree of control over a woman's right to abortion access. However, *Webster* did not overturn *Roe*'s holding that a woman has a right to an abortion free of state interference in the first trimester.

With a conservative majority on the U.S. Supreme Court, there may well be further erosion of *Roe v Wade* in the 1990s through state legislation or other court decisions. Marked differences between states in their abortion statutes are now to be anticipated.

The American Legal System

The majority of legal claims between physicians and patients arise from alleged professional negligence (medical malpractice). Such claims are *torts*, or wrongful acts to persons or their property in which the law permits the awarding of money damages. A tort is neither a crime nor a breach of contract and may result from either an intentional or an unintentional act.[2]

Most legal cases involving clinicians are brought under the rules of *common law*, as opposed to *statutory law*. In the United States, common law is the body of legal opinion based on English common law that is used in the settlement of torts. Common law depends on the precedent case method rather than statutory law. Statutory law, as the name implies, is law made by governmental agencies, usually state legislatures. The presumed advantage of precedent law is that the system is flexible, permitting new interpretations as society changes. Alternatively, from the point of view of the medical profession, it can be argued that this flexibility of common law has only resulted in an uncontrollable expansion of the grounds for potential patient litigation, especially as reflected in extensions in the statutes of limitations.

Whether changes in the statute of limitations and other alterations in the legal system to permit greater latitude for suits benefit society is controversial. No one involved in the current system for medical malpractice can argue that it is necessarily either equitable or rapid in the settlement of differences. In various jurisdictions, modifications of the current system for handling medical malpractice claims by requiring arbitration, setting limits to awards, and so forth, have been attempted, with varying success. In California the "fast tracking" of cases seeks to achieve resolution within 2 years of filing instead of 5. There is no national consensus concerning malpractice litigation except great dissatisfaction among most medical practitioners with the speed, fairness, and expense of the current system.

Medical Malpractice Liability

In order to recover damages in a medical malpractice suit, a deviation from accepted practice must be proved. Although the burden of proof in virtually all malpractice cases lies with the plaintiff, this burden is much less than for a criminal case. In a criminal case, the state must prove its case against the accused *beyond a reasonable doubt*. However, in a civil case, the plaintiff must only prove his or her case by *a preponderance of the evidence*. Thus, if the court concludes that the plaintiff's proof is at least slightly better than the defendant's, the plaintiff wins the judgment.

Uncommonly, in malpractice lawsuits, the doctrine of *res ipsa loquitur* ("the thing speaks for itself") is used by the plaintiff where there is no direct evidence as to how an injury occurred but the nature of the injury leads to the inference that it would not have happened without a negligent act. This is important because when courts permit use of the doctrine, the burden of proof shifts from the plaintiff to the defendant. The retention of foreign objects such as sponges, instruments, and needles after surgical procedures are situations in which this doctrine is usually applied.

Major Components of Malpractice Litigation

In order to prevail in a malpractice case, the plaintiff must prove each one of these following points:

1. A legal *duty* owed to the patient by the care provider
2. A *breach* of the duty (deviation from the applicable standard of care)
3. *Damages* (injury) due to the breach of duty
4. *Causation* (the injury was directly caused by the defendant's breach)

Duty

The legal duty owed to the patient can be simply stated: the provider cannot carelessly cause harm to the patient as he or she carries out patient care responsibilities. The facts are examined to determine whether or not the provider had sufficient control over the patient such that he or she owed this duty of care.

Practically, when patients have been admitted to an institutional setting, it is quite clear that the provider is obligated to use care as he or she performs medical responsibilities, and the issue of duty is simple. If a claim arises from outpatient management, the proof of duty is somewhat more complex and is related to the issue of whether a physician- patient relationship has been established.

Breach of Duty

Breach of duty is one of the most disputed areas in malpractice cases. The *key issue here is whether the physician adhered to the appropriate standard of care in management.* Put another way, what would a reasonable and prudent physician or nurse have done in the same or similar circumstances and what was the applicable standard of care?

Courts almost always require the testimony of expert witnesses to establish that a breach of duty has occurred. The defense attorneys use rebuttal expert witnesses to demonstrate to the jury that the provider did adhere to the applicable standards. Ultimately the jury weighs the evidence, considering the credentials of the expert witnesses and their credibility in reaching a decision.

Damages

For the plaintiff to recover financial compensation for injuries sustained, there must be discernible injury of at least a temporary nature.

Historically, courts required proof of an obvious physical injury before patients could recover damages. Today the situation is more complicated as patients in many jurisdictions can also recover money damages for nonphysical injuries such as anxiety and emotional stress caused by negligent or intentional conduct. Current trends, however, limit awards for "pain and suffering."

In unusual instances in which a defendant's actions are judged to be either reckless or grossly negligent, patients can recover *punitive* damages. Punitive damages are intended to punish the defendant for outrageous conduct. The awarding of such damages is distinctly uncommon. Such awards are above and beyond other compensable damages and are in general *not* covered by medical malpractice insurance.

Causation

To recover damages, the patient must incur an injury that is a *direct result* of the defendant's negligence or carelessness. The proof of causation (the *proximate cause*) can be difficult and almost always requires the use of expert physician testimony. Clinical medicine is an inexact science. Therefore, issues of causation consume much of the time of the attorneys and the expert witnesses.

The Problem of the Standard of Care

In a malpractice lawsuit, the standard of care is the issue that receives most attention. Such standards are a flexible yardstick by which the defendant's legal duty to the patient is measured. This standard is not a fixed measure but progressively evolves, reflecting advances in the science of medicine and in the theory of clinical practice. A physician or nurse is held legally accountable for conforming to the standard of care specific to that medical setting and *in effect at the time of the alleged patient injury.* Institutional policies and procedures as outlined in memoranda or protocol books often determine the standard of care as evidence of the applicable standards set by the hospital and/or the specialty nursing unit where the patient's injury occurred.

Journal articles, textbooks, and protocols and guidelines promulgated by various professional organizations also establish the standard of care. This is especially true now that courts have moved away from the "locality rule." In effect, this means that there is a national minimum standard of care for the evaluation and treatment of many conditions.

Injuries and the Statute of Limitations

The statute of limitations is the legal rule that specifies the period within which a lawsuit can be filed. Although the statute is established by an act of the legislature, the state's highest courts have variously ruled either to extend or limit the statute of limitations in various ways unique to a specific jurisdiction.

A key question for the provider is when the statute of limitations begins to expire. The date of incident, the date of the patient's last contact with the provider, and the date of the patient's discovery of the injury are all events that might trigger the statute of limitations rule.

A major controversy in this regard is the issue of discovery and other types of legal liberalization that extend the statute of limitations beyond the usually stated time period. The so-called discovery rule has been denounced as unfairly exposing physicians to liability essentially without limit. In rebuttal the representatives of injured plaintiffs argue that the right to recovery of damages should not be compromised in instances when the patient could not have known that an injury was caused by malpractice.

The statute of limitations also varies depending on the patient's legal status. All states give minors a longer period to file lawsuits than adults. Statutes of limitations also give the estates of deceased patients the right to file lawsuits within legislatively established time frames.

The statute of limitations in the provider's state has great significance, especially whether the individual's professional liability insurance policy provides coverage. Inflation and inflated jury verdicts can substantially reduce the adequacy of insurance protection purchased years or even decades before. In obstetric practice this has partially been a problem in suits brought by the families of cerebral palsy victims as many of these cases were filed many years after the child's birth when the alleged injury is thought to have taken place.

The Problem of Consent

General Consent

The right of privacy is the foundation for the law of consent. In general, under the right of privacy, individuals under treatment as patients have the right to control their bodies.

The doctrine of general consent requires that the acquiescence of an individual be obtained before examination or treatment. In a hospital setting, written or express consent to treatment is commonly obtained in the admitting department or emergency room. In outpatient settings or in physician's offices, written consent to treatment is frequently omitted. Here the patient's general consent is either given orally or is considered to be implied by the patient's action in seeking care. The patient's consent can be implied in two ways: implied *de facto* by the patient's actions, as when a female patient visits the obstetrician's office with medical questions and voluntarily submits to examination, or implied *de jure* as in the event of an unresponsive patient brought to a hospital for true emergency care.

Informed Consent

The law of informed consent varies with jurisdiction, reflecting both case law and legislation. In general, courts impose on physicians specific obligations for disclosing information to the patient. Unless the physician imparts certain information to an individual before performing a treatment or procedure, the patient is entitled to damages even though the treatment or procedure was performed correctly. Although the amount of disclosure required for informed consent varies among jurisdictions, most courts require that the patient be informed of the nature of the proposed procedure; the risks and benefits; the alternatives, if any; the risks and benefits; and the risk of nontreatment. In 1990, the majority of states followed the "professional standard" rule for disclosure, based on customary practice for that specific medical community.

Exceptions to Consent: Emergency Doctrine

Under the emergency doctrine, consent is implied in a true emergency if the patient is incapable of giving consent. The doctrine encourages treatment to preserve the patient's life in those unusual circumstances in which delay would jeopardize the chances of either survival or a successful outcome.

The urgent or emergent circumstances are the primary requirement for the application of this doctrine. If time permits, consent can be sought from next of kin or other legal representatives such as guardians, but a clinician must never jeopardize the success of treatment through the delay caused by such attempts to obtain consent. However, a *prior* refusal of treatment by a competent patient is virtually always binding on the provider even though that individual subsequently becomes incapacitated through a change in clinical condition.

Many states have statutes that provide specific authority and/or procedures for emergency medical and surgical care for minors and mentally ill persons. Practitioners need to be aware of the specifics of the legal restrictions for emergency care within their own jurisdiction.

Exceptions to Consent: Therapeutic Privilege

Embodied in case law and legislation, therapeutic privilege permits the clinician to withhold information that under other circumstances would be required to be given to the patient when disclosure or access to the information would be detrimental to the patient's health. The doctrine has been frequently cited to deny psychiatric patients access to medical records during the course of therapy.

In clinical settings this doctrine should rarely, if ever, be invoked because of the potential for abuse. For example, it is not permissible to withhold information in an attempt to alter a person's decision with which the provider disagrees. In almost all circumstances the provider should assume that the patient has the mental and emotional capability to deal with the information disclosed. To do otherwise violates the principle of patient autonomy.

Exceptions to Consent: Waiver

Patients have the right to waive the requirement that the provider must disclose information concerning informed consent and have the right to decide that they do not wish to be given information about treatment or wish to delegate decision-making authority to the physician or a third party. So long as the waiver is voluntary, it is an expression of patient autonomy. However, any such waiver should be carefully documented in the medical record.

Documentation of Consent

For malpractice defense purposes, it is important that there be evidence of consent to examination and treatment. In the institutional setting a general or "blanket" consent form is commonly obtained in the admitting or emergency department. In general, clinicians need to be more concerned with the forms used to document informed consent for specific procedures. Such consent forms must reflect applicable statutes or case law as well as readability. Not only must medical jargon be avoided, but the document should be reviewed by a communications specialist who can gear the consent form to the average patient. Such forms will also need to be provided in other languages or a qualified interpreter used if clinicians commonly encounter patients who do not speak or understand English. Whether or not a form is used, the medical record must contain evidence of the patient's consent. If specific forms are not available, unless otherwise legally mandated, the physician can write an entry concerning the consent process in the medical record that the patient signs. Another alternative is for the clinician to develop a standard discussion of risks and benefits for a particular procedure. After obtaining a verbal consent, after this oral presentation, the physician then records in an abbreviated entry in the medical record the issues discussed and the patient's consent to the specific procedure. Obviously, it is prudent that such verbal consents be witnessed.

The consent process should not be lightly regarded and the standard forms should be completed correctly. This writer has seen claims for lack of informed consent dismissed on the basis of the presence of a signed consent form. At the very least the formality of the consent process is an opportunity to gain or reinforce communication with the patient and family.

Research and Consent

Regulation of human subject research is almost exclusively the responsibility of the federal government. The Department of Health and Human Services (HHS) and the Food and Drug Administration (FDA) have enacted rules and regulations that require approval of most research by institutional review boards (IRBs). Three states, California, New York, and Virginia, have enacted specific legislation concerning the regulation of human subject research. Other states have also enacted research laws.

Federal laws on human subject research require investigators to obtain the legally effective informed consent from a subject or the subject's legally authorized representative. The only exceptions are certain exempt activities and the so-called compassionate use exception.

Emancipation

The age of majority differs among states and an individual below the specified age limit is defined as a minor, with a corresponding limitation of certain legal rights. However, many states specify a condition of minor emancipation by statute. So-called emancipated minors may consent to medical care as if they had reached the usual age of majority. Depending on state statute, emancipation can occur when the child enters into a valid marriage, reaches the age of majority, serves on active military duty, or obtains a juvenile court decree that confers the status.

Many states give minors the right by statute to consent to specific forms of treatment, including pregnancy and therapy for sexually transmitted diseases. Many states have recognized the consent of the "mature" or emancipated minor by statutes or by case law. In those instances in which it is appropriate to seek consent from such individuals, the medical record should contain language indicating that the minor's developmental stage or maturity was adequate to enable him or her to consent to the treatment offered. The literature and case law on the "mature minor" frequently discuss such persons as being aged 14 years or older.

Emergencies: Minors

When neither parent is available, the law implies consent for treatment in the event of an emergency. The provider should make every effort to document in the patient's record the medical need for proceeding with treatment without consent. The treating physician may wish to seek a court order if it can be procured without a delay that would threaten life or seriously worsen the patient's condition. When time permits, attempts can and should be made to obtain consent by telephone. In any event, the medical record should reflect what occurred with all attempts, including those that were unsuccessful. When an emergency exists and parents refuse treatment, this refusal should also be noted. Under these unusual circumstances, the clinician must evaluate the clinical situation to determine whether the parental refusal constitutes child neglect. If so, a court order could be sought to permit treatment.

The Abused or Neglected Minor

The obstetrician must be prepared to recognize, diagnose, and report sexual abuse of minors. All states have enacted child abuse and neglect reporting laws that require physicians to report suspected incidents of child abuse and neglect to local child protective agencies or to the police. These statutes typically make the reporting professional (physician, nurse, social worker) immune from civil liability for defamation, breach of confidentiality, emotional distress, or invasion of privacy lawsuits. In the majority of states, *failure to report* could result in criminal sanctions. Further, there is potential liability for malpractice if a clinician negligently fails to diagnose and report suspected child abuse.

In cases of sexual abuse, including incest, careful interviewing and documentation of the interview and physical examinations are essential and should be closely coordinated with law enforcement and child protective agencies. Every institution should have a sexual abuse protocol, designating one individual to interact with the patient, gather information through interviews, complete forms, and report to the appropriate agency and law enforcement personnel. The provider must be willing to make the personal time commitment involved in the legal actions up to and including litigation that results from the reporting of abuse and neglect.

Incompetency

Courts have the power to declare a person "incompetent," removing his or her right to make decisions about business, finance, and other personal matters. Typically, in such a case, the court appoints a guardian to make decisions on behalf of the person (ward). However, guardianship does not automatically remove the patient's ability to make medical decisions on his or her own behalf. If questions are raised the assistance of an attorney is required.

Risk Management

Risk management is a series of measures that reduce the potential for the filing of malpractice claims and make those claims filed more defensible. Most risk management measures simply involve the use of competent practice techniques combined with good documentation and common sense.

During the prenatal course, the provider must know the current condition and at-risk conditions of the mother and fetus. For each visit the mother's weight, blood pressure, and urinalysis results as well as other pertinent clinical findings must be documented. The last menstrual period and the estimated date of confinement must be recorded in the chart and discrepancies between menstrual dating, physical examination results, and ultrasonic data somehow reconciled. Test results, including ultrasound examinations, electronic fetal monitoring strips, and laboratory tests, should be retained. All medications given should be carefully documented, especially those prescribed by telephone. All noncompliant behavior such as missed appointments should be carefully recorded. Key information that often is not entered on the chart may be conveyed during telephone calls. In certain instances, this information could be critical, eg, whether spotting versus hemorrhage was present in a case subsequently found to involve a abruptio placentae. Similarly, in prenatal care, the absence of findings can be legally significant and should be charted, especially when clinical findings are unclear, eg, no rupture of membranes, no discharge, no contractions.

The case law and medicolegal literature are replete with problems associated with the failure to diagnose various fetal conditions. Problems occur in the misinterpretation of or failure to perform ultrasonic examinations, as well as the presence or absence of a record of the scan.

Problems with the omission or misuse of ultrasound in obstetrics include failure to diagnose fetal anomalies or identify growth retardation, define the time limits for abortion, diagnose ectopic or abdominal pregnancy, diagnose multiple pregnancy, or diagnose placenta previa.

Many claims involve inadequate monitoring of the fetal condition, particularly during labor. If the external electronic fetal monitoring strip is ambiguous or unreliable, internal monitoring and/or scalp sampling is indicated. Alternatively, other biophysical tests may be indicated in women remote from term with uncertain fetal condition. Many suits that arise from intrapartum events and at delivery are related to the administration of oxytocin and monitoring of labor after the drug is administered. Availability of adequate anesthesia coverage is another issue. In general, in regard to performing an emergency cesarean section, a 30-minute interval from decision to delivery is considered a reasonable standard of care.

Cesarean delivery, especially emergent delivery, involves other potential risks to both mother and fetus. The clinician must have a competent assistant present to perform infant intubation when a high-risk delivery is anticipated.

Oxytocin use in labor is a common problem area. Dosages, method of administration, and uterine as well as fetal response should be carefully documented. Current hospital protocols should be up-to-date and carefully followed. Although oxytocin is usually an effective and safe drug, its misuse continues to plague obstetricians.

In addition, Apgar scores should be assigned by a designated individual who is perceived to have no vested interest in the result. Artificially inflating the score causes more harm than benefit and should be avoided. Plaintiff's attorneys will attempt to discredit high Apgar scores when there is inconsistency in scoring between the obstetrician and the nursing staff or gross discrepancies exist between the score and the infant's recorded condition. Apgar scores are often a focal point in malpractice cases, especially the scores at 5 minutes and beyond in "bad baby" cases.

At the time of at-risk delivery it is prudent to obtain an umbilical blood segment. Umbilical artery and vein pH analysis may be performed as indicated. Preserve the placenta for subsequent histological examination! Regardless of the ultimate outcome, an accurate record is the most useful means of reconstructing what occurred. In complicated cases or those involving serious and unforeseen injuries to mother or child, it is best to dictate an extensive note while the events are still recalled and immediately counsel the patient. In these circumstances, the case should be referred to the hospital risk management department for additional advice or assistance. Obviously, in complicated circumstances it is prudent also to notify one's own insurance carrier.

Table 2.3 The Emotional Response of the Defendant Physician to a Malpractice Action

Denial	Depression
Anger	Acceptance
Bargaining	Hope

After Kubler-Ross[43]

Physicians should not underestimate the emotional impact on themselves of an allegation of malpractice (Table 2.3). In some states, "support" groups exist to help the health care provider deal with this situation.

References

1. American College of Obstetricians and Gynecologists: *Professional Liability Insurance and Its Effect: Report of a Survey of ACOG's Membership.* Washington, DC, American College of Obstetricians and Gynecologists, 1985.

2. Newton M, Boyer R: Legal and ethical complications, in Newton M, Newton ER (eds.): *Complications of Gynecologic and Obstetric Management.* Philadelphia, WB Saunders, 1988, pp 503–519.

3. Schifrin BS: The patient as the plaintiff, in Eden RD, Boehm FH (eds.): *Assessment and Care of the Fetus.* Norwalk, CT, Appleton and Lange, 1990.

4. Nelson KB, Ellenberg JH: The asymptomatic newborn and risk of cerebral palsy. *Am J Dis Child* 1987;141:1333–1339.

5. Nelson KB: What proportion of cerebral palsy is related to birth asphyxia? *J Pediatr* 1988;112:572–574.

6. Quilligan EJ, Uhrig Vu R: The expert medical witness, in Eden RD, Boehm FH (eds.): *Assessment and Care of the Fetus.* Norwalk, CT, Appleton and Lange, 1990.

7. *Pratt v University of Minnesota Affiliated Hospital and Clinics*, 403 N.W. 2d 865 (Minn Ct. App. 1987).

8. Wynstra N: Reproductive issues, in Younger P, Conner C, Susan L, et al (eds.): *Hospital Law Manual—Administrator's Volume* 1988;115:51–60.

9. *Curlender v Bio-Science Laboratories,* 165 (Cal 1980;477).

10. *Procanik v Cillo,* 478 A. 2d. 755 (NJ 1984).

11. Wynstra N: Reproductive issues, in Younger P, Conner C, Susan L, et al (eds.): *Hospital Law Manual* 1989;122:52.

12. *Becker v Schwantz,* 386 N.E. 2d 807 (NY 1978).

13. *Jackson v Bumgardner,* 347 S.E. 2d 743 (NC 1986).

14. *Hickman v Group Health Plan, Inc.* 396 N.W. 2d 10 (Minn 1986).

15. *Morris v Sanchez,* 746 P. 2d 184 (Okla 1987).

16. *Wafford v Davis,* 61. 424 (Okla 1988).

17. *Speck v Finegold,* 439 A. 2d 110 (Penn 1981).

18. Baby "M," A-39-87 (NJ 1988).

19. Utah Code Ann 76-7-204, H.B. No. 129, New Laws (1989).

20. *Griswald v Connecticut,* 381 U.S. 479, 85 S. Ct. 1678 (1965).

21. *Hathaway v Worcester City Hospital*, 475 F. 2d. 701 (1973).

22. *Buck v Bell,* 274 U.S. 200, 47 S. Ct. 584 (1927).

23. *Mildred G. v Valerie N.,* 219 Cal. Rptr. 387 (1965).

24. Grady, A. 2d. 467 (NJ 1981).

25. Crouitz L: Offenses against the rule of law: This year's winners. *Wall Street Journal,* Dec. 26, 1990.

26. Elkins T, Anderson H, Barclay M, et al: Court-ordered cesarean section: An analysis of ethical concerns in compelling cases. *Am J Obstet Gynecol* 1989;161:150–154.

27. 40 Am Jur 2d Homicide Sec. 9.

28. 40 Am Jur 2d Homicide Sec. 434.

29. LaFave WR, Scott AW: Criminal Law 607 (ed. 2). 1986.

30. Perkins RM, Boyce RN: Criminal Law 50 (ed. 3). 1982.

31. 40 ALR 4th 724.
32. *Goldsmith v State,* 344 So. 2d 793 (Ala 1977).
33. *Harvard Law Rev* 103:7:1560.
34. Rhoden N: The judge in the delivery room: The emergence of court-ordered cesareans. 74 *Cal Law Rev* 1951 (1986).
35. *Roe v Wade,* 410 U.S. 113 (1973).
36. *Griswold v Connecticut,* 381 U.S. 479 (1965).
37. Kolder VE, Gallagher J, Parsons MT: Court ordered obstetrical intervention. *N Engl J Med* 1987;316:1192–1196.
38. *Jeffersons v Griffin Spalding County Hospital,* 274 S.E. 2d 457 (Ga 1987).
39. *Carder v George Washington University,* 573 A. 2d 1235–1252 (Washington, DC, 1990).
40. Ruling in cesarean section case brightlights maternal- fetal conflict. *Med Ethical Adv* 1990;6:65.
41. Legal intervention during pregnancy: Court-ordered medical treatments and legal penalties for potentially harmful behavior by pregnant women. *JAMA* 1990;264:2663–2670.
42. *Webster v Reproductive Health Services,* 109 S. Ct. 3040 (1989).
43. Kubler-Ross E: *On Death and Dying.* New York, MacMillan, 1969.

Chapter 3

Ethics and the Practitioner

Mary B. Mahowald, PhD

> Elegance is inferior to virtue, . . . the first object of
> laudable ambition is to obtain a character as a human
> being, regardless of the distinction of sex.
> —*A Vindication of the Rights of Woman,* 1792
> Mary Wollstonecraft
> 1759–1797

As public support for the goal of sexual equality has grown, so have criticisms and mistrust of medical power and technology. Criticisms have been directed especially toward the practice of obstetrics and gynecology, which seems to epitomize the paternalistic model of the physician's role towards women.[1] Recent manifestations of such criticisms and responses to them include the growth of the women's health movement, along with books such as *Our Bodies, Ourselves*[2]; *Immaculate Deception*[3]; *Of Woman Born*[4]; *Men Who Control Women's Health*[5]; and *A Woman in Residence.*[6] More philosophical accounts have surfaced recently. These include *Ethics and Human Reproduction: A Feminist Analysis,*[7] and a special issue of *Hypatia,* a journal of feminist philosophy, devoted to "Ethics and Reproduction."[8] As with any critical movement, there are excesses, inaccuracies, inconsistencies, and vagueness. But the women's movement may provide clinicians with an opportunity for growth in self- understanding and professional sensitivity through an analysis of these criticisms.

This chapter discusses moral issues that occur in the practice of obstetrics, some of which are unique to this speciality. I offer an overview of the main ethical principles through which the issues have been addressed, and suggest questions that may guide their application in specific cases.

Role of the Obstetrician

The traditional model of the physician-patient relationship is paternalistic. Independent of whether the physicians are men or women this relationship mimics the parent-child relationship in which one party is powerful and autonomous, while the other is vulnerable and dependent.[9] Because the father figure is assumed to know and promote the child's (patient's) best interest, he has not only the right, but the responsibility to override the wishes of the

Portions of this chapter will also appear in Mahowald M: *More Last Than First: Women, Children, and Healthcare.* New York: Oxford University Press (in press).

child in certain circumstances. However, the father's decisions are made not simply in behalf of an incompetent child (since some children are surely competent), or in behalf of an unconscious or extremely ill child (since most children are neither), but mainly in behalf of normal healthy children.

The image of the parent-knows-and-does-what-is-best physician is especially applicable to the role of the obstetrician towards the patient. Obstetric patients are ordinarily healthy, competent, and conscious, yet their relationship to the physician is one of vulnerability. Because our socialization process tends to encourage men to be dominant and women to accept that dominance, the fact that the physician is usually male whereas the obstetric patient is always female reinforces the inegalitarian aspects of the relationship.[10]

As more women enter medicine and as many of them choose obstetrics and gynecology as a specialty, it is possible that the nature of the physician-patient relationship will change. However, studies comparing personality traits of male and female medical students, and traits of female medical students with those of other women suggest that paternalistic tendencies of doctors will continue even if most doctors are women.[11]

Further compromising the situation of the woman as patient is the fact that matters routinely discussed with an obstetrician/gynecologist are often quite intimate (lifestyle, sexual practices, and relationships). However, no similar personal revelations are required or expected on the part of the physician. Such topics are more integral to the patient's concept of self than are the conditions treated by other specialties. Not infrequently, these issues also raise important moral questions for both patient and clinician. Moreover, when the patient is pregnant, her situation is complicated by the fact that her physician views his or her primary responsibility as extended to *two* individuals whose interests and needs are occasionally incompatible.

Precisely because the obstetrician is traditionally perceived as having two patients, the woman and the fetus, from the beginning (if not before) to the end of the pregnancy, ethical decisions in this specialty are inseparable from legal and social questions. For example, the *Roe v Wade* decision of the U.S. Supreme Court (1973) challenges the traditional two-patient concept of obstetrics by affirming the legal right of a woman to terminate a pregnancy during the first two trimesters.[12] Thus, to some extent the role concept of the obstetric professional is at odds with the legal system. Further, if the fetus is judged viable, the states retain the authority to override the autonomous decision of a woman to terminate her pregnancy. As the recent *Webster v Reproductive Health Services* decision suggests, the technology that has advanced potential fetal viability into the late second trimester will almost certainly result in changes to the laws currently permitting relatively unrestricted access to abortion prior to the third trimester.[13]

A major portion of the ethical decisions made by patients and clinicians in the practice of obstetrics/gynecology concerns fertility and infertility. Such decisions have greater impact on women's lives than on men's, even if fathers are equally responsible for their children. It is inevitably and exclusively women's bodies that are affected by pregnancy, childbirth, and lactation; it is not inevitable but empirically true that the majority of women bear most of the responsibility for raising children.[14]

Historically, the medical assistance of men in childbirth is a comparatively recent event. It is not surprising that some women view the medicalization of childbirth as an assertion of masculine control over an essentially female process. Indeed, some women believe that the motivation for men choosing the specialty of obstetrics/gynecology is a way of reducing the lack of power they experience in confronting the origin of life.

The rise of obstetrics as a medical specialty reveals a drive on the part of a predominantly male medical establishment to replace the previously dominant role of women in assistance at childbirth. Possibly the worst example in this regard is the secretive use of the forceps by three generations of male members of the Chamberlen family in England during the 17th century.[4,15] Although the Chamberlens attempted to dominate male practitioners as well as women, and were largely motivated by the desire for economic gain and enhanced prestige, their practice also usurped the role of women who had served as midwives.

Despite the gains of the women's movement, there still exists a double standard regarding the social responsibilities and expectations of women and men. Women who work outside the home return to domestic responsibilities in which some men assist, but few share equally.[16] That women's work, whether in or outside the home, is viewed as less important than the work of men is reflected in salary discrepancies between the sexes and in low pay and regard for child care and housework.[17,18] This attitude is indirectly expressed in the physician-patient relationship through disregard for women's time; eg, by assuming that women who accompany patients (eg, children or parents) or who are patients themselves must wait because the physician's time is more valuable. Men who are patients or accompany patients must wait also, but this occurs less frequently because fewer men are either patients or primary caregivers.

It is frequently assumed that women are more concerned about their physical appearance than are men. When the assumption proves true, whether the trait is natural or nurtured, it may negatively affect a woman's self-concept during the course of a pregnancy, and can exacerbate the psychological toll of surgical interventions such as breast removal for metastatic cancer. A double standard is also evident in the still surprisingly common use of first names for patients, who address their physicians by both title and last name. Admittedly, this practice is often reinforced from both sides of the relationship.

In support of the double standard it may be argued that the physician-patient relationship is necessarily inegalitarian, and that the practice of obstetrics is one aspect of the relationship that has no ethical implications, sexist or otherwise. In other words, the fact that most obstetricians are male and their patients female does not imply sexism. Inequality, if based on fact, does not constitute a moral problem. The soundness of this argument hinges on the concept of equality, which it assumes.[19–21] If equality is construed as *sameness* (and inequality, correspondingly, as *difference*), then obviously the physician-patient relationship, or obstetrician's relationship to a patient, or for that matter any person's relationship to any other person, is inegalitarian—because all of us are different. Surely the differences in themselves are morally neutral; it is the *values* assigned to them that move us into an ethical context, where moral conflicts may arise. Thus equality means that either the same or different traits and accomplishments have the same value; inequality means that they have different values.

On such an account, inequality in the physician-patient relationship presents a moral problem only if relevant differences between the two are not respected, or either party is not valued by the other as a person. Where sexism occurs, it means that sexuality is used irrelevantly as a criterion for distinguishing between people. Indeed, in this age of antimedical backlash,[22] reverse sexism is also a distinct possibility.

Persistent Ethical Issues

Ethical issues in obstetrics run the gamut of those issues raised in other medical specialties, eg, questions regarding disclosure, confidentiality, consent to experimental therapy, criteria for determination of death, and allocation of scarce medical resources. The ethical issues peculiar to obstetrics have mainly to do with either the curbing or enhancing of reproduction. Recurrent themes include the right and responsibility to assist others to reproduce or not to reproduce, and rights and responsibilities concerning sexual expression and gender identity. Complicating these themes are special cases. The fact that the physiological capability for reproduction is present at times in children, as well as in retarded or mentally ill adults, expands the responsibility of care for them to their potential offspring. Motherhood constitutes legal emancipation for some minors, but clearly does not establish that the new mother is mature enough to assume total responsibility for her newborn.[23]

Ethical questions concerning curtailment of pregnancy, especially abortion, have been dealt with extensively in philosophical literature. With regard to sterilization and contraception, the concerns invoked are often based on (1) the principle of informed consent, (2) the right to express one's sexuality without risk of pregnancy, and (3) responsibility to the larger society, including other family members and future generations.[24] "Natural law" arguments, ie, those which assume that reproduction is a natural process that ought not to be obstructed, are also offered.[25] On the issue of abortion, the moral status of the fetus is usually perceived as crucial to ethical assessment, and the right of the pregnant woman to control what transpires within her own body is also stressed.[26] It is the last issue that challenges the practitioner to confront the apparent contradiction between his or her professional commitment to both fetus and pregnant woman.

As individuals, obstetricians may wish to separate their own moral stance from those of their patients, allowing patients to make choices at variance with their own. This implies some tolerance for what the clinician perceives as wrong, or at least ambivalence regarding what he or she believes is right. Unless we posit a dichotomy between professional and moral responsibility (by which the physician sheds one skin for another in commuting between hospital and home), there surely is a need to reconcile the two positions. In other words, it is necessary to determine how to act both morally and professionally with patients with whom one has ethical disagreements. Typically, such disagreements reflect moderate rather than extreme positions on the part of clinicians; for example, one who considers early abortion for an unwanted pregnancy morally justified, but considers it wrong to choose or perform a second-trimester abortion solely because the fetus is not of the desired sex.

There is admirable consistency on the part of the anti-choice physician who not only refuses to perform abortions but organizes lobbying efforts to eliminate liberal abortion statutes. There is similarly admirable consistency on the part of the pro-choice clinician who operates a free abortion clinic and lobbies against restrictive abortion laws. But consistency is not a sufficient basis for honoring the practices of either individual. Beyond consistency, each of us needs to confront and evaluate the reasons that support our practice.

Legally, there are limits to what patients and clinicians may do, but these do not resolve the moral dilemmas of individuals. Even for those who consider the abortion issue settled, other related ethical questions are inevitable. For example, how should a physician respond to the queries of the mother of a sexually active teenager, also a patient, concerning the daughter's possible practice of contraception? Or how should a clinician deal with a patient's request to sterilize his or her moderately retarded child? In such situations, there are no predefined, fixed, or exclusive ways of acting morally; yet this does not imply that whatever one does is morally acceptable.

Recent critics of contemporary biomedical ethics have rejected methodologies based on traditional ethical theories and principles. Clements and Sider,[27] for example, have accused philosophers of using the "autonomy principle" as "a way of separating ethical thinking from the empirical world and placing it in the rationalist realm of metaethics" (p. 2011). Such an approach, they maintain, constitutes an assault on the traditional medical values of adaptation, and the best interests and function of the patient. Clements and Sider attribute the latter values to a "naturalistic ethics" consistent with the Hippocratic tradition; this competes with the "formalist ethics" of Kant and contemporary bioethicists.[27] The model they propose to replace the formalist emphasis on patient autonomy is one that proceeds *inductively* from an examination of specific cases, or a posteriori rather than *deductively* from a priori principles. The choice of the individual patient is defined as one among other biological functions to be promoted through clinical expertise.

More recent critics of "philosophical ethics" are Jonsen and Toulmin,[28] whose study of casuistry entails not so much a rejection of traditional theories and principles as an exposition of a more practical method for addressing the ethical quandaries that arise in specific situations. Apparently, the authors learned the method from living it. While working on the President's Commission for the Study of Ethical Problems in Medicine and Biomedical and Behavioral Research, they discovered that the commissioners "often disagreed seriously over the formulation of principle, while they quickly reached agreement on particular cases"[29] (p. 71). This experience spurred the two to examine the history and practice of casuistry more carefully. They eventually compiled a contemporary version applicable to issues in medical ethics. The main features of the method are reliance on paradigm cases, reference to broad consensus, and acceptance of "probable certitude." The precise relevance of principles to specific cases is seen mainly in analogies with the paradigm cases.

Such critics of reductionist theories seem to attack a straw person, viz, one who is purely deductive in approaching clinical or ethical dilemmas. In reality, neither deductive nor inductive reasoning is practiced exclusively in the clinical setting. Despite their emphasis on cases, Jonsen and Toulmin appeal to principles as maxims embodied in the applicable paradigms, and Clements and Sider apply the general principle of beneficence to cases they consider.

The more characteristic situation is one of straddling both case- based and theoretical approaches, utilizing whatever strategies are available to facilitate resolution. Such a method is in fact *pragmatic* in the sense that it is practically oriented, rejecting a dichotomy between theory and action. To the pragmatist, theory and action are inseparable.[30] This view is consistent with the emphasis on context and the critique of absolutism embodied in a feminine model of moral reasoning such as Carol Gilligan[31] elaborates. This is an ethic based on care rather than justice, stressing relationships rather than individual rights.[31] Classical pragmatists also point to the reality and relevance of relationships.[32] Clearly, both care and relationships are crucial considerations for ethical decision making in clinical practice.

While we realize that principles are not adequate to resolve particular questions, we assume that the application of reason to the nuances of the situation, especially when conjoined to the rational, collaborative input of others, will bring us closer to the correct solution. Working on that assumption, we can compare basic ethical principles, guidelines, and strategies with the different bodily systems that must be checked in developing a patient diagnosis or plan of treatment. Just as therapeutic prescriptions are never certain to be successful, although that is surely their intent, so ethical decisions are never certain to provide correct answers to the questions asked, although that is also their intent.

Applicable Principles

What are the ethical principles or "systems" to be checked in determining ethical "prescriptions"? In recent years, prominent biomedical ethicists have proposed various combinations of principles that they consider crucial. Veatch,[33] for example, considers six different principles: beneficence, contract keeping, autonomy, honesty, avoiding killing, and justice. Contract keeping involves the obligation of confidentiality in the doctor-patient relationship. From differing ethical perspectives (utilitarian and deontological), Beauchamp and Childress[34] primarily deal with four principles: autonomy, beneficence, nonmaleficence, and justice; in addition, they consider veracity and confidentiality as important ethical components of the caregiver–patient bond. McCullough and Beauchamp,[35] Engelhardt,[36] and Jonsen et al[37] tend to focus on beneficence and respect for autonomy as the foremost ethical principles, dealing with justice as a necessary principle for situations requiring allocation of health care resources.

The meanings embodied in the broad list of principles can be encapsulated in three principles: *beneficence*, *respect for autonomy*, and *justice*. Honesty, veracity, and confidentiality may be viewed as essential to respect for autonomy; beneficence may be seen as encompassing nonmaleficence and the avoidance of killing. In teaching future doctors, I often compare these principles to the basic bodily systems that must be checked out if one is to conduct an adequate assessment of the patient's health before determining a specific plan of treatment. Unlike clinical principles, however, the ethical principles relevant to decisions of clinicians include consideration of patients, family members,

ETHICS AND THE PRACTITIONER   37

colleagues, and, occasionally, chaplains, lawyers, and administrators.

The first principle, beneficence, is essentially embodied in the Hippocratic imperative: "to help, or at least to do no harm."[38] Accordingly, this principle comprises both positive and negative duties towards the patient. The latter are sometimes described as nonmaleficence, which represents a more stringent obligation than simple beneficence. Practically, however, it may not only be difficult but unhelpful to observe this distinction. For example, the very "doing of harm" in accepting the risk of pain in surgical exploration may constitute the "doing of good." Insofar as medical and surgical interventions are therapeutic, they are all of this type. It remains the task of individuals to determine the expected proportion of harms to benefits, so that the minimal criterion of an equal balance between the two is observed. Beyond that point of obligation virtue invites the practitioner to do more good, that is, to do more than what is minimally required legally or morally in behalf of the patient as well as others.[39] Applying the principle of beneficence on the basis of either virtue or obligation involves the following question: "Is the proposed intervention (or nonintervention) justified on the basis of the good result expected primarily for the patient(s), and secondarily for others affected?" The answer to this question provides an important consequentialist or utilitarian input into the decision-making process.

Because benefits and burdens keep shifting, constant recalculation is required in order to apply the principle of beneficence faithfully. Burdens to be weighed include pain, medication, surgery, dietary restrictions, loss of privacy, incurrence of costs, loss of income, separation from one's family, etc. Expected benefits that may justify imposition of the burdens include maintenance, promotion, or restoration of health. However, an adequate ethical perspective calls for assessment of burdens and benefits to others besides the patient. In obstetrics, the calculation is complicated by concerns about the fetus and the pregnant woman's long-term reproductive capacity. The overall goal is to render the patient (or patients) free of any burden of health care interventions, ie, to make professional assistance no longer necessary.

The next principle, respect for autonomy, is essentially "deontological," that is, a priori, or based on nonconsequentialist rules or laws that arise from the very meaning of human nature or from divine command. Such principles are held to be discernible by human beings through their use of reason or faith (or both), and universally applicable and binding. In our own day, the principle of respect for autonomy embodied in the concept of informed consent has widely replaced the traditional paternalistic model of the physician's role. Important as it is, this concept applies the principle of respect for autonomy or self-determination to only one of those influenced by clinical ethical decisions, namely, the competent patient. In obstetrical and other reproductive decisions, however, there is always another autonomous individual affected, namely, the potential biological father. Moreover, clinicians themselves surely do not surrender their own autonomy at the door of the treatment or operating room. They are also responsible for what they do and do not do, regardless of what the patient chooses. To base decisions exclusively on the patient's "informed consent" is to ignore this continuous responsibility, and subscribe to a purely instrumentalist interpretation of the physician's role. To base decisions on the broader principle of respect for autonomy is to ask the question:

"What course is preferred by each of the individuals influenced by this decision?" Where there are conflicting answers, these should be weighed according to the degree in which the individual will be affected.

Since autonomous decisions can only be made on the basis of correct understanding of alternatives and their implications, respect for autonomy entails an obligation of disclosure or "truth telling." Absolute truth telling is an impossible goal because of the inevitable limitations of knowledge and ability to communicate. What remains possible is truthfulness, honesty, or veracity, ie, an attempt to communicate to others accurately and adequately. This does not imply that every individual has a right to all specific information in all circumstances. A clearly justified limitation to truthfulness or the obligation of disclosure is recognition of the right to privacy of the individual about whom information is known. In other words, there is also an obligation to observe confidentiality, which is especially applicable to the kinds of information that an obstetrician possesses. The relevant question for the clinician, therefore, is two-faceted: "What information do I owe my patient, those close to her, and other health professionals, and what information am I obligated not to disclose?" Another practical question immediately follows: "How might I most effectively communicate or refrain from communicating, where circumstances call for either approach?" Comparable questions apply to others who possess pertinent information, including nonclinicians, family members, and the patients themselves.

The third ethical "system" to be checked out in determining responses to ethical dilemmas is the principle of justice. This may be construed as deontological or utilitarian, and as applicable either to individual decisions or to social policy. In either case, it is the notion of distributive (rather than retributive) justice about which we are concerned. Inevitably, this entails an interpretation of equality as applicable (or inapplicable) to individuals or groups. Macroallocation decisions regarding distribution of health care resources are mainly a matter of social policy, but microallocation decisions are made every day through determinations regarding time, space, equipment, expertise, and medication.

If the principle of justice is to be applied in obstetrics, some determination needs to be made regarding the status of the fetus, so that conflicts that pit the alleged rights of the fetus against those of the pregnant woman may be addressed in that light. When fetus and pregnant woman count equally as patients or persons, justice requires that neither has the greater claim against the other, and a random way of determining care for one as opposed to the other may be acceptable.[40] Even then, however, duties towards and effects on others are morally relevant when the rights of persons are in conflict. On the other hand, justice does not require equal consideration of fetus and pregnant woman if either of the following positions is maintained: (a) rights to life and liberty are proportionate to the developmental status of the individual, whether that individual counts as person or not; or (b) the personhood by which an individual is judged worthy of equitable treatment with other persons commences at birth or some later point of life.

Since 1973 the U.S. Supreme Court has upheld a view not quite like either of the above positions.[12] According to that ruling, safe abortions are permissible on the basis of a woman's choice, prior to the point of fetal viability. When fetal viability is achieved, the pregnant woman's choice may be subordinated to the fetus's right to survive. The concept of justice invoked here is equal treatment for all who are legally persons. Despite the uncertainties inherent in prenatal determination of fetal viability, its achievement apparently bestows legal personhood. Thereafter, only when the life or health of the pregnant woman is threatened may the fetus be terminated or risked by preterm delivery. In other words, life and liberty are not viewed as equal values of those who count (or may count) as persons before the law. Justice implies that life is the more basic right or value, which cannot be denied in the name of another's liberty.

Newer Ethical Issues

The modern practice of obstetrics includes many other difficult ethical dilemmas. Court-ordered cesarean sections for pregnant women represent even greater restrictions to women's autonomy than do statutes prohibiting termination of pregnancy.[41] The apparent epidemic of crack use during pregnancy suggests the possibility of coercive interventions for the sake of the fetus. Again, an interpretation of justice as entailing equal treatment of all persons, extended to viable fetuses as "legal persons," may be invoked to justify the intervention. However, ethical positions affirming the rights of the pregnant woman over those of the fetus may also be maintained under the aegis of justice. In fact such positions seem more defensible in a society that upholds the rights of individuals to control their own lives and bodies. Although a recent decision regarding a dying pregnant woman in Washington supports this position, a survey of heads of maternal-fetal medicine programs in the United States suggests that the issue is far from settled among clinicians.[42] In deciding among conflicting interests, the pertinent question for clinicians and patients alike is the following: "Which approach is most likely to result in an equitable distribution of harms and benefits among those affected?"

Recent developments in fertility research have evoked recognition of ethical questions surrounding marital and sexual relationships, parenthood, and the right to biologically related progeny. Some of these issues have been with us for a long time without raising much public concern, perhaps because the relevant practices (such as artificial insemination by husband or donor) are usually implemented covertly. Newer means of facilitating reproduction tend to focus on infertility in women rather than men, and in that context, successful interventions can hardly be covert, eg, when a woman who has long been infertile is manifestly pregnant, or when a nonpregnant woman brings home the newborn of her husband and a "surrogate." In time, as techniques are refined and routinized, confidentiality may be better maintained in cases of ovum transfer and in vitro fertilization, as in artificial insemination. However, in all of these situations a rather new metaethical question is raised, namely, "Whose child is this?" (see Chapter 16).

In an individualistic society such as ours, the concept of parenthood is often traditional and biological: a heterosexual married couple who conceive a child through sexual intercourse, each contributing 23 chromosomes, one contributing her uterus, along with the physical and emotional costs of pregnancy and childbirth, and both partners contributing thereafter to the child's nurturance. In some respects, the child is then considered the property of the parents: he or she belongs to them, is named by them, is kept and cared for by them unless "given up" for adoption or until the child is "given" to another in marriage. Admittedly, parental rights over children have legal as well as moral limits, but they remain extremely significant determinants of children's lives and identities. Moreover, through the nuclear families which our modern transient lifestyle encourages, the family unit has come to represent an end in itself, a kind of self-justifying system. Within that framework it is difficult to appreciate a more complicated and extended concept of parenthood.

To grapple adequately with the ethical questions that advances in reproductive technologies present, and in light of the fact that in many cases it takes more than two individuals to create a child, we need to re-examine our traditional concept of parenthood. This latter fact points to rights and responsibilities on the part of the developers, and to conflicts in the exercise of those rights and responsibilities. Such conflicts might be resolved through examination of differing contributions of parent figures, including the duration, depth, and demands of their relationship to the child. A "priority among parents" could be determined on the basis of their contribution to the child, whether physical, psychological, or both. The nurturant input of those who care for a child beyond birth, regardless of their biological relationship, marital status, or sex, surely gives these individuals a higher priority than those who never actually cared for the child.

Justice is in a certain sense an extension of the principle of beneficence: an equitable distribution of harms and benefits. Applying this to reproduction entails examination of the costs of developing and implementing the technologies, and in examining the accessibility of the technology to the general population. As long as certain ways of facilitating reproduction are available only to a limited number of those in need (those who can pay for them) the claim that biological reproduction is a recognized universal right is hardly defensible. Limited application of technology may be justified on the basis of its experimental status, but the principle of justice demands that discrepancies in accessibility be reduced as much as possible. That the affluent receive the benefits of the research may be justified on utilitarian grounds: current discrimination is essential in order to make the technology eventually available to others. But this argument is inadequate so long as the ideal of justice might be approximated even now. Because the technology is of such great benefit to a wealthy few, part of what those few pay might be directed to the purchase of its availability to some of the poor. Although this view may be incompatible with the self-interested motivation of a free-enterprise system, it is not inconsistent with democratic principles. Similar arguments have been made regarding the availability of abortion and contraceptive procedures.

Assessing the Alternatives

At the beginning of this chapter I suggested that analysis of current criticism of the medical profession in general, and of obstetrics and gynecology in particular, might yield helpful insights for clinical practice. The same may be said for the women's movement. In fact, I believe the question "Whose children are they?" is crucial to the understanding and assessment of different versions of feminism, as well as for consideration of views opposed to feminism.[43,44] Advances in reproductive technologies have not only increased the capacity of individuals to control their reproductive lives, they have greatly complicated the expression of that capacity. Individualistic versions of feminism and medicine focus on the right of individual women or patients to control their reproductive lives; "communalistic" versions of feminism insist on concern for the larger community.[45] The question "Whose child?" is answered individualistically as "Mine." From a communalistic perspective, that answer is "Ours." The first response implies that the answerer has full rights and total responsibilities. Increasingly, the first answer is unrealizable. The second response is empirically unavoidable but morally questionable.

As medicine has moved toward a more socialized understanding of itself, and health care professionals have observed their responsibility to patients as extending to the broader society, feminism has reflected a critique of individualism, even while emphasizing respect for reproductive rights. Conflicting ideologies, whether in medicine or feminism, are not likely to be resolved any sooner than the perennial metaphysical problem of "the one and the many," but some of the tension between them may be reduced and rendered constructive through recognition of the validity and inadequacy of mutually exclusive positions. To the question "Whose child is this?" the answers "Mine" and "Ours" are both valid and inadequate if one subscribes to an ethic that stresses responsibilities as well as rights. "Mine" is least inadequately applied to the biological mother who has nurtured her child beyond pregnancy to some stage of self-sufficiency; but even here, the man through whom the child was conceived and who shares in the child's nurturance may also call the child "Mine." Thus the couple together, less inadequately, say "Ours." To the extent that others share the joy and burden of nurturing children, they too, even less inadequately, join in saying "Ours."

My own view, therefore, is that feminism is compatible with the physician-patient relationship, as long as the mutuality of rights and responsibilities among individuals is respected in both contexts. The emphasis on nurturance that characterizes health care practice provides further grounds for compatibility between the two sides. An emphasis on context or case-based reasoning eschews rigid adherence to unchanging principles, even those that have become well established in contemporary biomedical ethics. Like clinical concepts and generalized treatment plans, these provide a useful framework for understanding the complexity of a changing situation, but they cannot yield definitive answers to questions raised by unique cases. The cases themselves are instructive regarding interpretation of the concepts and modes of treatment. As already suggested, this interplay between theoretical and practical considerations illustrates the notion of pragmatism that William James wrote about in 1907.[46] Using an image proposed by the Italian pragmatist Papini, James compares the method of pragmatism to a corridor in a hotel:

> Innumerable chambers open out of it. In one you may find a man writing an atheistic volume; in the next some one on his knees praying for faith and strength; in a third a chemist investigating a body's properties; in a fourth a system of idealistic metaphysics is being excogitated; in a fifth the impossibility of metaphysics being shown. But they all

own the corridor, and all must pass through it if they want a practicable way of getting into or out of their respective rooms (p. 47).

Alternative theories, concepts, principles, and strategies are "owned" simultaneously but used discriminately in practical problem solving. An adage often used in the clinical situation is the following: "When all else fails, examine the patient." Obstetrics is a unique specialty in many respects, but each case within the specialty is unique as well, and different contexts raise issues that occur in other situations. Although general considerations are never adequate to the peculiarities of cases, it would be irresponsible not to draw on the meaning and relevance of basic principles and guidelines in addressing specific questions.

References

1. Holmes HB: The birth of a women-centered analysis, in Holmes H (ed.): *Birth Control and Controlling Birth*. Clifton, Humana Press, 1979, pp 5–6.
2. Boston Women's Health Book Collective Staff: *Our Bodies, Ourselves*. New York, Simon and Schuster, 1984.
3. Arms S: *Immaculate Deception*. New York, Bantam Books, 1975.
4. Rich A: *Of Woman Born*. New York, Bantam Books, 1977.
5. Scully D: *Men Who Control Women's Health*. Boston, Houghton-Mifflin, 1980.
6. Harrison M: *A Woman in Residence*. New York, Random House, 1982.
7. Overall C: *Ethics and Human Reproduction: A Feminist Analysis*. Boston, Allen and Unwin, 1987.
8. Purdy LM (ed.): Ethics and reproduction. *Hypatia* 1989;4,3:1–159.
9. Childress J: What is paternalism?, in Robinson J, Pritchard M (eds.): *Medical Responsibilities*. Clifton, Humana Press, 1979, pp 18–21.
10. American Medical Association, Division of Survey and Data Resources: *Physician Characteristics and Distribution in the U.S.* Chicago, American Medical Association, 1987, pp 8, 42.
11. Mahowald MB: Sex-role sterotypes in medicine. *Hypatia* 1987;2:22, 31.
12. *Roe v Wade*, 410 U.S. 113 (1973).
13. *Webster v Reproductive Health Services*, 109 S.Ct. 3040 (1989).
14. Rossi A, Breslau N: Care of disabled children and women's time use. *Med Care* 1983;21:620–629.
15. Ehrenreich B, English D: *Witches, Midwives and Nurses*. Old Westbury, CT, Feminist Press, 1973, pp 12–15.
16. Scott H: *Does Socialism Liberate Women?* Boston, Beacon Press, 1974, pp 199–200.
17. Illich I: *Gender,* New York, Pantheon Books, 1982, pp 24, 274.
18. Ratner RS: *Equal Employment Policy for Women: Strategies for Implementation in the USA, Canada and Western Europe*. Philadelphia, Temple University Press,1978, pp 20–23.
19. Blackstone W (ed.): *The Concept of Equality*. Minneapolis, Burgess Publishing, 1979.
20. Gutman A: *Liberal Equality*. New York, Cambridge University Press, 1980.
21. Walzer M: *Spheres of Justice*. New York, Basic Books, 1983.
22. Starr P: *The Social Transformation of American Medicine*. New York, Basic Books, 1982, pp 379–419.
23. Leikin S: Minors' assent or dissent to medical treatment. *J Pediatr* 1983; 102:169–176.

24. Petchesky R: Reproductive freedom. *Signs* 1980;5:661–685.
25. Curran C: *Contemporary Problems in Moral Theology.* Notre Dame, IN, Fides Publishers, 1970, pp 97–188.
26. Sumner LW: *Abortion and Moral Theory.* Princeton, NJ, Princeton University Press, 1981, pp 26–33, 40–123.
27. Clements CD, Sider RC: Medical ethics assault upon medical values. *JAMA* 1983;250:2011–2013.
28. Jonsen AR, Toulmin S: *The Abuse of Casuistry.* Berkeley, University of California Press, 1988.
29. Jonsen AR: Casuistry and clinical ethics. *Theor Med* 1986;7:71.
30. Thayer HS: *Meaning and Action: A Critical History of Pragmatism.* Indianapolis, Bobbs Merrill, 1968, pp 424–430.
31. Gilligan C: Moral orientation and moral development, in Kattay E, Meyers D (eds.): *Women and Moral Theory.* Totoway, NJ, Rowman and Littlefield, 1987, pp 19–33.
32. James W: The thing and its relations, in McDermott JJ (ed.): *The Writings of William James.* New York, Modern Library, 1967, pp 214–226.
33. Veatch R: *A Theory of Medical Ethics.* New York, Basic Books, 1981, pp 141–287.
34. Beauchamp T, Childress J: *Principles of Biomedical Ethics,* New York, Oxford University Press, 1983, pp 59–220.
35. McCullough L, Beauchamp T: *Medical Ethics.* Englewood Cliffs, NJ, Prentice-Hall, 1984, pp 13–51.
36. Engelhardt HT: *The Foundations of Bioethics.* New York, Oxford University Press, 1986, pp 66–103.
37. Jonsen AR, Siegler M, Winslade WJ: *Clinical Ethics.* New York, Macmillan, 1986, pp 11–127.
38. Hippocrates: Selections from the Hippocratic Corpus, in Reiser S (ed.): *Ethics in Medicine.* Cambridge, Massachusetts Institute of Technology Press, 1977, p 7.
39. Callahan D: Minimalist ethics. *Hastings Cent Rep* 1981;11:19–25.
40. Childress J: Who shall live when not all shall live?, in Munson R (ed.): *Intervention and Reflection.* Belmont, WA, Wadsworth, 1983, pp 501–504.
41. Annas G: Forced cesareans: The most unkindest cut. *Hastings Cent Rep* 1982;12:16–17, 45.
42. Kolder V, Gallagher J, Parsons M: Court ordered obstetrical interventions. *N Engl J Med* 1987;316:1192–1196.
43. Jaggar A, Struhl P (eds.): *Feminist Frameworks.* New York, McGraw Hill, 1978, pp 206–259
44. Tony R: *Feminist Thought.* Boulder, CO, Westview Press, 1989.
45. Mahowald MB: Feminism: Individualistic or communalistic?. *Proc Am Cathol Philos Assoc* 1976;219–229.
46. James W: *Pragmatism.* Cleveland, OH, Meridian, 1955, pp 47, 89–108.

PART II

Normal Gestation

Chapter 4

Psychological Adjustments to Pregnancy

Miriam Rosenthal, MD and John P. O'Grady, MD

Behave in *Words and Action*, with all imaginable tenderness. . . . Their pain, both in regard of the *Mind and Body*, are at that time very hard upon them, and . . . calls for the softest manner in the necessary assistance.
—*A Treatise on the Improvement of Midwifery*, 1733
Edmund Chapman

Pregnancy is a major developmental event with accompanying biological, psychological, and social changes.[1,2] Classically, clinicians have been trained to identify the biological abnormalities of gestation and focused their attention on detection of these abnormalities. Yet, in many instances psychological problems may cause equal if not more distress to pregnant women. All too frequently their distress is not addressed.[3,4] Social changes with rapid shifts in societal norms for sexual expression, the meaning of reproductive health care in general and of pregnancy in specific, and pressures on the traditional physician-patient relationship combine to make modern management difficult.[5] In clinical management the obstetrician is not expected to be a psychiatrist, but he or she needs to (1) be able to effectively communicate with patients for data gathering and to assure compliance; (2) be prepared to recognize norms and changes in behavior, mood, and thinking that may suggest a psychiatric disorder; and (3) know how and where to refer patients to mental health providers when required.

The aim of this chapter is to outline the psychological events of pregnancy. As will be emphasized both in this chapter as well as throughout the text, while the physiology of human gestation establishes the basis for clinical events, the pregnancy experience is a complex mix of individual personality, prior life events, and cultural and social influences.

Pregnancy: A Developmental Transition

Traditionally, pregnancy has been considered the fulfillment of deep and powerful wishes of a woman—a chance for creativity and self-realization, providing the opportunity for new growth and direction.[2] Today, however, due in part to modern technology, many women choose not to experience pregnancy or to delay conception. Still others are unable to have children. Some women learn to fulfill their personal and sexual potentials in ways other than child-bearing, while some may experience substantial emotional difficulty.[6]

While pregnancy may bring a sense of joy, well-being, and fulfillment, it is also a potentially stressful time.[1,7-9] New conflicts arise and old ones are reactivated from the past. Long-term psychological issues that are important include the relationships with one's own mother and father; the arrival of siblings in one's childhood; role issues; and the responsibilities of being a mother, career woman, wife, and partner. How one copes is related to early experiences of being nurtured, personal coping mechanisms, personality, lifestyle, life situation, the extent of emotional support received, and the physical care provided by the clinician.

The father-to-be is also presented with many conflicts. Today, fathers share much of the pregnancy experience with their partner. Not suprisingly, many men have an increase in physical symptoms during their wives' pregnancies and visit physicians more often with a variety of complaints.[10] More severe psychological reactions are also possible.[11] These symptoms reflect the fathers' own anxieties and concerns about their new role. They too may feel envy toward their partner's new condition, which can lessen the attention the couple formerly paid to each other. Marital satisfaction is important to the successful adaptation of a woman to the postpartum state. Sexual behavior is an important component of satisfaction that may be substantially altered by pregnancy[12] (see Chapter 7).

The obstetrical clinician-physician, nurse, or midwife has an unusual opportunity to help the individual woman and her partner mature and develop throughout pregnancy. Further, a good prenatal and birth experience increases the chances for the baby to have a good start and can influence family dynamics in the long term.[13] Conversely, the stresses associated with pregnancy may, on occasion, precipitate severe emotional reactions, confuse the identification of physiological abnormalities, interfere with "standard" therapies, and perhaps contribute to obstetric complications.

Motivations for Pregnancy

There are complex reasons why women seek pregnancy beyond the strong wish for a child.[2,14] Many pregnancies (about 50%) are either unanticipated and/or unwanted.[15] There is increased vulnerability to an unwanted pregnancy at times of transition, such as beginning sexual life, engagement, leaving school, moving to a new community, change of job, beginning a new educational opportunity, when a youngest child enters school, and perimenopause. Many of these undesired pregnancies result from errors or accidents of contraception or ignorance of birth control methods, especially among adolescent women. Some couples seek the advice of their obstetrician/gynecologist prior to planning their first or subsequent pregnancy, but the majority do not.

The wish for a pregnancy may not be the same as a wish for a baby or a child. A pregnancy can be desired to assure that one's body works adequately, that one is a female with a functioning reproductive system. This may be the situation for some young women with chronic illnesses who have been warned that pregnancy would be dangerous or undesirable. Unfortunately, some of these women have not received adequate counseling in regard to birth control.

Jane is a 17-year-old single high school student with myasthenia gravis of 2 years duration. She is 12 weeks pregnant. Her disease is progressive. She understood she might improve or get worse with a pregnancy and that she should not get pregnant. She was not given birth control advice by her physician. She wants to have a baby. "Maybe I will get better." "If I die, at least some part of me will be left."

When pregnancy occurs among unmarried adolescents, many factors may exist: concern about sexual identity, rebellion against parents, peer pressure, a response to loss of a parent or close person or attention, or a response to loneliness, with the idea that "the baby will love me." Identification with a fantasized child, or concern about maintaining a partner in a relationship may also occur. Pregnancy may be a way to separate from one's parents or to resolve competitive feelings concerning parents, or the pregnancy may represent a wish to fulfill the parents' or grandparents' desire for more children or grandchildren. For older women, the feeling of the pressure of a "biological clock" limiting the time left to achieve pregnancy has increasingly become a factor.

Ms. B is a 39-year-old banker. She wants a child before her "biological clock runs out." She has been very successful in her career, is heterosexual, and hopes to marry some day. She is requesting donor insemination to become pregnant now.

Some pregnancies, especially in adolescence, are the result of incest or forcible intercourse. Patients and their family are often reluctant to accept or discuss such events and the true state of affairs may not be immediately recognized by even an astute clinician.

Economic and social reasons are also commonly an influence on reproduction. In many cultures, children represent more than immortality; they are old age security and a reliable family work force. In these settings where the family unit is the work unit as well, reproductive failure has potentially disastrous consequences.

Sources of Stress in Pregnancy and the Puerperium

Endocrine, somatic, and psychological changes occur in all pregnant women but are manifested in varying fashions. The confirmation of pregnancy may be a great joy for some and devastating for others, although all women commonly experience at least some ambivalence.[2,8]

For some women with preexisting health problems, their primary concern is for sufficient resources to withstand the additional physiological demands of gestation. Even healthy women are not free from physical discomforts. Virtually all experience some physical distress due to abdominal enlargement, nausea, heartburn, or urinary frequency, independent of the anticipated discomforts of labor and delivery. Some level of psychological distress from worries about genetic risks, role changes, the effect on husband or partner, career, education plans, finances, personal attractiveness, and the ability to be a mother—like her own, or different—are also common. A worry frequently not voiced, especially for the nullipara is: Will I live through this experience?

Interpersonal relationships with the partner, mother, co-workers, and friends change during and after the pregnancy. Marital satisfaction often declines during pregnancy, which is probably related to the woman's turning more inward, especially in the first trimester. This is accompanied by a progressive decline in sexual interest but an increased desire for affection as pregnancy advances[12,16,17] (see Chapter 7). Pregnancy is a public statement of a woman's sexual activity and thus can be a source of either pride or embarassment. In general, women who react positively to their own sexuality will experience pregnancy more positively.

Normal Psychological Processes in Pregnancy and Puerperium

Anxiety, emotional lability, and worries are normal during gestation.[18] The basic developmental and psychological tasks for a woman during pregnancy are[8] (1) to incorporate and integrate the presence of a fetus (part of herself and partner) as an integral part of her body and self; and once fetal movement is present, (2) to perceive the fetus as a separate entity, to begin to visualize a fetus as a baby with needs of his/her own; and (3) to see herself as a mother, and to establish a caretaking relationship with an infant. In order to mother adequately, a woman needs to have had the experience of being nurtured herself as an infant. In the absence of such a positive experience she can have serious difficulties.

First Trimester

The initial psychological task of pregnancy is acceptance.[19] In the first trimester in a wanted pregnancy, when the diagnosis is confirmed, there is usually a sense of excitement and joy mixed with anxiety and ambivalence.[20] Even the most wanted pregnancy is often accompanied by ambivalence by both parents, who perceive that a major life transition is at hand. In an unwanted pregnancy, there may be a sense of despair and of life being out of control. However, an unplanned pregnancy is not necessarily unwanted and may become accepted once the initial unhappiness passes. A woman needs time to process her thoughts and feelings with her partner and family. If ambivalence concerning pregnancy is a major issue, she needs counseling concerning termination as soon as possible following a firm diagnosis. The woman's delays combined with the health care staff's own ambivalence may turn a technically simple first-trimester procedure into a traumatic or difficult second-trimester termination.

Physiologically, the first trimester of pregnancy is characterized by rapid elevations in chorionic gonadotropin and high estrogen and progesterone levels. Accompanying physical symptoms include fatigue, breast tenderness, and nausea and vomiting.

High progesterone levels likely contribute to feelings of sedation or mild depression noted in many pregnant women.[21,22] Yet, some women feel fulfilled and many have an increased sense of well- being while pregnant, especially after the first 8 to 10 weeks. Psychologically, there is a turning inward and more preoccupation with the self and the new inner growth. During the first trimester, the woman may be more emotionally labile, and feel discouraged at the fatigue and nausea. As pregnancy progresses, sexual interest declines, but there may be more of a wish to be held.[12,16] Fears concerning miscarriage, the health of baby, and role changes are common.

Thoughts giving magical reasons for occurrences are often present in early pregnancy. There is a belief in the cause-and-effect relationship of unrelated events such as "I am going to give birth, someone may die." If a close person does die or becomes seriously ill, this is often quite disturbing. This is not psychotic thought, as the individual realizes that this thinking is irrational. However, the person still finds such thoughts to be profoundly disturbing.

The frequent use of ultrasound during pregnancy is generally perceived by women as helpful.[20] The experience often leads to an earlier type of "maternal bonding" of both father and mother to the unborn child. Such parental involvement is important and can be used to predict later feelings toward the infant.[13] Knowing the sex of the fetus by chromosomal analysis or direct observation also assists the couple in adapting to that baby. The discovery that the woman is carrying a child of the "wrong" sex presents its own problems and such a woman should have counseling to resolve some of those feelings.

Second Trimester

During these weeks there is often a feeling of relief as the woman feels better physically. The sensation of nausea declines. There is a resuming of interest in outside events. Quickening provides a sense of reality concerning the pregnancy, reinforcing the idea of the fetus as a separate entity. This often leads to a focus on realistic planning for the remainder of pregnancy and delivery. At this point, women commonly fantasize about how the baby will appear and parents assess their own upbringing. Late in this period, there is increased sense of passivity and dependency. Sexual desire may increase or decrease. Changes in body image due to the increasing abdominal girth may be disturbing to the woman and to her partner. The main task of this period of pregnancy is the recognition of the baby as an individual, a part of herself, yet separate.[19]

Third Trimester

During the last trimester, there is increased anxiety and fear concerning labor and delivery combined with the desire for pregnancy to end. Anxieties develop about the possible pain or injury at delivery, the health of the baby, being a mother, and how relationships may be altered. Women worry about the possible death of both herself and her unborn child. Sleep is often difficult and there may be increasing somatic preoccupations as the increasing uterine bulk provokes new symptoms of pressure and general discomfort. A common preoccupation during the last trimester is preparation for the expected delivery. The major psychological task for these latter weeks is to prepare for physical separation from the child and for the child's life thereafter.[19] This is also the time when there is a preoccupation with childbirth and nest building. Childbirth education is widely available in special classes, videotapes, or films. In general, such education should occur in a setting where the woman feels free to ask questions regardless of how unconsequential they may seem.

Today, with progressive liberalization of hospital procedures, there are numerous birth options. These have proven to be a mixed blessing. Considerable psychological difficulties occur when women consider themselves a "failure" if they do not fulfill their own delivery expectations, eg, without anesthesia or surgical interventions. A problem that the profession has helped to create is the increasing expectation that with modern technology nothing can or will go wrong. Unfortunately, the human birth process is imperfect and complications are common. Prenatal counseling for labor and delivery is an important responsibility which clinicians should not entirely abandon to childbirth classes. Obstetricians sometimes believe they must protect themselves from lawsuits by telling the women everything that could possibly go wrong during the pregnancy or delivery. This is usually an error.

While medicolegally, perhaps, this is correct, such "disaster discussions" are at best psychologically suspect. Under such stresses communication between a woman and her physician can break down. As always, the art of medicine is best seen in patient interviews. If a pregnancy faces real and specific risks, then it is mandatory that these risks be openly discussed. On the other hand, an encyclopedic review of all possible complications is both unnecessary and potentially harmful, creating fears rather than relieving them.

Paradoxically, good communication does not require extra time. In fact, many physicians who spend much extra time with patients do so to patch up problems. They have not communicated or actively listened at the beginning of the relationship and are trying to backpedal and correct the situation. Active listening, an appreciation of what is going on at home and work, in addition to attention to physical symptoms, are an invaluable aid to lessening patient anxiety and fear. The problem of poor communication is particularly difficult for the consulting obstetrician who may be called into case management only very late in the clinical course when the mother and/or baby may be acutely ill and little time exists to permit the establishment of a relationship. The other partner to the interaction, the patient, can also be the problem, leading to severe stress for both the physician and the patient. (See Chapter 5.)

Labor and Delivery

Labor and delivery is a potentially frightening, but paradoxically desired experience for the pregnant woman. The goals of obstetric labor management are to ensure the safety and health of the mother and infant, and free the mother from excessive pain and complications. As recent research suggests, the events of labor/delivery and the responses of parents and care givers influence the long-term relationship between mother, infant, and the rest of the family.[13,23,25,26] Ideally, labor management occurs without complete loss of the excitement of the experience or great distress. Needless to say, such a happy combination of events is not always achieved and can never be guaranteed.

Today, there is emphasis on active mastery of birth with as much family participation as possible.[26] Fear and unfamiliarity increase pain and tension and can interfere with normal uterine activity, probably by elevating maternal catecholamines. Distress and anxiety are reduced in several ways. A good prelabor relationship between the woman and her obstetrician and/or midwife helps as does the judicious use of analgesics and/or epidural anesthesia.

Discomfort or pain perceived during parturition is related not only to the physiology of birth but also to fear; training, such as childhood preparation classes; past experiences with pain; general personality; style of expression; cultural factors; and the reassuring presence of a labor companion.[14] In general, women who do admit their complaints do better than passive individuals who suppress their concerns and feelings. Heightened maternal anxiety commonly leads to the increased use of medications during parturition for pain control and/or sedation. While properly administered, low-dose continuous epidural anesthesia has little or no demonstrable effects upon newborns, the same cannot be said for sedatives and narcotics.[27]

However, a woman's psychological state and anxiety level during pregnancy may not always be a good predictor of her condition in labor. Giving up the unity, the oneness, with the child through delivery is reported by some women as acutely stress provoking. Not surprisingly, labor evokes fears about dying, bodily damage, losing control, exposing one's bodily functions, and inadequacy that may be suppressed until the event actually occurs.

Bonding

Bonding refers to a sensitive period that exists after birth where psychological interactions between mother and infant occur and a special relationship develops.[14,28–30] While attachment begins long before birth, it is strengthened by the interactions occurring soon after delivery. Although there are critics of the concept of bonding, there is little doubt of the positive effect of a newborn on parents and other adults, including even the most outwardly blasé of obstetricians. Most clinicians believe that early visual and physical contact between mother and baby facilitates emotional attachment. Appropriate behaviors include fondling, kissing, cuddling, and face gazing, with continuous physical contact between mother and infant. The long-term benefits of bonding are less certain, but there is little question that early mother-infant interaction has favorable effects on parental feelings about infants and may have positive effects in later life as well.[25]

Bonding is an early process, commencing soon after birth. Factors that may interfere with bonding include lack of instinctual response, psychological problems in the mother, inadequate preparation, physical illnesses in the mother or baby, drugs administered in hospital, drug abuse, and, uncommonly, hospital practices that arbitrarily separate mother and infant.[14] In general, maternal sedation for labor/delivery and maternal-newborn separation should be minimal, within the limits necessary for the safety of both.

However, attachment is complex and not simply related to the immediate postpartum period. While separation has potential physical, biological, and emotional consequences, bonding obviously occurs in mothers with premature infants or in those undergoing cesarean section when some period of separation from the neonate following birth is common. A mother should never be led to believe that she will be a failure with her child because something has interfered with the first minutes or hours of mother-infant interaction following delivery. Overemphasis on the necessity for immediate interactive experiences is unnecessary and incorrect.[14]

Bonding is especially important for women and babies at risk for attachment problems. This includes mothers who are very young; older; or ill; or those who are ambivalent about pregnancy. Other problems exist among families with a history of child abuse, abusive relation with partner, or psychiatric disorders, including alcohol and substance abuse and depression. Infants who are acutely ill, premature, or handicapped are a particular problem.[14,31,32]

While the father's presence in the labor and delivery room contributes to father-infant bonding, the fathers must be prepared for the experience. The sights and sounds of delivery may be profoundly disturbing to the uninitiated. Whether the father should be present at delivery if complications occur, or during an unanticipated cesarean section, should be discussed in advance and the hospital ground rules well understood. Clinicians should recall that fathers undergo a process of attachment similar to maternal bonding. This consists of an early series of interactive patterns developing a complex psychological tie of parent to infant.[30]

Nationally, approximately 1% of all deliveries are out-of-hospital births. While some of these are accidental, others are planned deliveries in homes or birth centers. A continuing concern for practitioners in elective home births is maternal or fetal complications occurring after a normal pregnancy. In general, one third of infants requiring immediate intensive care come from what appear to be normal pregnancies. While there are definitely other issues, safety of mother and infant is the first priority for practitioners. If pregnancy and labor have been uneventful, serious maternal or fetal problems are distinctly uncommon, yet they still occur. A partial response to the demand for less encumbered delivery procedures has been the development of free-standing birth centers, new anesthetic techniques for less interference with the normal course of labor, liberalization of hospital policies, short- stay programs with early discharge, and the development of labor/delivery/recovery rooms. Hospitals are striving with varying success to create a less institutional climate not only architecturally, but through a warm atmosphere and psychologically trained personnel. Obviously, much remains to be done, but much has changed in the last 10 years.

Electronic fetal monitoring is commonly practiced during labor to evaluate fetal condition. Such monitoring is more likely to be positively accepted if there is an initial adequate explanation of the technique and if the clinician expresses a willingness to respond to questions and be flexible in the use of alternatives, specifically intermittent auscultation. Women who have had prior fetal loss are often more accepting of the use of continuous monitoring. A problem, however, is that monitoring sometimes leads women to believe that with the device in place nothing can "happen" to the baby. Again, adequate communication is necessary, and institution of a treatment philosophy in which the mechanical equipment is not a replacement for human skills, but only an adjunct, is critical.

Puerperium

The puerperium is a time of tremendous readjustment involving (1) physical problems (eg, pain postcesarean section or episiotomy); (2) hormonal changes; (3) emotional lability; and (4) support from family or friends and health care personnel. The obstetrician's responsibility does not end with the delivery of the baby and mother. The obstetrician, as a primary care physician, is expected to manage the emotional, social, and sexual problems that occur postpartum. If maternal emotional distress occurs after delivery, even if it is apparently unwarranted, it needs further investigation. Recognition of difficulties, counseling, and, if needed, referral to a competent social worker, nurse, psychologist, or other specially trained counselor are needed (see Chapter 8).

In the hospital setting, if possible, it is important for the clinician to note the progress of mother-infant interaction and feeding. If this cannot be done by direct observation, then attention to the written observations and verbal comments of the nursing staff is essential. Reassurance concerning neonatal problems should not be given until the physician has accurate data. To reassure a woman whose baby is ill or who herself is having difficulty without full information makes her feel more, not less, insecure. Some simple techniques are helpful. Open-ended questions are best. Sitting down in the hospital room during a routine visit is a good interpersonal technique. A physician who visits and sits rather than stands for an equal amount of time is perceived by the patient to have stayed longer. It also keeps one from towering over a patient who is in bed.

Transition to Motherhood

While pregnancy and birth are biological functions, human mothering is largely a learned skill. Attachment of mother to infant begins in utero often strenthened by ultrasonic visualization of the fetus. This attachment grows with interactions during the first few months of life and is learned by observation of other mothers and through classes, books, and organized instruction.[14] Early life nurturing experiences enable a woman to have the capacity to nurture. She needs to have people in her environment who share her ideas and support her emotionally while she is learning and getting used to her new role. In prior generations in the United States, and still today in other cultures, women learn a great deal about mothering from older relatives and are not so dependent on instinct or ideas derived from researching books or magazines. Mothers of young infants today are often isolated from family and from other new mothers. Thus, they are limited in both information and in assistance.

Major shifts occur in a woman's relationship with her own mother during and after gestation, especially postpartum.[7] The new mother reassesses her relationship with her own mother. If she felt her mother was a good or adequate mother, this is helpful. If she felt her mother was not a good mother, then she may have fears that she too will prove inadequate. Some writers believe that a disturbed relationship with a woman's own mother as a role model is a risk factor for peripartum depression, but this is at best controversial.[7,33] Women need reassurance that they are unlike their own mothers and will develop patterns and responses to their infant which are different.

Breast-feeding has both definite psychological and physiological advantages if the mother is both willing and able. Supportive and experienced staff facilitate this experience. However, a woman who decides to bottle feed should not be made to feel guilty or inadequate because of this choice.

Home-going instructions should be individualized. Activity, bathing, sexual intercourse, and mood changes should all be addressed in the routine discharge discussion. A physician should have some sense of the new mother's personality style and how she reacts. Ideally, recommendations should reflect an understanding of the family's economic circumstances and their religious and cultural practices related to reproduction, sexuality, nursing, and motherhood. For example, does the couple live with family or by themselves? When does the woman have to return to work? Are maternity or paternity leaves available from the respective employers? Can someone help the woman at home or is she totally alone with the new baby?

In the puerperium, somatic complaints are the ticket to admission to health care for a woman who is distressed and developing psychological problems. Thus, various physical ailments are common in individuals with mood disturbances (see Chapter 8). Such complaints need careful assessment and, generally, this is not best done over the telephone. Here is the situation where the physician or nurse does not think in terms of psychological versus organic, but, rather, what are the organic contributions, what are the psychological contributions, and what are the social contributions to the patient's distress and what can be done about each? A home visit to assess the situation as is practiced in England and in some special programs is helpful, but rarely feasible. A woman in whom a psychiatric disorder is possible may need referral, discussion with a liaison psychiatrist or psychiatric clinical nurse, or consultation with a social worker with special mental health training.

Routine management decisions need reconsideration and revision. A good example is the classic 6-week postpartum examination. We feel that it is better to see parturients initially at 2 weeks after delivery. What is needed before treatment is recognition of the problem! The majority of medical problems and the initial adjustment problems are usually present by this time, at least in their preliminary stages, and early intervention is still possible. Further, the majority of women resume sexual intercourse well prior to the traditional 6-week visit, often without contraception.[34] If a visit is not possible, a telephone call by the physician or nurse at about 2 weeks oftens identifies major physical and psychological adjustment problems before they become major issues. Such contact keeps the lines of general communication open, improving the chances for future contact if problems do develop.

Special Problems

Psychological High Risk

Some patients are at enhanced risk for psychological dysfunction. Hopefully, at least some of these individuals can be identified before major difficulties develop and increased observation and/or early consultation can be initiated. Warning signs include but are not necessarily limited to[7,35] (1) a prior psychiatric history; (2) a history of psychological problems that accompanied a maturational period, such as puberty; (3) a history of early maternal deprivation or mother's death; (4) reports of difficulty separating from parents; (5) conflicts about mothering; (6) marital or family difficulties including separation, divorce, or abuse; (7) past difficulty with pregnancy, delivery, or postpartum depression; (8) recent deaths in family or close friends; (9) familial or congenital disorders; (10) history of infertility; (11) history of repeat abortion; (12)

history of pseudocyesis or hyperemesis; (13) prior fetal death, miscarriage, or congenital abnormality; (14) extreme age range; (15) history of sexual, physical, or emotional abuse; (16) premenstrual syndrome; (17) poor coping skills; and (18) serious financial problems.

High-Risk Pregnancies

There is usually increased anxiety in pregnancies that follow infertility, a congenitally malformed or defective child, a child given up for adoption, or spontaneous abortion (see Chapter 16). Women fear their bodies may not work correctly or feel guilt and fear from losing a prior pregnancy. This anxiety may be manifest by extreme preoccupation with somatic complaints and/or not planning or making arrangements for the new baby as a form of denial (see Chapter 12).

Virtually all pregnant women experience some degree of anxiety or other psychological symptoms. The importance of such symptoms should not be overemphasized, as the range of normal is wide. For the hospitalized high-risk patient, anxiety and depression are often significant factors and can effect outcome.[10] Some, but not all, of these effects are due to patient compliance. Diabetic and toxemic patients also have psychological problems, especially depression. Such women need additional support. A team approach with staff that are sensitive to the patient's physical problems and feelings of discouragement is helpful.

The Adolescent Mother

Each year in the United States, there are approximately one million pregnancies of young women, 19 years and under, a statistic that has changed very little since 1973.[36] Of these, 16.6 per 1000 are girls 14 years and younger, and 109.8 per 1000 are girls ages 15 to 19 years. About half of these pregnancies go on to term, while the other half are terminated by abortion, mostly induced, although some are spontaneous. Most of the pregnancies are unintended.[37] The United States has a higher rate of teenage pregnancy, childbearing, and abortion than most industrialized nations, even though the rates of teenage sexual activity are the same as those in other countries.[36] This is at least partially due to the fact that access to and knowledge of contraceptives are restricted among American youth.[38]

Adolescence is a time of major developmental change and when it is combined with a second and later developmental task such as pregnancy, there can be serious consequences.[39] Health care workers have a major challenge in caring for these patients.

Adolescence needs more precise definition since girls at various ages vary tremendously. Three societal constructs of age can help. There is *chronological age*, that from date of birth to present. There is *biological age*, related to the onset and physical maturity of puberty (gynecological age is defined as time from menarche to pregnancy). Finally, there is *social age* at which time cultural milestones are achieved, such as marriage, birth of first child, and adult work roles. Generally, these age measures are synchronized, but for the long period of adolescence there may be a great discrepancy.[40] Hamburt[40] describes subsets of school-age mothers: (1) those who are problem prone, truant, and beset with behavioral difficulties; (2) those who cope adequately, finish school, and proceed with their lives; and (3) those who are depressed and the pregnancy has occurred in response to the depression. Social complications are common. A study of adolescent mothers showed a significant number had had losses in the year prior to the pregnancy.[41] Understanding to which group a given patient belongs is an important task for the clinician.

While the average age for menarche is now 12.8 years, there is wide variation. The timing of pubertal changes has important psychological influences on girls and boys. Early maturity may have advantages for boys, but disadvantages for girls. For boys it may mean more popularity, more leadership, and more self- confidence.[42] For girls, achieving biological maturity "on time" is the most gratifying, but early and late maturers see themselves as having less positive body images and self-esteem.[40]

Most early adolescents have not developed mature cognitive styles. In decision making, they do not see the wide range of alternatives, often overlook long-term consequences of their actions, and accept peer advice without doubting it. They tend to overgeneralize and to feel invulnerable in circumstances such as the risk taking of unprotected sexual intercourse.[40]

There has been an increasing number of young adolescents engaging in sexual activity at earlier and earlier ages. The data on 15-year-olds show a marked increase in sexual activity, with black women having a rate twice that of whites and initiation of sexual activity about a year earlier than whites. Contraceptive use by early adolescents is especially poor, but there are many other forces involved in whether or not teens get pregnant, bear a child, or have an abortion. Other reasons for pregnancies are peer pressure, rebellion against parents, fulfillment of parents' unconscious or conscious wishes, to test one's bodily functions, to have a baby to love and be one's own, and unfortunately, incest and sexual abuse. A survey in Illinois showed that over half of teenage mothers had been sexually abused as children.[43] Many pregnant teenagers come from a background of poverty, with poor educational goals, have relatively little involvement in social institutions such as church, and have less family involvement and good communication, especially about sex.[36] Some of the factors related to use of contraception are age, educational goals, sex education, accepting one's self as a sexual person, and having good self-esteem and independence. Girls who do well in school are more likely to delay sexual activity and to use contraception.

Women who become pregnant during adolescence are more likely to have larger families and unwanted pregnancies than women who delay childbearing.[44] Not surprisingly, women with such adolescent pregnancies are disadvantaged in terms of both eventual adult income level as well as educational attainment. Doctor and patient interactions are often strained when the doctor is frustrated at the girl's sexual activity, inability to use contraception, and immature attitudes toward sex, abortion, and mothering. Denial of the pregnancy, fear, or lack of knowledge may cause the girl to come in late for prenatal care, increasing her chances for obstetrical complications.

Pregnant teenagers who continue their pregnancies have more complications of pregnancies such as toxemia, anemia, premature labor, and low-birth-weight babies. However, good prenatal care may lead to as good an outcome as with older women, especially with attention to nutrition, control of anemia and blood pressure, and general health measures. Since many teenagers are late to recognize their pregnancy, early diagnosis through educational efforts is important.

The economic costs of such early childbearing are enormous with public assistance (Aid to Families with Dependent Children, food stamps, and Medicaid), costing over 19.27 billion dollars in 1987 to families established by a teenage parent. The psychological costs relate to depression, lack of education, and despair at having considerable responsibility, while virtually children themselves.

The children of teenage mothers have a wide range of outcomes depending on their culture, family supports, and care givers, but many offspring are less healthy, do less well in school, and have less verbal skills, and the daughters are more likely to get pregnant as adolescents.

In addition to taking good care of adolescent mothers in prenatal clinics and offices, obstetrical staff should have a major interest in thinking about prevention. While many programs are encouraging teens to delay sexual activity or to consider sexual interactions that do not include intercourse, a society such as ours presents sexual activity as very desirable in television advertisements and movies. It would be helpful for teenagers to have more access to contraceptives not only to prevent pregnancy, but also to provide protection from sexually transmitted diseases. The use of the pill would be beneficial for many girls, but many myths abound about its dangers, and it is often avoided. Abortion is sought and obtained by about half the adolescents who become pregnant. The encouragement to use contraception in many European countries has been a move to try to decrease the number of abortions.

There needs to be more attention paid to the adolescent father, and to his drive to have children. This is one of the many areas of adolescent pregnancy that needs further research.

In caring for the adolescent patient, the staff needs to try to understand at which developmental stage a particular girl is. Teenagers have a language of their own, which it is helpful to understand, but not necessarily to use. Adolescents are very labile and change from time to time. They fear getting out of control, although they may appear to look fearless and to be risk takers. When they come for care, they need an accepting and listening attitude on the part of the health providers, as well as education in various creative ways. It is often helpful to include the father of the baby in prenatal visits to get to know him. Support groups for pregnant teens have been established in some clinics with services that teach assertiveness, decision making, and strengthening of communication between parents and children, which help teens to see into the future with some hopefulness.[37]

Finally, for the practitioner, there are legal problems of treating minors since in most situations a girl under 18 years of age cannot consent to medical treatment. The exceptions are: emancipated minors who are either married or earning their own living and retaining most of their earnings; or, in certain states, treatment for sexually transmitted disease, drug or alcohol abuse, or any condition caused by such abuse or suspected sexual abuse. In most instances this should not be a problem, since family may be involved, but it may be and the practitioner must seek legal advice about the treatment of minors in his or her office or clinic (see Chapter 2).

Adolescents present a very special challenge to the health care practitioner. They can be frustrating, but working with them can also be satisfying. Seeing them gain some control in their lives and have a beneficial effect on their offspring is rewarding. To prevent further unintended pregnancies and to improve their mental, as well as physical, health are the goals.

The Older Mother

The number of women postponing childbearing is steadily increasing with more women having their first child beyond the age of 30 years.[45–48] There are complex sociocultural reasons for this trend including career planning with more women in the work force, later marriages, and increased infertility which may take years to treat. In general, women over 35 years, in good health, and with good medical and obstetrical care are at only minimal risk for serious complications of pregnancy.[46,47] Some problems that are related to increased age are decreased rates of conception, increased incidence of spontaneous abortion, fetal and chromosomal abnormalities, and an increased likelihood for medical problems such as chronic hypertension and diabetes. In thinking about chromosomal abnormalities such as trisomy 21, a fetal malformation that occurs in 2% of pregnancies in women aged 40 years, the risk must be put into perspective. While the risk is higher than for younger women, more than 95% of these mothers will not bear such an infant. Fortunately, current antepartum testing can detect many fetal abnormalities with high accuracy.[49] There is no evidence that older women experience any unique type or increased frequency of psychological disturbances during pregnancy in comparison to younger women. Genetic counseling can be very important to the older patient, as can general discussions relating to the realities of pregnancy for women over 35.

The Lesbian Mother

Pregnant patients may have a lesbian sexual orientation and may wish to have children and raise them with a same sex partner. It is important that clinicians be aware of their own attitudes and behaviors and be able to care for patients in a nonjudgmental manner. The patient's sexual orientation may not be known to the medical staff and its revelation may be anxiety producing for the patient, who may not know what sort of bias the clinician has. The clinical interview should be conducted in a neutral fashion. It is helpful to use the same language as the patient does, for example, referring to lesbian patients as lesbian rather than homosexual, which they may see as more pejorative.[50] Excessive curiosity about sexual details or psychiatric referral without adequate reason are inappropriate.

Some knowledge about homosexuality is helpful to all clinicians.[51–54] Gartrell[50] points out that men and women attracted to the same sex are not necessarily homosexual and that there is a continuum from exclusive heterosexuality to exclusive homosexuality with varying proportions in between. There is no evidence or data for increased psychiatric problems in lesbians, or endocrine or other physical abnormalities. There are also little data concerning etiology of heterosexual, bisexual, or homosexual orientations.[50]

For the pregnant lesbian patient, a supportive network of family and friends is important, as well as medical care given in a nonjudgmental and expert manner (see Chapter 7).

Denial of Pregnancy

In unusual circumstances the existence of pregnancy may be denied, resulting in the failure to seek early care. *Denial* of pregnancy is usually an unconscious psychological process in which a woman keeps an unpleasant reality, ie, unwanted pregnancy, out of awareness. She can be joined in this denial by family and even physicians. She may go through pregnancy believing herself to have menstrual periods—probably irregular spotting—and outwardly be unaware of breast changes or fetal movements. Such women present at emergency rooms in labor, not knowing that they are pregnant, or deliver the baby at home unaided, at times in the toilet! When the denial is removed with the appearance of the baby, temporary severe psychological reactions such as depersonalization can occur. While some of these women are demonstrably psychotic, most are not. More often, they are young, and experiencing their first pregnancy. For those whose denial is lifted *prior* to delivery, they commonly present very late for prenatal care. The issue of pregnancy denial is entangled with infanticide as the immediate neglect of a newborn can result in its death. The accompanying legal and ethical entanglements are obvious (see Chapter 12).

References

1. Bibring GL: Recognition of psychological stress often neglected in OB care. *Hosp Topics* 1966;44:100–103.
2. Nadelson CC: "Normal" and "special" aspects of pregnancy: A psychological approach, in Nadelson CC, Notman MT (eds.): *The Woman Patient, Medical and Psychological Interfaces*, vol. 1. New York, Plarium Press, 1978.
3. Chalners B: Psychological aspects of pregnancy: Some thoughts for the eighties. *Soc Sci Med* 1982;16:323–331.
4. Bradley CF, King JF, Effer SB: Psychology in obstetrics: Extinct or extant? *J Psychol Obstet Gynecol* 1987;6:49–57.
5. Stotland NL: Social change and women's representative health care. *WHI* 1990;1:4–11.
6. Valentine DP: Psychological impact of infertility: Identifying issues and needs. *Soc Work Health Care* 1986;11:59–69.
7. Atkinson AK, Rickel AU: Depression in women: The postpartum experience. *Iss Mental Health News* 1983;5:197–218.
8. Cohen RL: Some maladaptive syndromes of pregnancy and the puerperium. *Obstet Gynecol* 1966;27:562–570.
9. Stearn M: Social and psychological aspects of pregnancy. *Nursing* (Lond) 1986;3:17–19.
10. Kliot DA, Kliot H: Emotional components of labor and delivery, in Zatuchi GI, Laferla JJ, Sciarra JJ (eds.): *Gynecology and Obstetrics*, vol. 6. Philadelphia, JB Lippincott, 77; 1990, pp 1–13..
11. Cavendar JO, Butts NJ: Fatherhood and emotional disease. *Am J Psychiatry* 1977;134:429–431.

12. White SE, Reamy K: Sexuality and pregnancy: A review. *Arch Sex Behav* 1982;11:429–444.

13. Valentine D: Adaptation to pregnancy: Some implications for individual and family mental health. *Child Today* 1982;11:17–20.

14. Anselmo S: *Early Childhood Development: Prenatal Through Age Eight.* Columbus, OH, Merrill, 1987.

15. Forrest JD, Singh S: The sexual and reproductive behavior of American women 1982–1989. *Fam Plann Perspect* 1990;22:205–214.

16. Hollander MH, McGehee JB: The wish to be held during pregnancy. *J Psychosom Res* 1974;18:193–197.

17. Tolor A, DiGrazia PV: Sexual attitudes and behavior patterns during and following pregnancy. *Arch Sex Med* 1976;5:539–551.

18. Jarrahi-Zadeh A, Kane FJ, Van de Castle RL, Lachenbruch PA, Ewing JA: Emotional and cognitive changes in pregnancy and early puerperium. *Br J Psychiatry* 1969;115:797–805.

19. Galinsky E: *Between Generations: The Six Stages of Parenthood.* New York, Times Books, 1981.

20. Hyde B: An interview study of pregnant women's attitudes to ultrasound scanning. *Soc Sci Med* 1986;22:587–592.

21. Kane FJ: Psychiatric reactions to oral contraceptives. *Am J Obstet Gynecol* 1968;102:105–133.

22. Kyger K, Webb WW: Progesterone levels and psychological state in normal women. *Am J Obstet Gynecol* 1972;113:759–762.

23. Leboyer F: *Birth Without Violence.* New York, Knopf, 1975.

24. Buka SL, Lipsitt LP, Tsuang MT: Birth complications and psychological deviancy: A 25-year prospective inquiry. *Acta Paediatr Jpn* 1988;30:537–546.

25. Siegel E: A critical examination of studies of parent-infant bonding, in Klaus MH, Robertson MO (eds.): *Birth, Interaction, and Attachment: A Round Table.* Skillman, NJ, Johnson & Johnson, 1982.

26. Beck NC, Geden EA, Brouder GT, Anderson JS, Kennish ME, Shivvers NL: Techniques of labor preparation, in Zatuchi GI, Laferla JJ, Sciarra JJ (eds.): *Gynecology and Obstetrics*, vol. 6. Philadelphia, JB Lippincott, 78; 1990, pp 1–10.

27. Yang PK: Maternal attitudes during pregnancy and medication during labor and delivery: Methodological considerations, in Smeriglio VL (ed.): *Newborns and Patients: Parent-Infant Contact and Newborn Sensory Stimulations.* Hillsdale, NJ, Lawrence Erlbaum, 1981.

28. Klaus MH, Jerauld R, Kreger NC, McAlpine W, Steffa M, Kennell JH: Maternal attachment: Importance of the first post- partum days. *N Engl J Med* 1972;286:460–463.

29. Klaus MH, Kennell JH: *Maternal-Infant Bonding.* St. Louis, CV Mosby, 1976.

30. Klaus MH, Kennell JH: *Parent-Infant Bonding*, ed. 2. St. Louis, CV Mosby, 1982.

31. Brazelton TB: Behavioral assessment of the premature infant: Uses in intervention, in Klaus MH, Robertson MO (eds.): *Birth, Interaction, and Attachment: A Round Table.* Skillman, NJ, Johnson & Johnson, 1982.

32. Helfer R: The relationship between lack of bonding and child abuse and neglect, in Klaus MN, Leger T, Trause MA (eds.): *Maternal Attachment and Mothering Disorders: A Round Table*, ed. 2. Skillman, NJ, Johnson & Johnson, 1982.

33. Uddenberg N: Reproductive adaption in mother and daughters: A study of personality development and adaption to motherhood. *Acta Psychiatr Scand* [Suppl] 1975;254.

34. Mabray CR: Postpartum examination: A re-evaluation. *South Med J* 1979;72:1433–1435.

35. Friederich MA: Emotional aspects of pregnancy, in Benson R (ed.): *Current Obstetric and Gynecologic Diagnosis and Treatment.* Los Altos, CA, Lang Medical Publishers, 1982.

36. Children's Defense Fund: *Teenage Pregnancy: An Advocate's Guide to the Numbers.* Washington, DC, 1988.
37. Federman D: The dilemma of teenage parenthood, in *Science and Babies. Private Decisions, Public Dilemmas.* Washington, DC, Institute of Medicine, National Academy Press, 1990.
38. Jones EF, Forrest JD, Goldman N, Henshaw SK, Lincoln R, Rosoff JI, et al: Teenage pregnancy in developed countries: Determinants and policy implications. *Fam Plann Perspect* 1985;17:53–62.
39. Youngs DD, Marean AR: The pregnant adolescent patient, in Zatuchi GI, Laferla JJ, Sciarra JJ (eds.): *Gynecology and Obstetrics*, vol. 6. Philadelphia, JB Lippincott, 75; 1990, pp. 1–7.
40. Hamburt B: Subsets of adolescent mothers: Developmental, biomedical, and psychosocial issues, in Lancaster J, Hamburg B (eds.): *School Age Pregnancy and Parenthood.* New York, Aldine de Gruyter, 1986, pp 115–145.
41. Rosenthal M: Sexual counseling and interviewing of adolescents. *Primary Care* 1977;4:291–299.
42. Clausen J: The social meaning of differential physical and sexual maturation, in Dragastin S, Elder GH Jr (eds.): *Adolescence and the Life Cycle.* New York, Wiley, 1975.
43. Teen mothers report abuse as children. *Plain Dealer* (daily newspaper, Cleveland, OH), September 15, 1987.
44. Scott-Jones D, Turner SL: The impact of adolescent childbearing on educational attainment and income of black females. *Youth Soc* 1990;27:35–53.
45. Resnik R: Pregnancy in women aged 35 years or older, in Hollingsworth DR, Resnik R (eds.): *Medical Counseling Before Pregnancy.* New York, Churchill Livingstone, 1988, pp 14–18.
46. Resnik R: The "elderly primigravida" in 1990. *N Engl J Med* 1990;322:693–694. Editorial.
47. Berkowitz GS, Skovron ML, Lapinski RH, Berkowitz RL: Delayed childbearing and the outcome of pregnancy. *N Engl J Med* 1990:322:659–664.
48. Touleman L: Historical overview of fertility and age. *Maturitas* 1988;suppl:5–14.
49. Fleischer AC, Romero R, Manning FA, Jeanty P, James AE (eds.): *The Principles and Practice of Ultrasonography in Obstetrics and Gynecology*, Norwalk, CT, Appleton and Lange, 1991.
50. Gartell N: Gay patients in the medical setting and in treatment interventions, in Nadelson C, Marcotte D (eds.): *Human Sexuality.* New York, Plenum Press, 1983, pp 395–409.
51. Hetrick ES, Martin AD: Developmental issues and their resolution for gay and lesbian adolescents. *J Homosex* 1987;14:25–44.
52. Isay RA: *Being Homosexual.* New York, Farrar Straus Giroux, 1989.
53. Green R: Childhood cross-gender behavior and subsequent sexual preference. *Am J Psychiatry* 1979;136:106–108.
54. Kirkpatrick M, Smith C, Roy R: Lesbian mothers and their children: A comparative survey. *Am J Orthopsychiatry* 1981;51:545–551.

Chapter 5

Interview Techniques

Dennis H. Smith, MD and John P. O'Grady, MD

> Ask, and it shall be given you; seek, and ye shall find; knock and it shall be opened unto you.
> —*Matthew:7:7*

The primary purpose of medical interviewing is to form a working relationship with another individual who comes seeking aid or advice. Additional aims are the exploration of problems, the clarification of issues, and the establishment of an initial approach to evaluation and possible treatment.[1,2] Both the technique and, ultimately, the success or failure of interviewing reveal the style and personality of the clinician. The first or initial interaction between an obstetrical patient and a physician or other practitioner is one of the most important and often underemphasized aspects of obstetrical and gynecological practice. There is no single or correct way to proceed. However, there are a number of principles of interviewing that are worth review.

The current chapter presents an approach to interviewing as applied to obstetrical/gynecological practice. The ability to talk to the patient is an integral part of the art of medicine and a critical component in successful practice, whether one functions as a primary physician or as a consultant.

The Basics of Interviewing

The Physician/Patient Relationship

The relative positions of the patient and the physician have changed a great deal in the last half of this century. Thirty years ago I recall being the resident responsible for the admission of a woman for a hysterectomy. "Why are you having a hysterectomy?" I asked. "Because Dr. R. told me I needed one," she answered. This paternalistic style of telling patients what is best for them is now unacceptable to most patients, and rightly so.[3] By and large, to use such an approach at present would prompt the majority of potential patients to seek care elsewhere.

Recently, the opposite extreme has occurred. The patient may present a contract, drawn up with the assistance of her attorney, stating what she will or will not permit in terms of her care. Obviously, a middle ground is preferable. Most potential patients want a physician who is knowledgeable and skilled and who evidences appropriate self-confidence. At the same time, patients have a need and a right for information concerning their care. Thus, a partnership is formed: the trained professional, who may educate and advise or perform specialized interventions, and an informed patient, who has the final control of saying yes or no to any proposed plan of treatment or diagnosis.[4]

The Initial Approach

While an informal, almost familiar approach may come easily to some practitioners and be received pleasantly by the women they interview, this is risky, particularly with a new patient. It is best to begin by addressing an individual with a proper title and her first and last name. A good rule of thumb is that if the care giver is not ready to be called by his or her first name only, neither is the patient. With the more formal approach, if the woman needs to maintain some distance to bring up a sensitive issue, no compromise has occurred by jumping to a familiar first-name basis. Thus, respect for the individual is conveyed early on. One must truly be interested in people, interested in important aspects of their lives, and respectful of their dignity in order to be a good interviewer.

Each age-group will have its own sensitivities, often hidden from the physician at first encounter. For example, the elderly woman being seen in the hospital is already in a compromised position. Being addressed as "young lady" or "grandma" she is further stripped of her dignity and may respond to questioning with uncooperative monosyllables. Younger individuals are often a problem for practitioners. For example, adolescents are struggling with their own identity from day to day and need gentle but firm reassurance that they are important individuals, worthy of respect. The young professional may be sensitive about her new title and resentful if it is omitted when she is addressed.

It is important to speak in a vocabulary that the individual understands. Yet, this must not be perceived as demeaning or patronizing. Even when speaking, the physician must "listen" and watch for signs showing that the patient understands or, possibly, does not understand, what is occurring. Body language may communicate a special or hidden message much different from that conveyed by the actual words that are used.[1,5] Observing the patient's body positioning and facial expression may provide hints which convey her concerns more powerfully than what she says directly. If she sits on the edge of her chair and wrings her hands, despair and fear are evident although she states that she only has a "little problem." The woman who frowns while her physician is talking may be evidencing disapproval or misunderstanding while a smile may indicate you are right on target. The physician who fails to carefully observe the patient may miss all these and other more subtle clues. Similarly, the patient will observe the doctor's expressions and body language. A distracted look out the window will be interpreted as disinterest. Interrupting the patient to take phone calls may be perceived as rudeness or disinterest. Similarly, sitting with arms crossed conveys either hostility or defensiveness.

Evaluation of Patient Personality

During the course of the interaction between doctor and patient it is helpful to develop some knowledge of the patient's basic personality type. It is not necessary to develop a formal psychiatric character diagnosis but it is very useful to know what kind of a person one is dealing with. Personality is the style used in interpersonal relationships and the veil through which the medical history comes. Knowing something about how the patient views herself and the world in general is a powerful tool in gleaning kernels of useful clinical information.

Is the woman lonely and always seeking affection but never quite getting enough? Is she a self-confident, well-adjusted woman who takes stress in her stride? Is she a rigidly controlled person who regards her feelings as private information, or a person who floods the listener with many words and few facts? Is she a compulsive person who will insist on continuing to work even against medical advice? Does she communicate with the world through physical expressions, thus somatising her feelings resulting in many physical complaints and visits? Is she given to dramatic expression and dress, concealing her true feelings or even symptoms? Such traits can be useful in understanding the dynamics of a doctor/patient relationship. For example, patients with borderline personality characteristics tend to split everything into black or white distinctions: you are either for them or against them. Understanding this characteristic helps with management choices for such women and assists in how such choices are presented. In sum, an awareness of personality traits assists the physician in understanding the needs of the individuals who come for care and in predicting their responses to proposed plans of treatment or evaluation.

Understanding a woman's way of dealing with people can assist the obstetrician to work with her in the best way to obtain compliance with a difficult treatment regimen. An example is the woman who becomes diabetic and insulin dependent for the first time in her life during pregnancy. Now, in addition to the psychological tasks of dealing with pregnancy, she must deal with the concept of chronic illness. The feeling that she is set apart from normal, that she is somehow defective, can be perceived as a devastating loss. This is a problem with which she must come to grips. If the physician knows something of the patient's personality and past ways of dealing with such losses, he or she can help the patient deal with the present crisis. The general obstetrician who elects to refer such a patient to the maternal-fetal specialist may still be the best person to help the patient deal with the psychological manifestations of her disease. Thus, the referring physician can work with and reinforce the perinatal team.

In the initial interview, it may be useful to order one's thinking along the lines of major physical complaints or illnesses, personality traits, psychiatric disease states, if any, severity of psychosocial/sexual stressors in her life, and an overall assessment of functioning. This is an adaptation of the five axes method of diagnosis set forth in the *Diagnostic and Statistical Manual,* ed. 3, revised (DSM-IIIR).[6] A general outline of the important axes is presented below.

1. *Axis I.* Clinical syndromes: This includes the diagnoses of psychiatric disease states, if any are present. Most commonly, major affective diseases such as depression or manic- depressive disorders as well as the psychoses would be listed here, as well as substance-abuse disorders.

2. *Axis II.* Personality disorders: These are specific developmental disorders including histrionic personality, obsessive-compulsive personality, borderline personality, etc, as well as developmental disorders including mental retardation.
3. *Axis III.* This includes the various physical conditions or disorders that are present.
4. *Axis IV.* This section evaluates the severity of psychosocial stressors.
5. *Axis V.* This axis includes a clinical estimation of the overall level of functioning.

The physical disorder section, Axis III, is the one usually presented to the clinician. Most frequently, in obstetric practice, this is not a disease diagnosis but a diagnosis of pregnancy. It is important for the obstetrician to adopt such a framework of systematic assessment to the pregnant patient. This is not so much to emphasize disease as to form a complete concept of the patient, her environment, and how the two interact.

At times, much important data is not directly volunteered. For example, an Axis III diagnosis of a previous severe depression requiring hospitalization or drug therapy may not be something the patient readily reveals. However, a warm, nonjudgmental interviewer can put her at her ease and usually learn more about the course of the illness than the simple recounting of the diagnosis and medication administered. In all probability this apparently peripheral information will prove to be of more importance than first recognized.

Other Issues: Psychosocial Milieu

As one tries to learn about how the patient deals with her world one must also ask about the nonmedical stresses in her life. Once rapport is established a simple question as to how things in general are going may reveal stresses in her life which affect the course of pregnancy and, especially, her compliance with treatment regimens. The functioning of her marriage, home, and professional life may thus be approached. In one case, for example, a woman suffering with apparent depression stated there might be problems between she and her husband but she guessed it was "just the pregnancy." Such a hint was the only clue to a larger problem that required exploration. The physician does not have to treat all social and psychological problems but has to make certain that they do not go undetected if these issues can adversely effect the pregnancy. In this case, consultation with a social worker revealed that the patient's husband was drinking on a daily basis. To the patient, whose father had been an alcoholic, this represented a tremendous threat. The couple continued in family therapy and the patient's depression progressively lifted.

Assessment of Functioning

At some point in the interview it is important to learn the educational work background of the woman. Has there been a recent change? If the woman works outside the home, how long has she held the same position? It is also important to ascertain during the interview the relatives and friends the patient considers to be her support system. Is she able to make and to maintain close friends? What she says about her love for her mate will also give you much information. A simple definition of mental health is the ability to love and to work well. The ability or inability of the woman to integrate all aspects of her life and pregnancy may be determined by relatively simple questioning if one remembers to ask.

The Patient/Practitioner Interaction

In the interview process it is equally important for the care giver to have equal sensitivity to the subtleties of body language as it is to have insight into his or her own personality. It would be ideal if every physician could undergo some personality analysis as part of medical school or residency training. While this is not possible for the majority of physicians, practitioners can profitably indulge in a little introspection. Such a simple thing as knowing what you admire or dislike about yourself is immensely useful in relation to others and their perception of you.

For example, if one has stopped smoking only at great expense of energy and willpower, it is not unusual to be intolerant or even rejecting of a patient who continues to smoke. Likewise, a patient who has trouble with self control may be an emotional threat to the clinician who has to maintain a rigid behavior profile in order to control his or her own feelings. Similarly, women who indulge a passion for eating may arouse hostility in the obstetrician who maintains weight control only by strict dieting. Also, the free expresssion of anger or joy by some individuals may be far from the style of the physician and hard for him or her to deal with. Nowhere is this more difficult to deal with than in relation to reproductive functions and sexual behavior. Yet it is essential to be able to nonjudgmentally gain knowledge of the patient's sexual partner or partners. Social arrangements may be very complex. The biological father of the pregnancy may not be her mate or her mate may be either a man or a woman. In sum, the obstetrician must know his or her own feelings in order to deliver appropriate care.

If the physician's beliefs prohibit abortion he or she may fail to recognize the ambivalence a woman has regarding pregnancy and wonder why she is neglecting herself or even being self-abusive. Beliefs must sometimes be held aside in order to listen to the patient. One need not agree with her, but she must be heard and understood. If irreconcilable differences exist, she can be referred to someone else. At least both the patient and the clinician have options when communication is straightforward.

The obstetrician must have an ethical code underlying practice. Unfortunately, such issues are often not critically examined by physicians. They make judgments, express opinions, and initiate actions reflecting preconceived ideas, largely on a subconscious level. It is a valuable exercise for each of us to take a period for reflection concerning the ideals on which we think our actions should be governed. The developments in reproductive technology alone necessitate such introspection. Even though a general obstetrician may not be called upon to perform certain complex and controversial procedures such as multifetal pregnancy reduction, he or she will be called upon to discuss the situation with a patient with a multiple gestation. The woman carrying such a pregnancy commonly looks to her generalist, who may have originally referred her for infertility treatment to help her work through the difficult decisions necessary in such cases. In these and other circumstances, the obstetrician must know his or her own feelings and standards before beginning to explore those of the patients.

The physician must also know something about the ethical and religious systems under which his patients operate. Unless one's obstetrical practice is limited to a community with a markedly homogenous population, at least some knowledge of the tenets of major religious groups is necessary. Judaism, Christianity, and Islam all have major beliefs concerning sexual practices and reproduction. Further, every community will have ethnic groups who also have special concerns. To at least be aware of these customs and ask the woman if there are specific concerns is to allow oneself to be educated and it conveys to the patient one's capability of functioning at a level beyond that of a simple technician.

A part of every interview needs to include questions concerning her religious preference, if any. How much dependence does she place on her religion? Is religion a help to her in the handling of her everyday problems? There are religious directives concerning reproductive life and conduct in pregnancy and delivery that differ between groups. Individuals will also differ in their adherence to these dictates. Some understanding of this background will assist the clinician in planning the care of such individuals.

This knowledge of self and of the people in the community helps an interviewer to not impose personal values on others. For example, years ago a patient who was a long-standing infertility patient approached her physician, asking for contraception. It would have saved the physician's time to simply prescribe it. However, when he questioned her about why she now wished contraception after spending several years trying to get pregnant at great expense and considerable discomfort, a frightened response occurred. She stated at length that she had become greatly physically attracted to her best friend, and was concerned that she might be a lesbian. Therefore, she wanted to try to have intercourse with men other than her husband to see if that might in some fashion rekindle her heterosexual feelings. When psychiatric help was suggested, she said she had visited a psychiatrist several times. Every time she tried to bring up the issue of homosexuality and her fears about it the psychiatrist would change the subject. Almost certainly he was not consciously aware of so directing the conversation but the net result was to block her ability to discuss what had become the central dilemma of her life.

Significant Others

When to include others in the interview is often a dilemma. Obviously, one must ask the patient but many physicians are uncomfortable during intimate discussions with persons other than the patient present. Certainly her main support person, usually but not invariably her husband, needs to be present at some point. He or she will have questions and it is always best to answer them directly and in the presence of the patient. This is also an excellent time to observe their interaction. If, for example, they sit in chairs on opposite sides of the room they have told you a great deal about their relationship. Information which is likely to be distressing is best given to the couple together and at a time when they can ask questions and sort out their feelings.

Sensitive Issues

Some physicians like to have the patient fill out a printed history form and bring it in at the time of the first visit. This can be a great time-saver, but it is necessary to honestly and completely review the recorded responses. If she has replied "yes" to the query "Do you have any questions about sex?" and is not asked about them she will get the message that her doctor does not want to talk about sexual matters. In other sensitive areas, verbally repeating a question left blank can elicit additional valuable information, for example, a history of emotional illness in the family.

Taking a sexual history may be a stumbling block for an otherwise competent interviewer.[5] The old excuse that there is not enough time to ask all those questions usually means the interviewer has discomfort in talking about sex with a patient. The pregnant patient and her mate usually have a number of questions about sex and often are reluctant to bring them to the doctor's attention. A common question is, "Can we continue sex during the pregnancy?" What the clinician should immediately ask himself or herself and then the couple is what do they mean by sex? Other simple questions such as how has this pregnancy affected the couple's sex life gives them permission to talk about sex. This also tells them that here is a person who is also willing to discuss their sex life as it was before the pregnancy. The initial sexual interview is a private discussion with the patient alone. Her husband or mate should be included at some subsequent interview once the basics have been covered. In all interactions she must be reassured of the privacy of her replies.

Medical students frequently say, "What should I ask?" and residents complain, "There isn't time to ask about sex!" When sexual questions are posed in a relevant fashion there is rarely patient objection. Sexual questions should not be any more personal or difficult for an obstetrician than when asking someone about their last menstrual period. Simple questions will usually suffice: "Is your sexual life satisfactory?" "Are you able to reach a climax?" "How has pregnancy changed your sex life?" (see Chapter 7).

If the woman has a need for an extended interview concerning sexual matters, this can be scheduled at a later time or she can be referred if there seems to be significant dysfunction. The obstetrician is not called upon to be the sex expert, only an understanding physician who gives the patient permission to speak about sex and sexual problems. However, if the obstetrician does not have the time, experience, or training to treat such problems then the couple can be referred to an experienced counselor.

It is important that some record of baseline sexual function appear in the medical record. Patients may later believe sexual dysfunction is due to the course of the pregnancy or the result of medical intervention. With good records, one can refer back and document that certain problems were previously present.

A history of prior sexual assault or abuse is very important. There is an association between past sexual abuse and the potential for the victim to abuse her own children. If such information is obtained and she has never revealed such data before, this may be her first opportunity to get help in dealing with the emotions surrounding the event. In these circumstances, a referral to a psychologist or psychiatrist is a necessity.

As one takes the history of the timing of the last menstrual period it is equally important to ascertain if there was a positive intention to get pregnant or a more passive approach of just not using effective contraception. Could the pregnancy be the result of a contraceptive failure, a union outside of marriage or the primary relationship, or is it the result of assault? It is important to learn not only the present attitudes toward this pregnancy but also how the woman feels about her mate, the father of the pregnancy. Was there an initial thought to opt for abortion? Rarely is the woman unequivocally thrilled about being pregnant from the moment of conception. It is nonetheless important to understand her feelings about herself, her conceptus, and her mate at each stage of pregnancy (see Chapter 4).

Most of what has been said refers to the interview, or interviews, at the beginning of pregnancy. Unfortunately, subsequent prenatal visits tend to be a quick check of statistics having to do with the progress of the patient and the fetus with little opportunity for further in-depth evaluations. However, each visit should include a few minutes when the obstetrician sits down and asks the patient how things are going. It should be clear to both the physician and the patient that this part of the visit is different from the "housekeeping" requirements of the usual physical checks. All of the important areas of the first interview need to be followed up throughout the pregnancy in subsequent brief interviews. The patient's emotions and interpersonal relationships and even her ability to accomplish her goals will be significantly altered by pregnancy, and if there are difficulties, it is important to determine how she handles herself as circumstances change. It is to be hoped that her husband or mate can be present for a significant number of these visits so the adaptation of the couple can be judged.

Referral

When physical and obstetrical problems develop either the obstetrician is comfortable with dealing with them or the patient will be referred to a maternal-fetal or other specialist. But when the problems that the patient is facing are of an emotional nature, referral may be more difficult. After ascertaining that there is an emotional conflict, the obstetrician must inform the patient and family that specific treatment is needed. In the case of a psychotic break, the need for intervention is obvious. It is difficult to try to reason with a person whose reality testing is impaired. It is best to simply state to the patient and her significant support person that she is ill and a possible danger to herself and to her baby. If immediate help is demanded, referral to an emergency room facility which has psychiatric staffing is the first line of assistance, if a psychiatrist is not otherwise immediately available. The significant other and perhaps the members of the patient's immediate family must be informed of the need for immediate care and instructed to take the necessary measures.

More often the patient's emotional status is less unstable and emergent intervention is not required. Anxiety and depression are among the most common clinical problems. Recognizing anxiety and panic attacks is not difficult (see Chapter 8). The patient evidences fear and dread along with sweating, tachypnea, and tachycardia. Panic attacks appear suddenly and without apparent provocation. As these events are profoundly disturbing, patients are usually very willing to be referred to a psychiatrist or psychologist. The diagnosis of depression can be a great deal more subtle. The symptoms of depression are often expressed as multiple physical complaints in a patient who has not previously been given to complaining. When asked if she feels blue or depressed she will usually respond positively. Again, a sensitive explanation to her about what is happening will often result in compliance with a referral to a psychologist or psychiatrist. It is always best to explain that referral does not mean that two independent specialists will be caring for her but that there will be a *collaboration* between the doctors in assuring her best care. It is especially important to reassure her that she is not being abandoned or shuffled off to someone else.

With the patient who is hospitalized on an obstetrical ward for complications, depression and anxiety are often serious symptoms which can hinder her progress or compliance. Psychological support or intervention has been shown to shorten hospitalization in orthopedic patients.[7] Although this has not been formally demonstrated in obstetrical practice, many clinicians believe that consultation is helpful. The patient can be informed that a colleague is available who is especially skilled in helping to deal with emotions created by illness during pregnancy, and asked if she would be willing to see that person.

Sometimes, when an obstetrician calls a psychiatrist for assistance there is difficulty in reaching the consultant directly. The psychologist or psychiatrist usually works with a strict time schedule and commonly will not permit his or her staff to interrupt during a patient counseling session. Thus, it will be necessary to leave a message to call back. In such communications it is important to leave an accurate sense of urgency concerning the case in question. It is also helpful to the psychiatrist if the obstetrician writes in the consult request precisely what information is desired. These referrals are easiest when a psychiatrist works in liaison with a particular specialty. There is then a familiarity with obstetrical conditions and, usually, easy access to consultation.

The shoe is on the other foot when the psychiatrist calls the obstetrician for a consult on a patient hospitalized in the psychiatry services. Obstetricians need to remember that the threat of bleeding, miscarriage, or delivery from a pregnant patient is as anxiety provoking to the psychiatric staff as the out-of-control psychiatric patient is to the obstetrical service. Thus a rapid response to the request is necessary. A sit-down conference with the psychiatry staff regarding management is as important as a written consult. It is especially helpful to instruct the staff when to call for help while the patient remains on the psychiatry ward.

Conclusions

Interviewing is our initial and most important contact with new patients. This introduction to the patient is just as important as the introduction to a potential friend or business partner. In the interview, the physician must be skilled in hearing what the patient says and, in addition, must search out what has *not* been said. Interviewing must be performed not only in the context of the individual but in the context of the society in which we live. Both the patient's and the interviewer's background of education, family, and religious training are factors in the interview. This information is as important as the essential facts of physical well-being or illness. The physician must cultivate and continually practice the skills of listening and communicating. The interview not only reveals facts but also provides the opportunity to educate. This important and privileged opportunity to meet the patient must never be treated lightly. The ability to exchange ideas and information in the interview is essential to success in both the science and art of medical practice.

References

1. Bird B: *Talking with Patients*. Philadelphia, JB Lippincott, 1955, pp 1–65.
2. Friederick MA: History-taking and interview techniques and the physician-patient relationship, in Zatuchni GI, LaFerla JL, Sciarra JJ (eds.): *Gynecology and Obstetrics*, vol. 6. Philadelphia, JB Lippincott, 1990; 72, pp 1–8.
3. Editorial in Rosenthal MB, Smith DH (eds.): *Psychosomatic Obstetrics and Gynecology*. New York, Karger, 1985, pp 1–3.
4. Szasz A, Hollander J: The basic model of the doctor-patient relationship. *Arch Intern Med* 1956;97:585–590.
5. Good R: The third ear: Interviewing techniques in obstetrics and gynecology. *Obstet Gynecol* 1972;40:760–762.
6. American Psychiatric Association: *Diagnostic and Statistical Manual of Mental Disorders*, ed. 3, rev. Washington, DC, American Psychiatric Association Press, 1987.
7. Levitan ST, Kornfeld DS: Clinical and cost benefits of liaison psychiatry. *Am J Psychiatry* 1981;138:790–793.

Chapter 6

The Difficult Patient

Therese M. Madden-Fitzsimons, MB

Black and portentous must this humour prove,
Unless good counsel may the cause remove.
—*Romeo and Juliet* I,i,139
William Shakespeare (1564-1616)

Although physicians are reluctant to admit it, there exists a group of patients who evoke in them feelings of dread, anger, rage, irritation, despondency, and, at times, outright hatred.[1,2] Much of the medical literature has ignored this issue, and it has been left predominantly to the psychiatric and psychoanalytic literatures[9] to address this ubiquitous problem.[3,4] The value of scrutinizing this group, in the context of their relationships with physicians, cannot be overestimated, as difficult patients have a significant and undeniable impact on their clinician(s),[2] their milieu[5-7] (ie, the clinic or ward), and, ultimately, on their own treatment and care.

A review of the literature reveals attempts to unravel the various components involved in the development of "the difficult patient." Some of the components are the individual physician's personality, complete with idiosyncratic biases[8]; the individual patient's personality, complete with whatever constitutional and environmental factors that result in a maladaptive interpersonal style[1]; and certain behaviors, such as violent, acting-out, and/or suicidal, that promote feelings of impotence, anger, frustration, helplessness, and inadequacy in the would-be care provider. It is helpful to review each of these variables in turn.

The Individual Physician

In the context of our own practices it is clear that certain patient types evoke in us more intense reactions than others. By a usually unconscious screening, this commonly results in a uniformity of "types" in each of our practices over time. As Hackett[8] points out, "Look into your colleagues' waiting rooms. . . . Certain physicians attract certain types of people." Overall, this process benefits both the patient and the doctor. Illuminating these unconscious biases and understanding the basis for their decisions is of benefit to both the physician and the patient. Our own personal histories, subjective experiences, and perspectives enter into the physician-patient relationship just as the patient's individuality does. What we bring of ourselves contributes to that relationship—potentially to either enhance and enrich it, or, possibly, to disrupt or even nullify it.

Case 1

A patient, Mrs. G, was referred for psychiatric consultation because of "inability to accept infertility." The patient was a 32-year-old professional, married for 8 years, who had, along with her husband, endured exhaustive investigations and procedures for primary infertility with no definitive causal agent(s) found and no further avenues left to explore. The referring obstetrician, Dr. B, a tertiary care specialist in infertility, known for his tenacious and methodical approach to investigations, stated in the referral that the patient appeared unable to accept her infertility and clearly must be depressed and in need of psychotherapy and/or medications.

On psychiatric assessment, the couple appeared well-adjusted, supportive, and cohesive in their mutual plans and goals. Though both were tearful when discussing their infertility experiences and their sorrow at their inability to conceive, they were grieving openly and together, and spoke of mobilizing their emotional and physical resources to attempt adoption. Mrs. G, an intelligent, articulate, and attractive woman with a well-developed capacity for psychological insight and empathic relatedness, spoke of her impressions that the eminent Dr. B was angry with her because she had tried to "call off" further investigations. Dr. B wanted her to take part in a new research protocol. Mr. and Mrs. G, jointly, had decided that they had exhausted currently recognized investigative procedures and were keen to "move on," hoping for encouragement and support in their plans to adopt.

Further conversations with Dr. B revealed that Mrs. G reminded him of his revered older sister, an intelligent, attractive, verbal woman who, he had always felt, had "given up too easily" when discouraged from pursuing medical training by their authoritarian father. Dr. B frequently wondered if his sister suffered from depression and discontent because of this, and he himself felt pangs of guilt at being the "chosen one," particularly at times when he perceived his skill as a physician to be less than optimal. He would tell himself he "owed it" to her and to himself to ensure everyone got "all the possible chances." He had never fully discussed with his sister his belief that she should have "forced the issue," but would put critical thoughts of her out of his head, becoming even more determined to "protect" other people's opportunities for further development.

As he spoke of this, Dr. B became more aware of the unconscious bias he had harbored, and his perception of the G's as having "given up" because of "depression" or passive despondency began to waver. He was ultimately able to support them genuinely and accept their decision to forego experimental procedures as inappropriate for them and not based upon apathy or due to his "failure."

Case 2

Ms. K, a 28-year-old clerk, was referred for psychiatric assessment because of "tearfulness, query depression" following a myomyectomy. The referral source, a senior resident on gynecology who was following this patient, stated that the woman was "constantly crying in hospital" and had missed "two out of three appointments" postoperatively because of "weakness and nerves!" When Ms. K, a tearful and somewhat passive young woman, attended for consultation, the story became more complex. She disclosed a history of incest, and a date rape that resulted in pregnancy and therapeutic abortion (in another hospital) 3 months prior to the myomyectomy. She stated she was feeling weak and tired, was unable to "fight back" to confront and charge her assailant, and that the myomyectomy was "a very serious operation" that had scared her intensely. She felt afraid of most things in her life—particularly since the rape—and was ruminating that her inability to disclose the facts of the rape and subsequent termination may have complicated her surgery in some way. Because she withheld this information from the resident, she felt wracked with guilt and self-loathing. And she interpreted the referral to psychiatry as confirmation that she had, indeed, "cheated" in that relationship. She also felt that her cheating explained her physician's reluctance to believe the severity of her symptoms—such as the fatigue (and guilt)—which rendered her incapable of attending appointments.

The physician, Dr. S, also a 28-year-old woman, when informed of these facts with the patient's consent, wondered if her initial (and ongoing) impression of this patient as "whining" and "never ending crying" had served to blind her to investigating other issues and concerns in this patient's case. Dr. S, the only daughter in a family of six, had long fought the "female stereotype" of "weak, clinging, crying women" and reacted to these characteristics with immediate impatience and chagrin. The bias to discount these symptoms as evidence of inherent weakness and to avoid clarification of underlying processes had served to promote a dysfunctional patient-doctor relationship in this case. Dr. S decided to continue caring for Ms. K when she became more self-aware, particularly of this specific "blind spot." Ms. K's relationship with Dr. S slowly became more consistent and she eventually was able to assume more control in her relationships in general.

The two examples above serve as illustrations of what we as physicians can contribute, via our idiosyncratic biases, to the creation of "the difficult patient." These biases can be understood as components of countertransference[14]: the process whereby we react to patients not only as the individuals they are, but also as reminders of persons and situations from our past. This definition of countertransference is in contrast to the classical Freudian view, which views the physician's countertransference as an unconscious reaction to the patient's transference. Epstein and Feiner,[13] in their *Introduction to Countertransference,* describe a "natural view." In this approach, countertransference is held to be the "natural, role-responsive, necessary complement or counterpart to the transference of a patient and to his state of relatedness." Taking this broadened, more natural, interpersonal view of what constitutes "countertransference" is more useful in understanding, and thereby dealing with, the difficult patient and the patient-physician relationship. It also facilitates our understanding of the patient's "transference" to us, which is also, by necessity, an emotional reaction not only to us but to people and situations we may evoke from their experience. Clarifying both these processes can help us negotiate any relationship, especially the "difficult" one.

The Patient

The next related variable in the difficult patient-doctor relationship is that of the patient.[9] Various attempts have been made to produce a typology of these patients. The most useful, in our opinion, is that of Groves,[1] who defines these patients as those whom most physicians dread. He groups them according to their predominant behavioral style and the responses they evoke in treating staff, emphasizing that awareness and scrutiny of the physician's negative reactions constitute important clinical data for the understanding and management of these patients.

Groves's first group is that of the "dependent clingers," [1] akin to the dependent, demanding patient described by Grete Bibring[3] in 1956. This is a group whose hallmark is overt insatiable neediness, coupled with a perception of the physician as an inexhaustible "mother," a bottomless well of resources. Their dependency may initially be gratifying, even seductive, and may evoke feelings of power and specialness in the physician, but sooner or later this is replaced by dread as the reality of one's limitations becomes clearer and the patient's behavior and demands escalate. The extent of these patients' neediness is such that the physician can ultimately respond with aversion, anger, frustration, exhaustion, and irritability, and be unable to deal with this patient's incessant demands any longer. As Bibring points out, it can help if we realize that for this patient, the satisfaction derived from attention and care is paramount, and covers underlying fears and terrors of abandonment and desertion. The extent of their neediness is such that their behavior and demands are often extreme.

Behavior can include overtly seductive and sexual behavior, which again should be understood as a reflection of their neediness and responded to by firmly reiterating and modeling appropriate and ethical physician-patient behavior. In dealing with this particular group of patients, early recognition and anticipation of difficulties is essential. This allows the physician to gently but firmly lay some ground rules—to set limits on specific behaviors—by emphasizing the nature of the physician's relationship with the patient. This should emphasize the physician's limitations, but also conviction that patients are receiving the best care, which they deserve. Regular appointments with definite instructions on individual policies regarding telephone calls and some extra visits are best. These patients benefit from scheduled visits, which serve to regulate their hunger for more and more help and attention versus their dread of isolation and abandonment. Psychiatric consultation can be made palatable if offered as an adjunct, but never as a substitute for the physician's care. In selected cases also, consultation with a colleague and even well-prepared transfer of care may be needed, particularly in cases of overtly and consistently seductive behavior.

Case 3

Mrs A, in the 39th week of her second pregnancy, was admitted in active labor. Her cervix was fully dilated, with bulging membranes. A singleton fetus was present in a transverse lie. She had undergone a first cesarean section 3 years prior for cephalo-pelvic disproportion and a large baby. In this pregnancy she desired a vaginal birth and had been counseled for a trial of vaginal delivery following cesarean section. She was followed by ultrasound scanning and electronic fetal monitoring in the last several weeks of her pregnancy. It was noted during examinations at both 36 and 38 weeks that while the fetus was in a longitudinal lie (cephalic presentation) the head was not yet engaged and the lie was unstable. Mrs. A labored at home without advising her physician. When admitted, she was quickly rushed to the cesarean section room after the fixed transverse lie was diagnosed. On the operating table she repeatedly questioned the need for a cesarean section, sitting upright to directly confront the obstetrician on call, Dr. D, about his judgment and view of the situation, saying things such as: "Do you mean I should not have labored at home?" or "Why am I not to deliver vaginally?" On the 4th postpartum day she called Dr. D and asked to meet with him (he was not her personal physician so he had not seen her the next day for her postpartum care). Mrs. A confronted him once again for several minutes with the situation, trying to elicit from him information he did not have, such as the possibility that she should not have been allowed to labor at all and that her prenatal care may not have been optimal. Dr. D tried to diplomatically explain that the presentation of her child had been cephalic prior to the onset of contractions, albeit with a high presenting part and that a trial of labor was a reasonable possibility under those conditions. Further, no one had expected her to convert to a transverse lie and labor at home for 10 hours before coming to the hospital. She was nevertheless still aggressive and pointed out to him that her father was an obstetrician and she understood very well the inherent risk of childbirth. She seemed to demand special care or favors because of her background, although she had truly not been aware of the risk she had taken on her own.

The second group Groves draws attention to are the *entitled demanders*.[1] These patients are as equally needy as the aforementioned group; however, they express this by means of intimidation, devaluation, and guilt induction rather than the naive flattery and seduction used by the "dependent clingers." This group attempts a vicelike grip on their physician by means of threat such as litigation or withholding payment. Their hostility is often coupled with a "repulsive sense of innate deservedness" and entitlement.[1] These patient behaviors may evoke a wish to counterattack in the physician, who feels enraged, devalued, and assaulted by these patients.[10] It is crucial in dealing with these individuals to maintain a constant awareness that they are needy and dependent, and it is this which underlies their hostile attack. These are patients who respond to fear of abandonment and their own neediness by shielding themselves from it in an attitude of deserving entitlement and superiority. Their devaluation, attack, and entitlement are means for them to preserve their sense of themselves when under threat, ie, during illness or some other crisis. Responding to them with defensive counterattack only serves to perpetuate and escalate their belief that they are, in fact, under threat and at risk, which in turn increases their dysfunctional behavior.[11]

Dealing with these patients is very difficult, particularly since as physicians we are inordinately sensitive to the fantasies of omnipotence we have had to relinquish.[1] It is hard, too, to deal with ridicule, obnoxiousness, and devaluation in the context of a hectic schedule and the realistic demands of patient care. It may often seem far easier to retort with a hostile, cutting defense, though as stated, this only serves to escalate the situation. An approach that is more useful is the following: avoid engaging in verbal battles, avoid defensive counterploys, and validate and support the realistic entitlement these and all patients have, which is (realistically) adequate care. Reiteration of this, and, if possible, redirection of their vehemence, anger, and energy into more appropriate channels (eg, to therapeutic compliance) is a fair treatment strategy. Consultation with colleagues is also frequently helpful, not only as a defensive maneuver from a medicolegal perspective, but also as a means to support one's own treatment plan, and, therefore, one's self- esteem, in the face of ridicule and verbal abuse from this patient group.

Case 4

Ms. J, a 22-year-old gravida 2 para 2, was referred to psychiatry on the 5th postpartum day. She was hospitalized for intravenous antibiotic treatment of an endometritis postcesarean delivery and was described as "impossible," "hostile," and "unmanageable" by the nursing staff. The attending obstetrician described her as "always difficult," but "worse" in this admission, which had been lengthy owing to a significant antepartum hemorrhage at 30 weeks, diagnosis of a complete placenta previa, and eventual cesarean delivery 8 weeks later. She was stated to have neglected her personal hygiene, verbally abused other patients and their spouses, engaged in frequent verbal battles with staff, and had been pulling out her intravenous line before it should have been removed.

On assessment, Ms. J was revealed to be an energetic, vocal, and somewhat defensive young woman who immediately berated the assessor for the "lousy care" the hospital provided and the "horrible, stupid" nursing staff attending her. She appeared angry and embittered, stating no one ever answered her call bell, and that "no one cares." She had been concerned her intravenous was "infected" but "no one would come" so she pulled it out, causing great uproar. She was adamant that she was "in the right," deserved better care, and that overall "they're going to pay." Further history revealed that Ms. J came from a chaotic and deprived background. She had lived alone from the age of 15 years on and was now trying to raise a newborn and 2-year-old with social assistance and little else. She was ambitious—wanting to "get off" Social Security and have a career—but was obviously aware of the difficulties ahead. With some direction, she could frame her immediate goals as discharge, "to get away from the lousy hospital," and "get better," disclosing her fear that "they don't know what they're doing" and that the infection may render her sterile.

Interventions began with validation of her immediate goals and recognition of her angry, hostile, frustrated feelings. It was then clarified that directing these feelings at the staff and acting impulsively, ie, by pulling out the intravenous line, were not compatible with ensuring the good care she deserved and to allow for full recovery and discharge. At the same time, interventions were implemented with the staff: to recognize and empathize with their frustration, to validate their experiences with the patient as difficult and self-denigrating; and to clarify that the drive behind her hostile and demeaning stance was an effort to maintain her sense of self and her integrity while experiencing hospitalization and illness as attacking and threatening. Completing their picture of her—not as just an angry, hostile woman, but a frightened, isolated woman faced with severe social stressors—also served to defuse the staff's mounting hatred and antipathy. It was suggested, and accepted, that every shift, her nurse would come by and see her for 10 minutes every 2 hours and then address her needs, concerns, and demands. This served to reduce the intensity of her demands, and the acting- out behavior of pulling out her intravenous ceased.

Groves's third group is termed the *manipulative help-rejecters*.[1] Again, they have a tremendous need for emotional support and an insatiable need for assistance. However, their hallmark is that no matter what the intervention, or so it seems, *no* regimen can help them. They tenaciously report therapeutic failures and/or symptom re-emergence (or new symptom formation). Their behavior initially evokes anxiety in the physician: a concern he or she has missed something. Next, irritation is felt and finally self-doubt and depression. The net result seems to be a seemingly endless litany of complaints, with ever increasing desperation in the physician as no remedy, interpretation, or intervention seems to work. As the physician's frustration mounts, treatments can begin to be implemented in an impulsive way, as a last-ditch attempt to quell the flood of complaints and to regain some measure of self-worth.

With this relationship, it is critical, as physician, to maintain a distance or an observing role to ensure the patient's (and the physician's) best interests. This type of relationship is marked by manipulative behavior—an extreme dependency where the patient tries to get these dependency needs met in an intense, contradictory, self-defeating, and indirect way. The conflict is between meeting these needs, and the concomitant fear of being overwhelmed by the other person. These patients need help in regulating emotional distance in their relationships. They are particularly vulnerable to extremes of distance, eg, easily prone to feeling engulfed or abandoned. In practical terms, this implies that a consistent patient-doctor relationship is best, with regular follow-ups specified by the physician and an approach of "therapeutic pessimism" shared with the patient, ie, making them aware from the outset that complete symptom cure is unlikely. This group is again difficult to refer for psychiatric assistance as they interpret referral frequently as the ultimate distancing ploy. Again, presented as an adjunct, it is more acceptable.[12]

Case 5

Mrs. NE, a 54-year-old woman, was referred by her gynecologist, Dr. F, for "depression." Mrs. NE had been a patient of Dr. F for almost 30 years, and he had delivered three of her five children. Though always a "difficult" patient, she had become progressively more problematic over the preceding 10 years, and in the months leading to referral had established a litany of complaints which she presented as due to "the change" but which were unremitting and unresponsive to conventional treatments. She would visit his office three, sometimes four times a month; would telephone his home on weekends and on evenings and seemed to take an inordinate pleasure in his inability to "sort things out." Dr. F felt frustrated and, at times, bewildered. He was not sure just how or when things had "got out of hand" but had an uneasy feeling he was "missing the boat" and was "fed up" with her. At times he felt like giving up—particularly when she would present with voluminous symptom lists and complaints of side effects to whatever treatment he had employed. He wondered if she was depressed and "somatizing." He also hoped, if that was the case, that psychiatric treatment would be all she needed and he could get a well-deserved rest.

Mrs. NE canceled her first two appointments with the psychiatrist. On the third, she recounted her symptom list and was redirected with great difficulty to the broader area of how she felt, given her symptoms and treatment failures. She appeared to be a woman focused on her symptoms and Dr. F's perceived failures, with marked reluctance to go beyond this. Suggestions that Dr. F, indeed, any doctor, could not cure all her symptoms, were met with disdain. She emphasized only a "real" doctor could do this, certainly not a psychiatrist, but that she was prepared to "stick" with Dr. F until he was, in fact, successful. She denied any role for psychiatric assistance and refused further psychiatric follow-up. She continues unabated in her ambivalent pursuit of Dr. F.

Case 6

Ms. N was a 27-year-old gravida, 3para0, referred by her obstetrician during an antepartum admission for septicemia due to using infected dirty needles. She was at 32 weeks of gestation, single, and a self-confessed multiple substance abuser and prostitute. She agreed to a psychiatric referral, although she was equally clear that her main goal was to be discharged and to resume her hazardous behaviors. She described in great detail her long- standing history of substance abuse—beginning at age 11 years with alcohol, culminating in 4 g of intravenous cocaine a day. She came from a disrupted family: her father was unknown, her mother an alcoholic and intermittent prostitute. Her younger siblings and herself had been apprehended at several points in their childhood by child welfare agencies. She was sexually abused from the age of 7 years, initially by a client of her mother's, then by a succession of foster parents. She "went on the streets" at age 13 years and returned to live with her mother when she was 17. She tested positive for hepatitis B and had three negative HIV tests. However, she continued to trade needles and did not always insist on using condoms when engaged in sex. Her pregnancy was unplanned, but she had decided to keep the baby as she did not want a third abortion. She commented that some of her clients found her pregnant state to be particularly appealing.

She agreed to a trial of desipramine while in hospital in an effort to reduce her craving for cocaine and thereby reduce the likelihood of her return to it. However, after 3 weeks of hospitalization she coerced a day pass from an unsuspecting intern and did not return to care until time for her delivery.

By then she had resumed her cocaine usage of 4 to 5 g per day, intravenously. She continued to abuse marijuana and alcohol. She had returned to live with her mother and planned to resume prostitution as soon as possible.

She had an uneventful delivery of a low-birth-weight, jittery baby who nonetheless was discharged to her care 10 days later under the supervision of a child welfare agency.

Groves's final category is that of the *self-destructive deniers*[1]: a group of patients who utilize denial in a chronic self-destructive way, and show behaviors which can be seen as unconsciously "self murderous," such as the alcoholic who persists in drinking even with a history of subdural hematomas and esophageal varices, or the pregnant woman with a placenta previa who persists in having intercourse and refuses admission to hospital. These are patients who tend to evoke feelings of malice, and even a wish they would "get it over with." It poses a conflict for the physician—between the ideal of rescue and the wish for the patient to die. The feelings of malice can further evoke guilt, self-reproach, dread, heroism, or an attitude of giving up. The issue again is one of realism in that the physicians' capability to help self-destructive patients is limited. If a treatable depression exists, this must be treated. However, in most cases these patients refuse psychiatric help and continue on their paths of self-destruction. These are patients who have renounced all hope of having their dependency needs met. However, an attempt to maintain them in the doctor-patient relationship must be made. Abandoning them only serves to enforce their position. The difficulties inherent in dealing with these patients can be helped by consultation with other colleagues and reminding oneself of one's own therapeutic limitations. The position of the obstetrician who, in fact, has two, not one, patient, to deal with, is further complicated in these situations. On occasion the physician must consider a legal action to preserve the life of the fetus, even if this may ultimately jeopardize the physician-patient relationship.

Conclusion

The care of the difficult patient is an integral part of any practice. This problem may be better understood as "the difficult doctor-patient relationship," as it refers to the interpersonal arena, and those events and behaviors which can evoke (in both parties) feelings of despair, futility, frustration, and hostility. To ensure adequate patient care in a therapeutic relationship, identification of our "blind spots" is essential. From there, consistent "good enough" care, with judicious consultations and, if necessary, well-planned transfers to colleagues, are reasonable measures to ensure both the patient's best interests and our own as care givers.

References

1. Groves JE: Taking care of the hateful patient. *N Engl J Med* 1978;298:883–887.
2. Smith RJ, Steindler EM: The impact of difficult patients upon treaters. *Bull Menninger Clin* 1983;47:107–116.
3. Bibring GL: Psychiatry and medical practice in a general hospital. *N Engl J Med* 1956;254:366–372.
4. Steiger WA: Managing difficult patients. *Psychosomatics* 1967;8:305–308.
5. Burnham DL: The special-problem patient: Victim or agent of splitting? *Psychiatry* 1966;29:105–122.
6. Friedman HJ: Some problems of inpatient management with borderline patients. *Am J Psychiatry* 1969;126:299–304.
7. Groves JE: Management of the borderline patient on a medical or surgical ward: The psychiatric consultant's role. *Int J Psychiatr Med* 1975;6:337–348.
8. Hackett TP: Which patients turn you off? It's worth analyzing. *Med Econ* July 21, 1969, pp 95–99.
9. Silver D: Psychodynamics and psychotherapeutic management of the self-destructive character-disordered patient. *Psychiatr Clin North Am* 1985;8:357–375.
10. Adler G: Helplessness in the helpers. *Br J Med Psychol* 1972;45:315–326.
11. Adler G, Buie DH: The misuses of confrontation with borderline patients. *Int J Psychoanal Psychother* 1972;1:109–120
12. Kris K: Psychiatric consultation in the management of patient ambivalence interfering with the doctor-patient relationship. *Am J Psychol* 1981;138:194–197.
13. Epstein L, Feiner AH: Introduction, in Epstein L, Feiner AH (eds.): *Countertransference*. New York, Jason Aronson, 1979, p 23.
14. Finkel JB: Physician countertransference: Impact on patients, treatment team, and adaptation to illness, in Finkel JB (ed.): *Consultation-Liaison Psychiatry: Current Trends and New Perspectives*. New York, Grune and Stratton, 1983, pp 53–57.

Suggested Reading

1. Adler G: Valuing and devaluing in the psychotherapeutic process. *Arch Gen Psychiatry* 1970;22:454–462.
2. Giovacchini PL: Characterological problems: The need to be helped. *Arch Gen Psychiatry* 1970;22:245–251.
3. Lipowski ZJ: Physical illness, the individual, and the coping process. *Psychiatry* 1:91–102.
4. Book HE, Sadavoy J, Silver D: Staff countertransference to borderline patients on an inpatient unit. *Am J Psychother* 1979;32:521–531.
5. Maltsberger JT, Buie DH: Countertransference hate in the treatment of suicidal patients. *Arch Gen Psychiatry* 1974;30:625–633.
6. Lipsitt DR: Medical and psychological characteristics of crocks. *Int J Psychiatry Med* 1970;1:15–25.
7. Winnicott DW: Hate in countertransference. *Int J Psychoanal* 1949;30:69–74.
8. Steiger WA, Hirsh H: The difficult patient in everyday medical practice. *Med Clin North Am* 1965;49:1449–1465.
9. Wise TN, Berlin RM: Burnout: Stresses in consultation- liaison psychiatry. *Psychosomatics* 1981;22:744–745, 749–751.

Chapter 7

Sexual Function

Max Chorowski, MD

Let copulation thrive.
—*King Lear IV*,vi,110
William Shakespeare (1564–1616)

Sexuality is a paradoxically difficult subject for women's health practitioners. Few areas in medical practice are so influenced by culture, folklore, religion, and life experiences of the obstetrician and of the couple. The inability and/or unwillingness of practitioners to discuss sexuality with their pregnant patients except to recommend an arbitrary peripartum period of abstinence is common, peculiar, and unfortunate. Unnecessary sexual restrictions undermine confidence in the physician, lead to increased distress, and contribute to male infidelity.[1,2]

The current chapter is written to enhance clinicians' ability to understand and discuss sexuality and sexual functions during pregnancy. Sexual feelings and sexual response are important parts of human functioning.[3] As an integral part of marital satisfaction sexual activity does not stop once pregnancy begins. An important task for clinicians is to be able to counsel couples appropriately concerning sexual expression during both normal and abnormal gestation.

Sexuality: Erroneous Assumptions

Pregnant Women Are Invariably Heterosexual

In fact, there is an increasing worldwide phenomenon of lesbian women's having babies, often by donor insemination.[4,5] Although we can expect more information about the sexual functioning of these women and their partners in pregnancy to emerge in the future, little is known to date. In general, sex therapists dealing with lesbians observe that these individuals are capable of the same sexual functions and dysfunctions as heterosexuals in the nonpregnant state. Thus, there is no reason to believe that sexual reactions in pregnancy are different among lesbian women. The conclusions resulting from the Zeidenstein[5] interviews are of particular value in counseling such patients. When traditional health history questions concerning marital status, sexual activity, and birth control were presented to lesbian women, inaccurate information was elicited. This was due to the content of the questions as well as to subtle overtones of disapproval emanating from the questioner that made the interviewees uncomfortable. Beyond sensitivity, the women in this study placed high value on practitioners with knowledge of lesbian sexuality and sexual practices.

The Majority of Pregnancies Are Planned

In fact, some 57% of the pregnancies conceived in 1987 and going to term were *unintended*.[6] Even among women who intend pregnancy, ambivalence is normal, especially in the first trimester.[7] Such uncertainty concerns both the issues of carrying the pregnancy and of raising a child. Many levels of desire for and acceptance of pregnancy exist. Such ideas affect the woman's perception of the sexual act that brought about the pregnancy (see Chapter 4).

Pregnancy Indicates Comfort with Sexuality and Its Consequences

In fact, many women who become pregnant are in conflict about their sexuality and its expression. Public knowledge that they are sexual beings (certainly by the time they "show" pregnancy) is a source of pride to some but of shame and humiliation to others. Such responses doubtless affect sexual behavior. The most extreme reactions occur in the syndrome of the denial of pregnancy (see Chapter 12).

In addition, the extraordinary number of relationships that do not survive pregnancy or the early years of the child's life belie assumptions of maturity, sexual and otherwise. Many pregnancies result from "inappropriate causes," including forcible rape, statutory rape, incest, "one-night stands," extramari-

Table 7.1 Influence of Pregnancy on Sexual Libido

Phase of Pregnancy	Facilitating	Inhibiting
I. Periconceptual	Lack of contraception Purposeful intercourse	Ambivalence toward partner and pregnancy Infertility
II. First trimester	Happy to be pregnant Increased pelvic vascularity Enlarged breasts	Nausea/vomiting Tiredness Fear of miscarriage
III. Second trimester	Increased vaginal lubrication Increased energy	Quickening Orgasm-induced contractions Fear of hurting baby
IV. Third trimester	Wanting to be close	Anxiety regarding birth process Large size/awkward
V. Postpartum	Joy of having child Evolving family identity	Episiotomy and/or lacerations Lactation-related dyspareunia Child care/fatigue Adaptation to parenthood

Reprinted from LaFerla,[39] with permission.

Table 7.2 Self-Reported Frequency of Coitus by Trimester of Pregnancy in 260 Normal Women

Coital Frequency*	1st Trimester (%)	2nd Trimester (%)	Term (%)
NONE	2	2	59
1×/WEEK	11	16	19
2–5×/WEEK	78	77	23
≥6×/WEEK	9	5	1

* 81% reported a baseline of 2 to 5 acts of coitus per week 1 year before conception.

Modified from Solberg, Butler, Wagner,[10] with permission.

tal affairs, and other human events that require a practitioner to be minimally judgmental but maximally open and available to listen. Clinicians who feel that this is beyond the scope of their training should employ staff members with these qualities to speak with these women about their concerns. Couples enjoy meeting all members of the prenatal care team and do not question why the office nurse, midwife, or associate is obtaining the initial history which includes the question: Was this a planned pregnancy? Further, such private opportunities to speak to the staff should recur throughout the pregnancy as new issues or concerns arise.

Sexual Expression during Pregnancy

Effects of Pregnancy on Sexual Function

Although most observations concerning pregnancy and sex hold true for parous patients, the functional changes observed are most dramatic among nulliparas attempting to conceive. Most of the following discussion pertains to the 50% or fewer of couples for whom pregnancy is mutually planned.[6]

Various studies of sexual interest, activity, and responsiveness have been conducted in gravid women as a way of summarizing the net effect of the enhancing and detracting factors (Table 7.1). Most have reported a slow, steady decline in both sexual interest and activity as pregnancy progresses[3,8–10] (Tables 7.2 and 7.3).

Thus, the preponderance of literature does not support the concept of a midtrimester rise in sexual interest, activity, or responsiveness as originally reported by Masters and Johnson,[2] although Reamy and co-workers[3] did find

Table 7.3 Women's Self-Rated Sexual Interest by Trimester as Compared with the Year before Pregnancy.

	1st Trimester (%)	2nd Trimester (%)	Term (%)
Increased	23	24	13
No Change	48	32	11
Decreased	28	44	75

Modified from Solberg, Butler, Wagner,[10] with permission.

a midtrimester increase in desire. Almost all studies concur that by the third-trimester there is little maternal sexual interest, activity, or orgasmic capacity.[3,11,12] However, a possible bias in studies of late third trimester sexual activity is the fact that about one-third of women are still instructed to stop coitus at some time during the third trimester.

The rate of return to prepregnancy levels of sexual functioning is variously reported. Aside from the Masters and Johnson[2] and Falicov[8] studies, a slow return to prepregnancy levels was found by Kenny,[13] Robson and co-workers,[14] and Ryding[12] among others. Improved interest and activity but not responsiveness was reported by Tolor and DiGrazia.[15]

In Solberg and associates' study[10] four major reasons were given by women for their change in sexual behavior during pregnancy. These included physical discomfort (46%), fear of injury to the fetus (27%), loss of interest (23%), and awkwardness during coitus (17%). Of interest, in this series of 260 normal women, 29% were instructed by their physicians to avoid intercourse from 2 to 8 weeks before the estimated date of confinement. Such physician prohibitions against intercourse are still common. The most recent (18th) edition of *Williams' Obstetrics* notes that it is "the custom" of obstetricians to suggest coital abstinence during the last 4 weeks of gestation.[16] This basic obstetric textbook does not make any specific recommendations concerning sexual restriction for normal pregnancies but does relate that risks and benefits "have not been clearly delineated." In contrast, Gabbe's obstetric text, another commonly used source, simply states, "No restriction need be placed on sexual intercourse" in normal pregnancies.[17]

Issues of Fertility and Conception

Currently, couples learn either from practitioners or from various lay literature sources when during the menstrual cycle conception is most likely. Sexual frequency is correspondingly increased, especially around the time of midcycle ovulation. A positive factor for the couple attempting to conceive is that they experience sex without contraceptive worries and are excited about the prospects of pregnancy (Table 7.1).

Under ideal circumstances with otherwise normal couples, the expected rate of conception with unprotected midcycle intercourse is approximately 30% per month. Thus, concerns about fertility may develop if conception does not occur within a few cycles.

For the man, the awareness that fertility problems involve male factors half the time increases performance pressure, perhaps leading to situational erectile failure. Another difficulty for males is "sex by the clock and calendar" as coached by an infertility consultant, perhaps affecting desire and/or erection. In addition, a man who is concerned about the quality of his sperm can be further distracted during lovemaking. Such pressures commonly worsen any preexisting sexual dysfunction.[18,19]

Women may find their premenstrual and intramenstrual symptoms more difficult to tolerate if they interpret them as indicating a failure to conceive. Disorders of the desire phase, or arousal phase, anorgasmia, and coital pain have been reported in such instances.[20,21] Another complaint is "skipping" foreplay.

Long-standing fertility problems challenge the couple's emotional and sexual stability, with in vitro fertilization representing this challenge taken to the extreme. Using strict criteria, 21% of the individuals making up the first 45 couples to request in vitro fertilization from Johns Hopkins University Hospital were found to have either a sexual dysfunction or a psychologic disorder.[22]

For these reasons, the clinician should regularly *retake* a sexual history from the couple as the fertility investigation progresses, reminding them that an important purpose of sex is the demonstration of affection toward each other.[19] An excellent resource for couples with fertility problems is Linda Salzer's book,[23] which contains a helpful chapter on sexual concerns and function.

First Trimester

With the pressure to conceive relieved and in the absence of miscarriage anxiety, sexual frequency improves. Some patients have described this time as the most carefree in their sex lives: not only are there no worries concerning contraception, there are also no additional pressures to achieve pregnancy. As pregnancy advances, the vascularity to the pelvis increases and female orgasm or multiple orgasm is progressively easier to achieve, aided perhaps by increased breast sensitivity.

Normal physiologic events of this trimester such as morning sickness and chronic fatigue can be quite distressing and not conducive to sexual activity.[24] Commonly for women who experience nausea and/or vomiting at several points during the day and night, sexual frequency declines markedly (Table 7.2). Couples who have previously lost a pregnancy in the first trimester often refrain from coitus because of concern of initiating another miscarriage. Finally, the breast tenderness most women experience in this trimester can be deleterious to normal foreplay. In later gestation and postpartum, the milk release associated with orgasm can be bothersome to either partner, although for some it is exciting. It can also provide a welcome moment of laughter, often the best medicine for sexual ills.

Second Trimester

The second trimester is the trimester of greatest sexual interest for pregnant women. How this translates into sexual frequency or satisfaction depends on the health of the relationship and each partner's self-image. Although a midtrimester peaking of sexual activity was found in a nulliparous group studied by Masters and Johnson,[2] most studies indicate a steady decrease in sexual activity throughout pregnancy, as previously discussed.

Key enhancing factors include a decline in earlier symptoms, including sensations of fatigue, and cessation of morning sickness. The fears of miscarriage are lessened once the 12th week is past and the emotional introversion or "regression" of the first trimester has ended. Further, by the second trimester the man has generally accepted the pregnancy and is showing enthusiasm toward joint future planning. For her part, the woman progressively accepts her bodily changes. Orgasm is at times achieved in a previously nonorgasmic woman, partially associated with additional vaginal lubrication accompanying advancing gestation.[25] The male partner may also be enthusiastic about his partner's more voluptuous figure, and she might be pleased to find him more sexually aroused.

These generally beneficial or favorable changes must be weighed against the progressive development of new physical discomforts such as urinary frequency, constipation, and heartburn from reflux esophagitis. There may be concerns of harming the fetus, especially if the now more friable cervix bleeds after coitus. The uterine contractions that frequently accompany orgasm are occasionally frightening and the woman might respond by holding back from achieving her climax. The increased vaginal secretions may not be welcome during oral sex.

At some point in the second trimester, as a result of increasing uterine bulk, it becomes difficult or impossible to have coitus in the male superior position.[3,10,24] Couples who are adept at alternative positions from their prior sexual experiences or who have been counseled regarding positions during pregnancy make this transition with little difficulty (Appendix 7.1). For couples with no alternative experience and no information, this elimination of the "missionary position" can prove disastrous to usual marital relations.

Third Trimester

There is little evidence of enhanced sexuality in the third trimester. Although the likelihood of pregnancy loss is low, some physicians still instill a fear of premature labor in their normal patients and suggest no sexual activity during at least a portion of this trimester. Usually, there is no clarification as to whether or not masturbation or other alternatives are included in the prohibition. Because of the increase in fetal size and pelvic instability, the fatigue that plagued the female partner in the first trimester now returns. Neither the pressure of the uterus on the bladder nor the back pain predisposes toward the desire for romantic interludes. The male partner may not accept his partner's weight gain and change in bodily contours graciously. A feeling of pelvic fullness from unrelieved vasocongestion can lead to chronic pain or dyspareunia despite orgasm. Thus, in the late third trimester fewer coital positions are comfortable. Two fifths of couples stop intercourse and another fifth report pain more than half the time in the late third trimester.[26] Tempers may be short as the couple feels they "have been pregnant forever."

Couples most adept at adjusting to this trimester recognize the mutual need to be close and to be held without always proceeding to sexual activity.[25,27,28] If one or both partners desire orgasm, this can be achieved by gentle oral or manual manipulation.

Postpartum

Unless proscribed by religious practice[29] the majority of couples resume sexual activity well before the traditional 6-week postpartum visit.[30] Surgical healing of the perineum is well advanced by 3 weeks post partum and pelvic tone usually recovered, aided by Kegel exercises. There is no longer any concern about "harming the baby" or premature labor. A method of contraception should be in use. The couple feels growth because of their pregnancy experience and the new person with whom to share intimacy.

However, many factors stand in the way of a return to prepregnancy levels of sexual activity as studied 3 months[2] and even 7 months postpartum.[8] The adjustment to new parenthood is a transition that is rarely easy or equal for both partners. Traditionally, the mother remains home with the newborn and is often fatigued by the end of the day.[31] Her affect can be altered by the transient postpartum blues or the longer-term more severe true depressions (see Chapter 8). She may be resentful of her partner's freedom and the loss of hers. The male partner may not be able to "share" her comfortably with the infant and may make demands that leave her conflicted.

In the psychoanalytic view when a woman becomes a mother, there is projected on her a special motherly persona, the characteristics of which are important to the development of that child. Her partner might find it difficult to accept her as both motherly *and* sexual,[32] with a resultant difficulty in functioning sexually with the mother of one's children. In severe cases the man may be functional only with casual partners; this is termed the "madonna-whore complex."[33]

The lactating mother faces additional issues. Can her partner use the same breast for satisfaction that her infant used a few minutes ago? Is breast-feeding sexually stimulating for her? Will the diminished estrogen in these mothers cause deficient libido as well as atrophic vaginitis, diminished lubrication, or dyspareunia?[25]

Even in the nonlactating woman postpartum dyspareunia is not unusual.[2,34] Perineal discomfort from the episiotomy may require a prolonged time to resolve.[35] Dyspareunia is more prevalent after a mediolateral episiotomy as these incisions require a longer healing phase than midline incisions.[36] Similarly, in terms of comfort, Pfannenstiel incisions are preferred to midline incisions for cesarean delivery.[31]

There is often anticipation of pain with the first lovemaking that contributes to dyspareunia by inducing spasm and inhibiting lubrication. After a few instances of painful coitus, the woman learns to expect discomfort, leading to and perpetuating psychogenic dyspareunia or possibly vaginismus. Preventative management at the time of hospital discharge includes a frank discussion in reference to first postpartum coitus (see Appendix 7.1). Recommendations might include the use of lubricants or an estrogen-containing cream or the female superior position. Sensate focus exercises are also helpful if dyspareunia persists despite simple measures.

Normal Pregnancy: Routine Management

Couples should be made to expect physical, emotional, and sexual changes during pregnancy. They should be asked, with some regularity, What changes have you experienced? to allow them to share their experiences and concerns.[34]

The clinician should meet with both partners early during prenatal care and discuss the rationale for his or her general recommendations about sexual practices during pregnancy so that these suggestions are not perceived as simply arbitrary and there is adequate time for discussion.[37] The couple should be encouraged to discuss their fears and concerns, allowing the clinician to assess whether his reassurances are premature or will create further ambivalence or conflict for the couple. If the recommendations about sexual prac-

Table 7.4 The Screening Sexual History

How often are you having coitus or other forms of sex?

If it were up to you, how often would you be having sex?

Is it pleasurable for you?

What has changed since the pregnancy? (omit for gynecologic patients)

What changes would you like to see in your sexual relationship?

Modified from Sloan,[78] with permission.

tices change, the partners should again be informed as a couple. If, in listening to the couple with a "third ear" one is left with the impression that the couple would benefit from either relationship or sexual counseling, this recommendation is made before further damage to the relationship occurs.

Appendix 7.1 includes a sample patient handout that has proved useful in our service. Other thoughts about speaking to couples may be found in the section Sexuality: Erroneous Assumptions, presented earlier in this chapter.

Differential Diagnosis: Sexual Dysfunctions

Although the anatomy and physiology of nonproblematic human sexuality is a required "basic science" for all practitioners, many choose to refer gynecologic patients who have sexual dysfunctions to others for resolution. Insofar as this pattern of referral reflects a lack of comfort with dealing with such problems, clinician discomfort will persist and may even intensify when pregnant patients seek counseling. This is particularly unfortunate since all couples, not simply the 50% who have either sexual dysfunctions or sexual concerns, could benefit from a clinician open to discussions concerning sexuality.[35]

Taking a sexual history is actually less difficult than many believe. For most gynecologic patients a screening history can be obtained in less than 1 minute; in most obstetric patients the average is 2 minutes (see Tables 7.4 and 7.5). Alternative approaches to such a brief inquiry abound.[38]

Once the dysfunction(s) is identified and a basic history obtained, a physical examination is carried out to determine whether physical factors are involved. For example, many chronic illnesses adversely affect sexual desire and an intact central nervous system is crucial to all stages of sexual function.[39] There are dozens of organic causes of dyspareunia and a careful pelvic exam

Table 7.5 Sexual History: Additional Questions If a Sexual Dysfunction Is Suspected

How long has this been occurring?

Has there been any period or episode of normal functioning?

Does the problem exist in all situations and with all partners?

How much has the problem affected the relationship (partners on the verge of breakup first need relationship therapy, not sex therapy)?

Modified from Shover et al,[79] with permission.

that looks for these causes (referred to as the sexological exam) is critical to evaluating any woman with any sexual complaint.[40] The partner should also undergo a complete physical and urologic examination to identify any physical abnormalities.

There are no specific laboratory tests for sexual dysfunction in the woman, except as indicated on the basis of the initial physical exam. Chronic illness is excluded by appropriate general examination and by relevant laboratory study results. Suspected atrophic vaginitis in the postpartum female can be confirmed by lateral vaginal wall cell maturation index. This study is a better and less expensive "bioassay" for local estrogen effect than serum steroid levels.

The final step toward a clear statement of the complaint is to assign the dysfunction to the appropriate phase of the sexual response cycle in which it occurs. A correct assignment of the dysfunction has both therapeutic and prognostic significance. The dysfunctions in human sexual response can be

Table 7.6 The Most Common Sexual Dysfunctions

DESIRE PHASE DYSFUNCTION: MALE AND FEMALE

    Low sexual desire

    Aversion to sex

    Desires change from current level of activity

AROUSAL PHASE DYSFUNCTIONS

    Female

        Decreased subjective arousal

        Decreased physiologic arousal

    Male

        Decreased subjective arousal

        Difficulty achieving erections

        Difficulty maintaining erections

ORGASMIC PHASE

    Female

        Nonorgasmic

        Painful orgasm (hypoestrogenic, inflammatory, etc)

    Male

        Premature ejaculation

        Inhibited ejaculation

COITAL PAIN

    Vaginismus

    Dyspareunia (psychogenic, ie, organic causes ruled out)

    Pain on or after ejaculation

    Pain exacerbated by sexual activity

Modified from Shover et al,[79] with permission.

Table 7.7 A Comparison of Therapeutic and Prognostic Factors in Sexual Dysfunctions

	Desire phase dysfunctions*	Arousal phase dysfunctions[†]	Orgasmic phase dysfunctions[‡]
Likelihood of success using short-term behavior modification techniques	Least likely	Intermediate	Most likely
Likelihood of needing additional individual psychotherapy to achieve success	Most likely	Intermediate	Least likely
Comparative length of therapy (and cost)	Longest-term therapy, greatest cost	Intermediate	Short-term therapy, lowest cost
Success rates	Lowest	Intermediate	Highest

* Patients who have been victims of sexual abuse (especially as children) seem to share many therapeutic and prognostic factors with the desire phase dysfunctions.

[†] Psychogenic dyspareunia seems to share many therapeutic and prognostic factors with the arousal phase dysfunctions.

divided into three emotional phases (Table 7.6): (1) the desire phase, (2) the arousal phase, (3) the orgasm phase.

The problem should be stated for each partner as the presence or absence of a desire, arousal, or orgasmic phase dysfunction and the presence or absence of coital pain. The specific dysfunctions should then be carefully enumerated.

Treatment

Once the dysfunction has been mapped, a plan for treatment and some general statements about prognosis become possible (Table 7.7). For example, the absence of a long-term desire phase dysfunction connotes a good prognosis. Arousal phase dysfunctions are easier to resolve than desire phase dysfunctions. Orgasm phase dysfunction and vaginismus are often treated in a limited number of sessions. Thus, obstetricians with training and interest in behaviorally oriented sex therapy can consider working with couples with orgasmic dysfunction or vaginismus. The more complex problems are usually referred to practitioners with extensive training in sex therapy, who are able to initiate long-term treatment programs (Table 7.8).

The mainstay in sex therapy, to which all other therapies are compared, is sensate focus training.[41] In the absence of an aversion to sexual contact by the couple, sensate focus exercises form the cornerstone of treatment, with other techniques serving as adjuncts.

Sensate focus therapy presupposes that the couple accepts the need for joint therapy. They must understand that it is the *relationship* that is the subject of treatment, not the "dysfunctional" individual. There can be no such thing as an "uninvolved" sexual partner.

Sensate focus training helps to diminish performance anxieties and pres-

Table 7.8 Therapeutic Modalities Available to the Sex Therapist

Sensate focus (pleasuring) exercises

Educational films (often as an adjunct to sensate focus)

Behavior modification exercises

Individual psychotherapy

Fantasy training

Sexual self-awareness techniques, including masturbatory techniques

Squeeze technique

Vibrator use

Vaginal dilator exercises

Adjunctive medication

Communication skills and other couple therapy techniques

Hypnotherapy

Paradoxical interdictions ("Don't have orgasms")

Bibliotherapy (educational books)

---

sures. Especially important for men, it moves the sexual focus away from the simply the pelvis and eroticizes the whole body. Such retraining restores confidence by starting with "can't fail" exercises. It emphasizes both giving and receiving pleasure. It teaches that "my pleasure is my own responsibility," diminishing blame and finger pointing in a couple's relationship.

An overview of the sensate focus exercises appears in Table 7.9. All exercises are performed privately at home by the couple. After completing approximately three exercises at each current level, the couple returns to the therapist and reviews the way the exercises went. The therapist makes suggestions if needed and assigns the next level of exercise, when appropriate.

The adjuncts to sensate focus training depend on the problem. For example, between exercises with her partner the nonorgasmic female should be practicing self-pleasuring, progressing on to genital self-stimulation. Once she is able to achieve orgasm manually, she instructs her partner on how to bring her to orgasm manually. This manual manipulation can then be added to level

Table 7.9 General Levels of Sensate Focus

Level One—Touching exercises with breasts and genitals "off limits"

Level Two—Add breasts; later add genitals. Exercises are still sensual, not sexual.

Level Three—Massaging, pleasuring. Sexual pleasuring allowed; orgasm is not.

Level Four—Vaginal containment in the female superior position, no thrusting, no orgasm attempted.

Level Five—Allow minimal thrusting, no orgasm from thrusting.

Level Six—Allow orgasm from thrusting.

Modified from Masters and Johnson,[41] by the Division of Behavioral Gynecology, Baystate Medical Center, Springfield, Massachusetts 1980–1985, with permission.

five and six training to bring about orgasm during vaginal containment.

If the difficulty is in male premature ejaculation, the couple is instructed to practice the squeeze technique between levels three and four.[41] In this technique his partner masturbates the man until just before the point of ejaculatory inevitability. A squeeze is then applied to the penis just below the coronal ridge, causing the man to lose some of his erection and blocking ejaculation. The squeeze is subsequently relaxed and the technique repeated. The start-stop technique permits the man to build up control and confidence before attempting the same technique during vaginal containment in the female superior position. The female lifts herself off the penis to allow her access for applying the squeeze technique. If this seems too "athletic," especially later in pregnancy, the original start-stop technique is employed.[42]

A woman with psychogenic coital pain is taught Kegel's exercises to increase her awareness of vaginal sensation. Next she begins self-dilation, using her fingers or vaginal dilators. The woman combines the dilators with Kegel's exercises, squeezing and relaxing around the dilators to enhance control of the pubococcygeus muscle as well as desensitizing the vagina and introitus to distention. When she has completed mastery of the fourth and largest dilator, she uses her partner's erect penis as dilator number five in the female superior position during level four's sensate focus exercises.

Do couples with sexual problems during pregnancy benefit from sensate focus training? The answer is a resounding *yes!* Since the need to be held or cuddled seems to increase during pregnancy[27,28] and the first three levels of sensate focus exercises seem to stress this area, it would seem that sensate focus exercises are tailor made for the couple with sexual concerns or problems that predate or emerge during pregnancy. Of course, the use of vaginal dilators would need the endorsement of the obstetrician (especially in the high-risk pregnancy) along with instructions to limit the depth of penetration.

If therapy is not completed by the time of delivery, the couple should not attempt puerperal vaginal intercourse until they have reviewed level one, proceeding at their own pace to where they left off and continuing progressively on to level six. This is especially valuable for individuals or couples fearful of the potential pain of the first intercourse.

Sensate focus is a skill all couples should have available to them for their lifetimes. It is inevitable that all couples will have a "glitch" in their sex lives at some point (eg, cessation of intercourse just before and after hysterectomy, a temporary bout of impotence, or adjustment to aging). The skills once learned will always be of value and should be applied with the couple's acting as their own therapists with little or no outside help.

Coitus: Possible Dangers

Concerns about the likelihood of pregnancy complications with coitus have largely surrounded the possible deleterious effects of uterine cramping with orgasm[43–45] and introduction of infection[1,46] or injury due to vaginal insufflation.[47,48] Although some of these risks are controversial and even to some extent theoretical, there are some clear dangers. For example, there are at least 10 reported cases of fatal air embolism in pregnant women resulting from the intravaginal instillation of air during sexual encounters.[47–49,51]

Presumably because of the increased vascularity of pregnancy and general tissue friability, during pneumovagina intravaginal air enters subplacental venous channels. This results in these gases passing into the general circulation. Air can then enter the arterial circulation either by passing across arterovenous pulmonary connections or by traversing a patent intracardiac septum. Potentially fatal cerebral air embolism follows.

Emergency treatment for suspected air embolism[48,49] includes (1) positioning of the patient with head and left side down, (2) administration of 100% oxygen, (3) treatment with high-dose steroid, (4) platelet aggregation inhibition with aspirin or a similar agent. Definitive therapy requires the use of a hyperbaric chamber.[50] Fortunately, this complication is rare, as this variant of cunnilingus is uncommon. However, couples should be warned against blowing air into the vagina, douching, and even vigorous rear entry intercourse during pregnancy.[51]

There have been attempts to link coitus in late pregnancy to untoward outcomes. Naeye[46,52,53] has questioned the relationship between vaginal intercourse and infection, perhaps leading to premature rupture of membranes, premature delivery, and even fetal aspiration of infected fluid. Goodlin and coworkers[44,45] observed fetal bradycardias after maternal orgasm from masturbation in late pregnancy and thought that women who delivered prematurely had a higher incidence of orgasm after 32 weeks of gestation.

These concerns should be weighed against the enormous evidence from the literature that repeatedly confirms the lack of premature deliveries and/or deleterious fetal outcomes in normal pregnancy (Table 7.10). Most impressive in all these studies were the 39,217 pregnancies studied in the Collaborative Perinatal Project, which found no association between coitus and adverse outcomes of pregnancy.[54]

Naeye's work can be best understood when we realize that his research has focused on the malnourished mothers in the third world whose amniotic fluid commonly lacks antimicrobial activity. Although this phenomenon approaches 90% in some countries, Naeye suggests that it occurs only 5% of the time in the United States.[71] What does emerge from his work is the observation that coitus should be stopped once genital tract infection is clinically suspected.

Goodlin[55] has softened his stance since his original work and now concludes that in the absence of infection, premature labor is rare, "especially

Table 7.10 Studies Confirming Good Outcomes in Normal Pregnancies When Sexual Activity Is Continued to Term

Pugh and Fernandez (1953)[77]
Solberg et al (1973)[10]
Perkins (1979)[65]
Rayburn and Wilson (1980)[64]
Mills et al (1981)[73]
Zlatnik and Burmeister (1982)[66]
Klebanoff et al (1984)[54]
Georgakoupoulos et al (1984)[76]

when related to orgasm."[56] Again, what emerges is a concern for the compromised pregnancy in which postcoital uterine activity takes longer to subside than in low-risk patients[57] or structural abnormalities predispose to membrane rupture.

In 1978 and 1979 at the University of Rochester, Labrum and LaFerla studied three couples at approximately 36 weeks of uncomplicated singleton gestation (personal communication). The women were healthy whites who agreed to stimulate themselves to orgasm with only their partners present in a private labor room. Electronic fetal monitors that these women wore recorded both the baseline fetal heart rate and the uterine activity both during and after orgasm (Figure 7.1).

No fetal heart rate decelerations were observed in any of these tracings. Further, in none of these patients did labor ensue, and all went on to term delivery of healthy infants. This experience and the uncontrolled experiments of a multitude of pregnant women over many years attest to the generally innocuous nature of sexual activity for the vast majority of gravid individuals. Thus, transient bradycardias can occur after coitus in pregnancies that progress to normal delivery of healthy infants.[58] At worst, coitus with orgasm can be looked upon as an unmonitored contraction stress test.

However, there are clinical circumstances in which coital activity may not

Figure 7.1 Fetal heart rate tracings (**A**) before orgasm and (**B**) during orgasm.

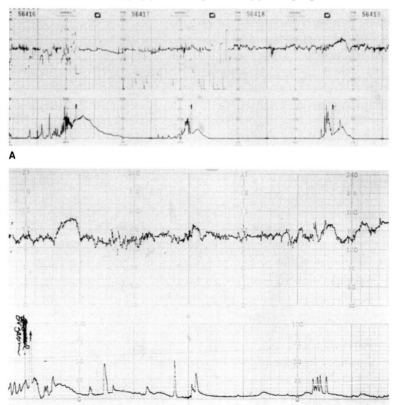

Table 7.11 Recommendations: Curtailment of Sexual Activity during Pregnancy

Recommend Suspension	Individualize Recommendations
Placenta previa	Stable cerclage
Premature membrane rupture	Prior history of abruptio placentae, premature rupture of membranes, preterm labor
Preterm labor arrested with tocolytics	Multiple gestation
Cervical incompetence with dilation/effacement	Friable cervicitis or other genital tract infections
	Uterine abnormalities (myoma, Müllerian fusion defects)

prove harmless.[24,53,56,57,59–69] In instances of premature membrane rupture, previously treated premature labor, and placenta previa or abruptio placentae, the majority of investigators would concur in interdicting sexual intercourse.

It is less clear what to recommend when a cerclage is in place, or when there is a prior history of premature membrane rupture, preterm labor, abruptio placentae, or miscarriage. In these instances there may be no immediate evidence of jeopardy, only a suspicion of higher than normal risk.

For some clinical situations, reasonable data exist. For example, otherwise normal twin pregnancies should not entail restrictions on coital activity. A prospective study of 126 women in Zimbabwe with twin gestations showed that coitus did not necessarily precipitate preterm labor.[69]

In high-risk patients, these risks for labor and membrane rupture are believed to result largely from episodes of increased uterine activity after coitus.[57] In theory at least, these contractions might risk membrane integrity or promote more extensive uterine irritability. Whether this increased activity is due to the maternal orgasm as discussed later, oxytocin release from associated breast stimulations, or absorption of seminal prostaglandins is moot. It is also potentially possible that coital pelvic manipulation could directly introduce either vaginal flora bacteria or venereal pathogens, leading to genital infections.[1,52,53,70] Naeye[53,71] suggests that the combination of coitus with occult chorioamnionitis is an important risk factor for preterm labor. In this view, uterine contractions from intercourse result in the rupture of membranes locally weakened by preexisting infection.

It may be that the risk factor in a number of these conditions is not the vaginal manipulations of coitus, but the uterine contractions accompanying orgasm.[64,72–75] In theory at least, recurrent cramping might create a risk to membrane integrity or predispose to placental separation. If so, then any activity leading to orgasm is what should be proscribed. However, the clinician should realize that spontaneous orgasms occur during the sleep of both men and women and substantial uterine activity accompanies breast stimulation. Thus, the attempt to limit or control "self-generated" uterine contractions is likely to prove futile.

Despite these uncertainties, some recommendations must still be made. Table 7.11 includes our general suggestions in reference to coital activity during pregnancy. If intercourse or orgasm is restricted for a medical indication, discussion should take place with the couple and options for the male (including intracrural intercourse) should be explored.

In sum, in otherwise normal pregnancy there is no indication beyond maternal comfort for restricting intercourse.[1,17,54,59,65,66,73,76] There is no clearly established association between coitus and preterm labor or premature membrane rupture in otherwise normal individuals. Although some uncertainty persists, the traditional and arbitrary admonitions against intercourse during pregnancy, except for those pregnancies at high risk, cannot be scientifically supported.

It takes little skill or knowledge to interdict sex during a normal pregnancy. It creates a false sense of protection for the practitioner at the cost of endowing the couple with an unnecessary burden of guilt should there be an obstetric complication and/or loss.

Conclusions

Both the physiology and the psychology of sexual activity change substantially during pregnancy. Sex is an important part of human function, and a mutually satisfying physical relationship is helpful if not critical to marital stability.[1] Recommendations for the curtailment of masturbation, sexual intercourse, or cunnilingus or proscribing of orgasm should be made on the basis of individual clinical findings, as modified by the requirements of individual clinical circumstances. Such recommendations should be uncommon. With appropriate education and counseling, clinicians can assist couples in understanding and safely expressing their sexuality during pregnancy.

The suggestions and critiques of my colleagues in the American Society for Psychosomatic Obstetrics and Gynecology, including Drs. John J. LaFerla, Richard P. Perkins, and Kenneth J. Reamy, in the preparation of this chapter are gratefully acknowledged.

References

1. White SE, Reamy K: Sexuality and pregnancy: A review. *Arch Sex Behav* 1982;11:429–444.
2. Masters WH, Johnson VE: *Human Sexual Response*. Boston, Little, Brown, 1966.
3. Reamy K, White SE, Daniell WC, et al: Sexuality and pregnancy a prospective study. *J Reprod Med* 1982;27:321–327.
4. Brewaeys A, Olbrechts H, Devroey P, et al: Counselling and selection of homosexual couples in fertility treatment. *Hum Reprod* 1989;4:850–853.
5. Zeidenstein L: Gynecological and childbearing needs of lesbians. *J Nurs Midwife* 1990;35:10–18.
6. Forrest JD, Singh S: The sexual and reproductive behavior of American women, 1982–1988. *Fam Plann Perspect* 1990;22:206–214.
7. Nilsson A, Almgren P: Para-natal emotional adjustment: A prospective investigation of 165 women: II. The influence of background factors, psychiatric history, parental relations, and personality characteristics. *Acta Psychiatr Scand* 1970;20(suppl):65–141.
8. Falicov CJ: Sexual adjustment during first pregnancy and postpartum. *Am J Obstet Gynecol* 1973;117:991–1000.

9. Elliott SA, Watson JP: Sex during pregnancy and the first postnatal year. *J Psychosom Res* 1985;29:541–548.

10. Solberg DA, Butler J, Wagner NN: Sexual behavior in pregnancy. *N Engl J Med* 1973;288:1098–1103.

11. Steege JF, Jelovsek FR: Sexual behavior during pregnancy. *Obstet Gynecol* 1973;60:163–168.

12. Ryding EL: Sexuality during and after pregnancy. *Acta Obstet Gynecol Scand* 1984;63:679–682.

13. Kenny JA: Sexuality of pregnant and breast feeding women. *Arch Sexual Behavior* 1973;2:215–229.

14. Robson KM, Brant HA, Kumar R: Maternal sexuality during first pregnancy and after childbirth. *Br J Obstet Gynaecol* 1981;88:882–889.

15. Tolor A, DiGrazia PV: Sexual attitudes and behavior patterns during and following pregnancy. *Arch Sex Behav* 1976;5:539–551.

16. Cunningham FG, MacDonald PC, Grant NF (eds.): *Williams' Obstetrics* (ed. 18). Norwalk, CT, Appleton & Lange, 1989, pp 268–269.

17. Johnson TRB, Walker MA, Niebyl JR: Prenatal care, in Gabbe SG, Niebyl JR, Simpson JL (eds.): *Obstetrics: Normal and Problem Pregnancies*. New York, Churchill Livingstone, 1986, pp 159–183.

18. Seibel MM, Taymor ML: Emotional aspects of infertility. *Fertil Steril* 1982;37:137–145.

19. Rantala ML, Koskimies AI: Sexual behavior of infertile couples. *Int J Fertil* 1988;33:26–30.

20. Debrovner CH, Shubin-Stein R: Sexual problems in the infertile couple. *Med Aspects Hum Sex* 1975;9:140–150.

21. Elstein M: Effects of infertility on psychosexual function. *Br Med J* 1975;3:296–299.

22. Fagan PJ, Schmidt CW, Rock JA, et al: Sexual functioning and psychologic evaluation of in vitro fertilization couples. *Fertil Steril* 1986;46:668–672.

23. Salzer LP: *Infertility: How Couples Can Cope*. Boston, G.K. Hall, 1986, pp 92–106.

24. Ling FW: Sex in pregnancy, in Sciarra JJ (ed.): *Gynecology and Obstetrics*, vol. 2. Philadelphia, JB Lippincott, 1985; 20:1–7.

25. Pion RJ, Delli Quadri L: Sexual function during gestation, in Iffy L, Kaminetsky HA (eds.): *Principles and Practice of Obstetrics and Perinatology*. New York, John Wiley & Sons, 1981, pp 703–706.

26. Reamy KJ, White SE: Dyspareunia in pregnancy. *J Psychosom Obstet Gynecol* 1985;4:263–270.

27. Hollender MH, McGehee JB: The wish to be held during pregnancy. *J Psychosom Res* 1974;18:193–197.

28. White SE, Reamy K, Southward GM: Nurturant needs of pregnancy. *J Psychosom Obstet Gynecol* 1983;2:243–249.

29. Leviticus 12:1–5.

30. Mabray CR: Postpartum examination: A reevaluation. *South Med J* 1979;72:1433–1435.

31. Reamy KJ: A management guide to postpartum problems. *Med Aspects Hum Sex* 1991;25:20–24.

32. Alder EM: Sexual behaviour in pregnancy, after childbirth and during breastfeeding. *Bailliere's Clin Obstet Gynaecol* 1989;3:805–821.

33. Levay AN, Weissberg JH, Woods SM: Intrapsychic factors in sexual dysfunctions, in Lief HI (ed.): *Sexual Problems in Medical Practice*. American Medical Association, 1981, pp 159–168.

34. Reamy KJ, White SE: Sexuality in the puerperium: A review. *Arch Sex Behav* 1987;16:165–186.

35. Frank E, Anderson C, Rubenstein D: Frequency of sexual dysfunction in "normal" couples. *N Engl J Med* 1978;299:111–115.

36. Thacker SB, Banta HD: Benefits and risks of episiotomy: An interpretative review of the English language literature 1860-1980. *Obstet Gynecol Surv* 1983;38:322–338.

37. Perkins RP: Sexuality during pregnancy. *Clinical Obstet Gynecol* 1984;27:706–716.

38. Backman GA, Leiblum SR, Grill J: Brief sexual inquiry in gynecologic practice. *Obstet Gynecol* 1989;73:425–427.

39. LaFerla JJ: Inhibited sexual desire and orgasmic dysfunction in women. *Clin Obstet Gynecol* 1984;27:738–749.

40. Chorowski M: Pelvic pain, in Nichols DH, Evrard JR (eds.): *Ambulatory Gynecology.* Philadelphia, Harper & Row 1985, pp 175–192.

41. Masters WH, Johnson VE: *Human Sexual Inadequacy.* Boston, Little, Brown, 1970.

42. Semans J: Premature ejaculation. *South Med J* 1956;49:352–356.

43. Fox CA: Recent studies in human coital physiology. *Clin Endocrinol Metab* 1973;2:527–543.

44. Goodlin RC, Keller DW, Raffin M: Orgasm during late pregnancy. *Obstet Gynecol* 1971;38:916–920.

45. Goodlin RC, Schmidt W, Creevy DC: Uterine tension and fetal heart rate during maternal orgasm. *Obstet Gynecol* 1972;39:125–127.

46. Naeye RL: Safety of coitus in pregnancy. *Lancet* 1981;9:686. Letter to the editor.

47. Aronson ME, Nelson PK: Fatal air embolism in pregnancy resulting from unusual sexual act. *Obstet Gynecol* 1967;30:127–130.

48. Bray P, Myers RAM, Cowley RA: Orogenital sex as a cause of nonfatal air embolism in pregnancy. *Obstet Gynecol* 1983;61:653–657.

49. Bernhardt TL, Goldmann RW, Thombs PA, et al: Hyperbaric oxygen treatment of cerebral air embolism from orogenital sex during pregnancy. *Crit Care Med* 1988;16:729–731.

50. Van Genderon L, Waite CL: Evaluation of the rapid decompression–high pressure oxygenation approach to the treatment of traumatic cerebral air embolism. *Aerosp Med* 1968;39:709–713.

51. Lipshultz BD, Donoghue ER: Air embolism during intercourse in pregnancy. *J Forensic Sci* 1983;28:1021–1022.

52. Naeye RL: Coitus and antepartum haemorrhage. *Br J Obstet Gynaecol* 1981;88:765–770.

53. Naeye RL: Factors that predispose to premature rupture of the fetal membranes. *Obstet Gynecol* 1982;60:93–98.

54. Klebanoff MA, Nugent RP, Rhoads GG: Coitus during pregnancy: Is it safe? *Lancet* 1984;2:914–917.

55. Goodlin RC: Sexual activity during pregnancy. *N Engl J Med* 1973;280:379. Letter to the editor.

56. Goodlin RC: Can sex in pregnancy harm the fetus? *Contemp Obstet Gynecol* 1976;8:21–24.

57. Brustman LE, Raptoulis M, Langer O, et al: Changes in the pattern of uterine contractility in relationships to coitus during pregnancies at low and high risk for preterm labor *Obstet Gynecol* 1989;73:166–168.

58. Chayen B, Tejani N, Verma UL, et al: Fetal heart rate changes and uterine activity during coitus. *Acta Obstet Gynecol Scand* 1986;65:853–855.

59. Reamy K, White SE: Sexuality in pregnancy and the puerperium: A review. *Obstet Gynecol Surv* 1985;40:1–13.

60. Neilson JP, Mutambira M: Coitus, twin pregnancy, and preterm labor. *Am J Obstet Gynecol* 1989;160:416–418.

61. Kitzinger S: Intercourse during pregnancy. *Br J Sex Med* 1973;1:22–30.

62. Mills JL: Should coitus in late pregnancy be discouraged? *Sex Med Today* 1982;6:32.

63. Grudzinkas JG, Watson C, Chard T: Does sexual intercourse cause fetal distress? *Lancet* 1979;2:692–693. Letter to the editor.

64. Rayburn WF, Wilson EA: Coital activity and premature delivery. *Am J Obstet Gynecol* 1980;137:972–974.

65. Perkins RP: Sexual behaviors and response in relation to complications of pregnancy. *Am J Obstet Gynecol* 1979;134:498–505.

66. Zlatnik FJ, Burmeister LF: Reported sexual behavior in late pregnancy: Selected associations. *J Reprod Med* 1982;27:627–632.

67. Herbst AL: Coitus and the fetus. *N Engl J Med* 1979;301:1235–1236.

68. Grover JS: Coitus during pregnancy for women with a history of spontaneous abortion. *Med Aspects Hum Sex* 1977;5:113–114.

69. Neilson JP, Mutambisa M: Coitus, twin pregnancy, and preterm labor. *Am J Obstet Gynecol* 1989;160:416–418.

70. Rehu M: The effect of education, marital status and sexual behavior on the incidence of puerperal endometritis and bacteriuria. *Ann Clin Res* 1980;12:315–319.

71. Naeye RL: Functionally important disorders of the placenta, umbilical cord, and fetal membranes. *Hum Pathol* 1987;18:680–691.

72. Naeye RL, Ross S: Coitus and chorioamnionitis: A prospective study. *Early Hum Dev* 1982;6:91–97.

73. Mills JL, Harlap S, Harley EE: Should coitus late in pregnancy be discouraged? *Lancet* 1981;2:136–138.

74. Fox CA, Wolff HS, Baker JA: Measurement of intra-vaginal and intra-uterine pressures during human coitus by radio-telemetry. *J Reprod Fertil* 1970;22:243–251.

75. Fox CA, Knaggs GS: Milk ejection activity (oxytocin) in peripheral venous blood in man during lactation and in association with coitus. *J Endocrinol* 1969;45:145–150.

76. Georgakoupoulus PA, Dodo SD, Mechleris D: Sexuality in pregnancy and premature labour. *Br J Obstet Gynaecol* 1984;91:891–893.

77. Pugh WE, Fernandez FL: Coitus in late pregnancy. *Obstet Gynecol* 1953;2:636–642.

78. Sloan D: Primary care for sexual dysfunction. *Network Contin Med Educ* 1980:343.

79. Shover LR, Friedman J, Weiler S, et al: The multi-axial problem-oriented diagnostic system for the sexual dysfunctions: An alternative to DSM-III. *Arch Gen Psychiat* 1982;39:614–619.

Appendix 7.1

Information Sheet on Sex During Pregnancy and After

As we have discussed during your visits, just as your body changes during pregnancy so will your emotions and sexual feelings, for both you and your partner. We would like to hear about these changes at each visit and perhaps guide you if there are concerns or questions. It is also helpful for you and your partner to talk about these changes in an effort to come closer together.

The fetus is not harmed by sex, so unless yours is a high-risk pregnancy, we endorse your having intercourse with your partner all through pregnancy. We emphasize staying with one partner—this is not an opportune time to expose yourself to infectious agents from outside. Should we express concern about your health or the health of the baby later on in pregnancy, please ask us whether sex is to be stopped because of that concern.

As the pregnancy progresses, you may find that comfort will dictate trying new positions such as a side by side ("spoon") position (Figure 7.2). We have enclosed some diagrams of positions to consider. *Hint: be generous with pillows!* There are times you may want to consider masturbation, manual manipulation, or oral sex. All of these are fine. The only activities to avoid are douching, blowing air into the vagina, or vigorous rear-entry sex. Any activity that pushes air into the vagina is considered dangerous to maternal health.

It is important to realize that even if you are not having sex, the need to be cuddled or held doesn't go away during pregnancy. In the final weeks and right after delivery, you might have fewer options for sex but the need to be loved and loving might be strongest at that time.

After the baby comes it might take a while for desire to return, perhaps from fatigue or from the efforts you both are putting into this new role. Continue the discussions of feelings with your partner—this is a difficult time for most couples. It takes about 3 weeks for a midline episiotomy to heal, longer for other incisions, including those used for cesarean delivery. During those weeks you should be practicing the Kegel exercises as you will be instructed before leaving the hospital. When you are ready to try, the female superior position will allow you to control the depth of thrusting if concern about pain is an issue. Expect to need a lubricant (saliva and K-Y jelly are examples; avoid petroleum jelly) the first few times, longer if you are breast-feeding. Make sure a method of contraception is used. Most of all, *take your time*, especially with foreplay.

Again, changes in desire, arousal, and/or ability to experience orgasm are to be expected during pregnancy and post partum. The staff is available to you should you or your partner have questions or concerns.

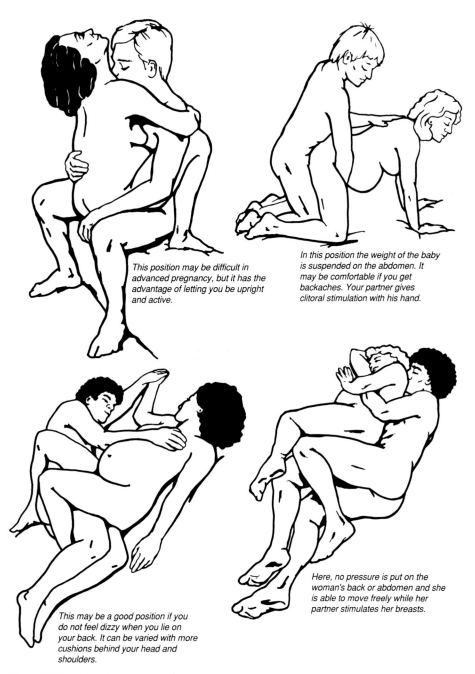

This position may be difficult in advanced pregnancy, but it has the advantage of letting you be upright and active.

In this position the weight of the baby is suspended on the abdomen. It may be comfortable if you get backaches. Your partner gives clitoral stimulation with his hand.

This may be a good position if you do not feel dizzy when you lie on your back. It can be varied with more cushions behind your head and shoulders.

Here, no pressure is put on the woman's back or abdomen and she is able to move freely while her partner stimulates her breasts.

Figure 7.2 Positions for intercourse during pregnancy.

PART III

Psychological Disorders in Pregnancy

Chapter 8

Affective and Anxiety Disorders

Miriam Rosenthal, MD and John P. O'Grady, MD

> In sooth, I know not why I am so sad.
> It wearies me; you say it wearies you;
> But how I caught it, found it, or came by it,
> What stuff 'tis made of, whereof it is born
> I am to learn.
> —*Merchant of Venice*
> William Shakespeare (1564–1616)

Psychological disturbances of varying severity are common postpartum events. In the first few days after delivery mothers commonly report mood swings, anxiety, tiredness, ready crying, negative feelings, anger at times at the baby's father or at the baby, or fear and guilt about having any negative or hostile thoughts. This period of adjustment is commonly termed the baby "blues."[1-7] So frequently does this condition occur as to require its identification as normal behavior. Other potentially serious psychological conditions also occur, primarily in the first month post partum but with a lower incidence than the blues. These conditions include, among others, severe clinical depressions, psychoses, and pathologic grief reactions (see Table 8.1).

The literature on these conditions is complex and often contradictory, reflecting the controversies and uncertainties concerning both the cause and the clinical presentation of these disorders.[8-12] Much in the literature is anecdotal and many reports deal with only small numbers and often control groups are inappropriate or absent.[13-16] Further, because of the lack of agreement concerning the criterion for diagnosis, there is great variety in the patients chosen for inclusion in an individual study, making cross-comparison of results difficult.

There is still disagreement whether true postpartum depressions and the occasional postpartum psychotic reaction are the same or different from those occurring in nonpregnant women. The consensus of opinion is that these disorders of the puerperium are the same as those seen at other times during life.[16] Yet, postpartum depression does have several characteristic features and, in comparison to nonpuerperal depressed patients, individuals with peripartum disturbances tend to display more liability, agitation, and disorientation.[4,17] Despite controversy, most clinicians recognize that an increased frequency of psychological disorders occur—or at least clinically present—postpartum and that most of these problems are affective disorders, especially depressions.[7,10,18-20]

Of the postpartum affective disorders, the following are generally recognized[4,7,14,16,24]: (1) the maternity blues, (2) postpartum depression, and (3) psychotic depression/mania with delusions (Table 8.1 and 8.2). Although these mood disturbances are described as clinically distinct entities, there may be many gradations between them. The blues are common and usually transitory but can be a precursor to a true depression. True depressions are usually differentiated from the maternity blues by their persistence and severity and from the psychoses by the absence of delusions and hallucinations.

The existence of peripartum mood disturbances has been recognized since antiquity. Hippocrates considered the puerperal mood disturbances to be due to the effects of suppressed or sequestered lochia or, alternatively, blood collection at the breast, suppressing normal lactation.[4] Scientific study of peripartum mental abnormalities began in the mid-19th century when two French workers, J.E.D. Esquirol[25] and Louis V. Marcé[26] reported their clinical experience. They observed a group of mood and behavioral symptoms in women both in and out of institutions. These symptoms were sufficiently distinct to be characteristic of what they identified as a specific puerperal mental disorder in women both in and out of institutions who displayed symptoms characteristic of what they identified as a puerperal mental disorder. In his 1858 text, Marcé linked the disorder to an organic cause, at the time unknown to him. Such disorders arose, he recorded, because of the "modification organique et fonctionelle de l'uterus et de ses anexes," or, in modern terms, to the specific hormonal milieu of pregnancy. This is still the predominant view. Extensive study into peripartum mental dysfunction has occurred only during the last 20 years as a result of newer methods of clinical and laboratory inves-

Table 8.1 Clinical Classification and Incidence of Puerperal Mental Disorders

	Incidence*
Disorders of maternal-infant attachment	
Delayed attachment	1:10
Obsessions of hostility or newborn rejection	1:100
Child abuse	1:1000
Infanticide	1:50,000
The blues	≥ 1:2
Depressive disorders	
Puerperal depression	1:10
Dysthymic reaction	?
Grief, pathologic grief	1:100
Psychoses	
Psychotic depression	1–2:1000
Mania/schizophrenia	<1:1000

*Clinical approximations for women with third-trimester pregnancies. Modified from Brockington and Cox-Roper.[10] See Chapters 10 and 16.

tigation as well as a general reawakening of interest in the connection between neuroendocrinology and mental disorders.

In this chapter, the peripartum affective disorders are reviewed with special attention to their clinical recognition and treatment. These conditions are common and all too easily overlooked in busy practices. Early identification and prompt intervention are essential to reduce distress for the affected mother, her family, and her newborn.[24,27,28]

Clinical Presentation

Postpartum Blues

Postpartum "blues" is also termed the 3-day or 5-day blues, the maternity blues, postnatal blues, third-day depression, transitory syndrome, or baby blues.[1,3,13] This condition is a normal, transient set of characteristic mood disturbances that occur in 50% to 80% of women after vaginal or cesarean delivery.[1,2,3,5-7,13,14,29] The blues are characterized by maternal weeping, irritability, anxiety, general emotional lability, complaints of an inability to think clearly, fatigue, sleep disturbances, and ambivalence.[1,2,5,30,31] There is no cognitive impairment in these women, but they do report easy distractability, absentmindedness, and difficulties in concentration.[1,13,23,32] The individual symptoms do not have the same time course and usually do not persist without improvement beyond 7 days postpartum. As both the onset of the symptoms and their spontaneous improvement are usually abrupt and occur at a time of profound physiologic change, there are a number of endocrinologic theories concerning cause.

The development of the blues is generally unrelated to the postpartum health of mother or baby, obstetric complications, hospitalization, social class, or breast- or bottle feeding, although those factors do affect mood.[13]

The blues occurs worldwide, although the manifestations are culturally patterned and may be less noticeable to outside observers. This is especially true where emotional expression is different and where family and friends surround new mothers offering care and support.[30,33-35] The validity of the blues as an entity separate from true depression has been confirmed by both multiple clinical observations over the years and prospective studies of mood using control nonpregnant populations.[17,36]

The vast majority of these mood disturbances are transient. However, most observers agree that in a small proportion of women with the most severe postpartum reactions a major depression develops, indistinguishable from depressions occurring at other times of life.[3,29] Unfortunately, the clinical distinction between the severity of individual cases is that of degree only, without sharp separation. Thus, the blues is difficult to define discretely or separate from forms of true depression in terms of severity, timing, or symptoms.[3-5,13] In the attempt to improve and clarify the diagnosis and distinguish the transitory blues from persisting depression, a number of rating scales and/or questionnaires are available to assist the clinician and researcher[1,22,24,29,37] (see Table 8.2).

Major Depression

It is estimated that in 10% to 15% of parturients a clinical depression develops

Table 8.2 The Edinburgh Postnatal Depression Scale Questionnaire*

Name:	Date:
Address:	Age:
	Date of Delivery:

As you have recently had a baby, we would like to know how you are feeling now. Please UNDERLINE the answer which comes closest to how you have felt IN THE PAST WEEK.

Here is an example, already completed.

> I have felt happy:
>
> Yes, all the time
>
> <u>Yes, most of the time</u>
>
> No, not very often
>
> No, not at all

This would mean: "I have felt happy most of the time" during the past week.

Please complete the other questions in the same way.

IN THE PAST 7 DAYS

1. I have been able to laugh and see the funny side of things

> As much as I always could
>
> Not quite so much now
>
> Definitely not so much now
>
> Not at all

2. People upset me so that I felt like slamming doors and banging about

> Yes, often
>
> Yes, sometimes
>
> Only occasionally
>
> Not at all

3. I have looked forward with enjoyment to things

> As much as I ever did
>
> Rather less than I used to
>
> Definitely less than I used to
>
> Hardly at all

4. I have blamed myself unnecessarily when things went wrong

> Yes, most of the time
>
> Yes, some of the time
>
> Not very often
>
> No never

5. I have been anxious or worried for no good reason

> No, not at all
>
> Hardly ever
>
> Yes, sometimes
>
> Yes, very often

6. I have enjoyed being a mother

> Yes, very much so

Table 8.2 (continued)

Yes, on the whole

Rather less than usual

No, not very much

7. I have felt scared or panicky for no very good reason

Yes, quite a lot

Yes, sometimes

No, not much

No, not at all

8. Things have been getting on top of me

Yes, most of the time I haven't been able to cope at all

Yes, sometimes I haven't been coping as well as usual

No, most of the time I have coped quite well

No, I have been coping as well as ever

9. I have been so unhappy that I have had difficulty sleeping

Yes, most of the time

Yes, sometimes

Not very often

No, not at all

10. I have felt sad or miserable

Yes, most of the time

Yes, quite often

Not very often

No, not at all

11. I have felt I might lose control and hit someone

Yes, frequently

Yes, sometimes

Only occasionally

Never

12. I have been so unhappy that I have been crying

Yes, most of the time

Yes, quite often

Only occasionally

No, never

13. The thought of harming myself has occurred to me

Yes, quite often

Sometimes

Hardly ever

Never

---

*Items omitted in the 10-item scale. Reprinted from Cox,[24] with permission.

postpartum that is severe enough to interfere with their usual functioning.[14,22,24,38–43] As with the maternity blues, these depressive reactions are not restricted to Western societies alone.[35] Recognition of such disorders by the obstetrician and suitable management and/or referral to a mental health professional are essential. Unfortunately, many dysfunctional women are never correctly identified or referred for treatment. Depression also has long-term family importance and has been related to subsequent behavioral disturbances in the child.[28,44]

The term *depression* is used imprecisely. It may refer to a transitory mood, a syndrome, or a clinical disorder characterized by a change in mood accompanied by vegetative symptoms, lasting 2 weeks or more. There is also confusion concerning the acceptable time limit after delivery for a depression to be considered childbirth-related. O'Hara and Zekoski[22] suggest an outside limit of 6 months. This issue is far from academic since the psychological and physiologic correlates thought to be causative factors of depression are clearly different the more distant onset is from parturition.

Since many writers accept or exclude cases on the basis of temporal conventions, comparison of studies is difficult. Although there are many descriptions of maternity blues and severe puerperal psychoses, there is less discussion in the literature of the moderate depressive disorders.[14,42,45] This is partly because of difficulties in describing the normal postpartum adjustment and the lability often noted in this period. In addition, there are disagreements over essentially every aspect of peripartum depression from its existence as a separate entity to its cause, associations, and appropriate treatment.[23] Such controversies are prominent now that an intense effort is being made to make psychiatric diagnoses more precise and to understand more of the biologic causes of such disorders. There is also considerable research on the epidemiology of psychiatric disorders that can be conducted more precisely when the entities are better defined.

Incidence and Prevalence

As O'Hara and others[10,22,42,46] caution, both incidence and prevalence rates for peripartum depression need critical review. The data establishing that there is a greater increase in depressive episodes after childbirth than at other times in life is not solid.[47] A number of the normal psychological signs and symptoms of the puerperium can be misidentified as those of depression, artificially inflating the incidence of this disorder. Unfortunately, prevalence rates for preconceptual mental dysfunction are unknown for most of the populations reported in the literature, indicating that caution is needed in the interpretation of the high rates of puerperal mood dysfunction reported by many writers.

As with the blues, there is no firm relationship established between but much speculation about the development of depression and obstetric complications, parity, maternal age, or social status.[22,23,48] However, a prior history of puerperal depression is clearly important as the recurrence risk can approach 50%.[4,23] There is also a significant risk that clinical depression will develop anew in such individuals independent of pregnancy if their cases are followed long term.[49]

A chronic affective disorder is an important risk factor for the development of peripartum disease.[50] Those individuals with bipolar (combining mania and depression) as opposed to unipolar (depression only) chronic disease are at increased risk for the development of a peripartum psychosis. Individuals with unipolar disease have a 5% to 7% risk of postpartum depression, with no greater risk for subsequent pregnancies. In contrast, individuals with bipolar disease have a 40% to 50% risk of postpartum mood dysfunction. There is also a hereditary risk as fully 20% of first- degree family members of those with bipolar disease develop postpartum affective disorders in comparison to 5% to 7% for unipolar disease patients.

Puerperal Psychosis

Puerperal psychosis is an uncommon but serious condition, occurring in approximately 1 in every 1000 births.[23,44] Early recognition and skillful management are important as the effects of psychotic behavior can be devastating on the newborn, the mother, and the family alike. Postpartum or puerperal psychoses are defined as psychotic reactions occurring shortly after delivery, meeting the standard definitions for mania, schizoaffective mania, or undiagnosed functional psychosis.[16,51] The majority of these disorders are affective, and schizophrenic reactions are uncommon: only 2% to 16% in most series.[23,52] These disorders begin within 2 weeks of delivery and occur irrespective of social circumstances.[10] The major feature is the temporal relation to pregnancy and delivery, and there are variations in the time frame, with periods varying from 2 weeks to 12 months after birth (see Table 8.3).

Confusion, visual hallucinations, and delirium are the classic symptoms.[9,10] Prodromal symptoms include weeping, sleep disturbances, and general irritability.[53] The manic phase is notable for restlessness, excitement, and grandiosity. Rapid alterations from depression to apparent elation can occur. Classically, the disorder does not commence in the first 3 days after delivery and although there is substantial clinical variation, the onset is usually acute. Untreated cases can persist for 6 months, but treatment shortens the course and the prognosis for full recovery is good. The more rapid the onset after delivery and the more florid the presentation, the *better* the overall prognosis.

These conditions occur in other cultures with slightly different patterns but with similar timing.[35] Women with a prior history of a bipolar affective psychosis, either puerperal or not, appear to have the highest recurrence risk.[52] If there is a prior nonpuerperal psychotic episode, the risk of disease with parturition is 20% to 50%.[7,9,23]

In the past, appreciable mortality was associated with puerperal psychoses, due either to general inanition, secondary infection, or "maniacal exhaustion," but this is no longer true. In modern times, death related to psychosis is virtually always self- inflicted. Although successful suicide in these patients is uncommon, attempts or gestures are not. Infanticide does occur in association with puerperal psychotic breaks but is rare (see Chapter 12).

A major controversy exists among researchers in this field about whether or not these conditions are the same as or different from psychoses developing at other times of life and whether pregnancy or delivery triggers a preexisting propensity for mental dysfunction.[10,16,20,53] At present, it is generally accepted, and reflected in the DSM-IIIR coding, that a separate entity of puerperal psychosis *does not exist*.[9] However, the role of parturition in triggering a break is accepted by most reviewers.[53–57]

Those who argue for a specific effect of pregnancy point to these data to suggest that pregnancy/parturition has a "particular and deleterious" effect on mental health.[58] Brockington and co-workers[59] have also described a menstruation-related pattern of relapse in a small series of individuals with puerperal psychosis implying a hormonal effect.

It is probable that puerperal psychoses are more common in primiparas, but study of the associations with race, social class, or obstetric disease has produced findings that are at best uncertain.[9,23,53,57,60] In sum, despite the complexities of the data, there is good evidence that there is an increased risk for psychotic breaks postpartum. It is estimated that the risk for the development of a psychotic break in the puerperium is some 15- fold greater than in the nonpregnant state.[23]

Differential Diagnosis

Management of an individual with a peripartum mood disturbance begins with a careful history and physical examination, with special attention to recent drug therapy and/or recreational drug use (see Chapters 11 and 12). Identification of a prior psychiatric history or a family history of mental dysfunction is essential. Beyond the physical examination and determination of basic vital signs, a laboratory screen (hemoglobin [Hgb], hematocrit [Hct], electrolytes, blood urea nitrogen [BUN], Cr., Ca/PO$_4$), including a thyroid panel (T$_4$, index, thyroid-stimulating hormone [TSH] level), is indicated to exclude easily identified causes of mental dysfunction or depression. If the history or presentation is suggestive, urinary or serum drug screens should also be ordered.

In selected cases involving dementia and/or psychotic behavior more extensive studies such as computerized axial tomography, nuclear magnetic resources studies of the central nervous system, or lumbar puncture may be indicated.

Establishing the diagnosis of depression during pregnancy or the puerperium

Table 8.3 Clinical Features: Major Affective Disorders*

	Blues	Major Depression	Psychosis
Occurrence	50%–70%	10%–15%	1%
Peak onset	3–5 Days Postpartum	2–3 Weeks Postpartum	1–2 Weeks Postpartum (90% within 4 weeks)
Duration	2 Days–2 Weeks	4–6 Weeks Treated 1 Year Untreated	6–12 Weeks Treated
Psychiatric Referral	No	Helpful	Yes
Therapy	Support	Support Medications Psychotherapy	Medications Hospitalization

*Estimates based on third-trimester, hospital-derived delivery statistics.
Modified from Cox.[24]

can be difficult. In many services, the clinician seeing a patient may not know what the individual is like under normal circumstances. Often, in the rush to treat and discharge parturients, there is little time for assessment of mood or mental functioning, especially as postpartum discharges often occur within 24 hours of delivery. Mildly depressed women often have numerous nonspecific somatic complaints or mood disturbances essentially undistinguishable from the blues. When the somatic symptoms are carefully evaluated, no abnormality is found, and the woman is commonly discharged as normal.

Medical Differential Diagnosis

In the evaluation of an individual case of acute depression and particularly psychosis, the possibility of a medical disorder or an atypical drug reaction must be considered in the initial differential diagnosis.[44,53,61] Drug or alcohol withdrawal reactions, moderate hypoxia, or early septicemia may be present with restlessness, agitation, or tachycardia. Spontaneous intracranial hemorrhage or cerebral edema resulting from hypertension can result in coma or stupor. Water intoxication or acute infection occasionally produces a clinical syndrome of apparent dementia. Cerebral vasculitis or steroid psychosis can be seen in individuals with lupus erythematosus or other collagen vascular diseases. Uncommonly, Sheehan's syndrome occurs with acute mental symptoms.[62] Atypical or dysphoric reactions to ergot derivatives, narcotics, or occasionally antibiotics and other commonly administered agents are possible. Rarely, Wernicke's encephalopathy, thyrotoxicosis, hyperparathyroidism, or other endocrine disorders manifests with acute signs and symptoms, confusing the unwary. Nothing substitutes for a good history, record review, and complete physical/neurologic examination at the time when the acute symptoms occur (see Chapter 20).

Clinical Evaluation

Depression

In general, the clinical diagnosis of depression in pregnancy or postpartum is the same as in nonpregnant individuals. However, many women are ashamed of revealing their depression, especially when the baby is healthy. They may consider their dysphoric feelings as a sign of weakness. They may only be able to report physical symptoms to physicians because such symptoms are acceptable. There should be a change in mood plus related somatic symptoms that persist for 2 weeks or more. Commonly, there are loss of interest or pleasure in life, and at least five of the following: weight loss or gain, appetite changes, sleep disturbances, psychomotor agitation or retardation, fatigue, energy loss, feeling of worthlessness or inappropriate guilt, diminished concentration, and suicidal ideation.[51]

In interviewing those possibly affected with a peripartum mood disorder the clinician needs to review a number of specific symptoms, recalling the difficulty in separating true depressive reactions from the routine postpartum symptoms and discomforts.[6,42] Women may not use the term *depressed*, but report irritability, anxiety, sadness, uncontrolled weepiness, or other evidence of emotional lability. They may appear tearful, sad, or withdrawn. *Sleep disturbances* are common, but these are often difficult to assess in a new mother with a frequently crying baby combined with her anxiety about listening for the child. Some clues may be difficulty in falling asleep, early morning awakening, and obsessive ruminations and worries when awake. *Appetite disturbances* are common. New mothers may find it difficult to have time to eat in the usual patterns. They may complain of lack of appetite or increased appetite with weight changes. *Mental concentration and memory* may be disturbed, and a mental status examination may be appropriate if a true cognitive defect is suspected. Complaints of *loss of libido* are common symptoms but difficult to interpret. Sexual interest is usually decreased in new mothers and in lactating women, but this is variable and often may relate to depression, physical problems, fatigue, role changes, and relationship with one's partner. *Obsessive ideas* about coping, self-blame, and guilt are quite common. Less common but extremely distressing to many women are ideas about harming the baby or oneself. If such symptoms are elicited it is important to be certain that there is no loss of reality testing.

Anxiety symptoms may be markedly increased in depressed individuals. Anxiety states are often accompanied by physical symptoms such as headaches, palpitations, and complaints of feeling shaky or extremely frightened. *Panic attacks* can indicate depression or anxiety and require prompt assessment and treatment. A *past history* of depression and/or a family history is important in establishing the correct diagnosis. Screening questionnaires such as the Edinburgh Postnatal Depression Scale can help in objectively evaluating patients and detecting postnatal depression[24] (Table 8.2).

If clinical depression is present or a more severe thought disorder is noted, it is essential to inquire about *suicidal ideation*. Specifically, the woman should be questioned about thoughts about harming her baby. These questions give considerable relief to the woman who fears these ideas but is ashamed to reveal them. The question does not serve as a suggestion. In the unusual circumstance in which the woman admits to suicidal ideation or fears she will harm her child, the clinician has performed an important service to both the patient and her family. Immediate referral to an individual or clinic capable of crisis intervention and hospital admission, if necessary, is, of course, indicated.

Postpartum Psychosis

Postpartum psychoses often do not occur in hospital populations as most parturients are discharged by the time acute signs and symptoms develop. Characteristically, psychoses involve an onset and acute symptoms after a normal lucid postpartum period of several days. Thought disturbances, mania, or, alternatively, severe depressive states with hallucinations usually cause family or friends to return these individuals to the hospital promptly for evaluation and treatment.

The symptoms that identify puerperal psychosis and should be noted by the obstetric clinician are (1) *insomnia*: this may be difficult to distinguish from the new mother's awakenings from a new baby, but a careful history of difficulty falling asleep or staying asleep or being able to rest at all should alert the staff; (2) *mood disturbance*: a persistence in mood lability, elation, or depression may be noted by asking about mood, observing facial expressions, noting ignoring of the baby, persistent crying, and inability to concentrate on any task after the first week or two; (3) *unusual behavior*: a change in the mother's usual personality, such as continued and excessive restlessness, excitement, hearing voices; (4) *unusual beliefs*: delusions or false beliefs about the baby, excessive guilt, persecutory ideas about staff or family, special powers; (5) *suicidal ideas*: harm to self and, more dangerously, ideas involving a plan of action.

Blues

In the blues, despite complaints of depressive symptoms and considerable emotional lability, spontaneous, rapid recovery of spirits is common. There is no true confusion. Maniacal behavior and hallucinations are absent. Symptoms virtually always disappear within 2 weeks of delivery and long-term or residual depression is uncommon.

Dysthymic Reaction

The dysthymic reaction (depressive neurosis [DSM-IIIR 296.2,300.40])[51] is a condition of depressed mood in which some depressive symptoms are present and persist for at least 2 years in the absence of mania, hypomania, or another chronic psychotic disorder. On occasion, this diagnosis is made post partum in a woman with a previously recognized disorder.

Anxiety Disorders

At times it is difficult to distinguish between the conditions of depression and anxiety, as both can coexist. However, using both clinical criteria and rating scales, the differentiation can usually be established. A certain degree of anxiety is expected in pregnancy and its total absence is abnormal. When anxiety is pathologic it is defined as a sense of doom or dread, unrelated to reality or out of proportion to the true threat with the source not recognized by the patient.[63] There are two major categories of anxiety disorders[51]: *phobic disorders* and *anxiety states* with panic disorders, generalized anxiety, obsessive-compulsive disorders, or posttraumatic stress disorders. Generally, in all of these conditions the individual recognizes the irrationality of her symptoms but is helpless to make changes. Such conditions have an incidence in the general population of 2% to 5%. *Phobic disorders* involve continuous and unreasonable fears of objects, situations, or activities. The individual avoids involvement or life events that would force her or him to face these feared objects or events. Usually the individual recognizes the fear as unreasonable. The DSM-IIR defines agoraphobia, social phobias, and simple phobias as the major types. Any of these subtypes can be present in the pregnant or postpartum patient.

Agoraphobia is defined as marked fear of being alone or being somewhere that escape might be difficult. This fear must interfere with the person's daily life and not be due to any other physical or mental illness.

Mrs A was 12 weeks pregnant in an unplanned and wanted pregnancy. She began to have increasingly incapacitating symptoms of being unable to leave her home or go to work. She would not drive her car unless someone else was with her.

Postpartum, a mother with agoraphobia may be afraid of leaving home, unable to go to the market or take her baby to the pediatrician.[24]

Social phobias are those in which individuals are fearful of situations in which they may be judged by others. They may be unable to speak in public, eat in public, use public lavatories. Again, they must be significantly distressed and have a condition not caused by other diseases.

Mrs B had significant anxiety when admitted to the hospital in labor. She felt staff was critical of her and other patients also. She wanted to be with her husband only. A supportive staff was able to understand her problem and help her through the delivery.

Simple phobias are persistent and irrational fears accompanied by a need to avoid the object or situation.

Mrs C had an irrational fear of intravenous needles and became extremely upset when admitted to the hospital in labor to have her baby. She became so disturbed that a psychiatrist was called. In discussing this fear, she recalled that as a child she had been in a terrible auto accident, in which her mother had been killed. The first memory she had on awakening in a hospital was having intravenous fluids administered to her. She was less fearful after this memory returned and she talked about it. She had not been in a hospital since those early days until she came to have her baby.

Phobias can be treated in various ways, including behavioral techniques (see Chapter 22).

Panic disorders are recurrent attacks of intense fear, terror, and impending doom. They may be accompanied by physical symptoms of dyspnea, palpitations, chest pain, sweating, choking, shakiness, paresthesias, dizziness, and other uncomfortable feelings. To establish the diagnosis there must be at least three attacks in 3 weeks occurring in the absence of other physical or mental disorders, physical exertions, life-threatening situations, organic illness, or phobic stimuli. Panic disorders occasionally occur in pregnancy and the puerperium though the exact pathophysiology is not yet clearly understood. Such attacks can be successfully treated with standard antidepressants such as the tricyclics or certain benzodiazepams such as alprazolam, raising the question of their relationship to depressive disorders (see Chapters 8 and 21).

Generalized anxiety disorders are defined as those occurring in individuals 18 years and older and persisting for at least a month. These disorders are characterized by motor tension, autonomic hyperactivity, apprehensive expectation, and vigilance and scanning. It is important to rule out other causes such as acute drug injection, hyperthyroidism, or depression. It is not known whether generalized anxiety disorders are more prevalent in pregnant women, but the presence of this condition should be known to the obstetrician as the condition has obvious implications for intrapartum and postpartum management.

Obsessive-compulsive disorders are characterized by intrusive thought, ideas, images, and behavior beyond an individual's voluntary control. Attempts to arrest the thoughts or behavior often result in anxiety and depression. These conditions may be present in pregnancy and the puerperium. The problem is often not shared with the medical staff because the patient is embarrassed about the existence of these feelings. For example, a pregnant woman may be ashamed of having recurrent depressive thoughts and consequently believe they may harm the baby but be incapable of escaping the ideas, with resulting agitation or depression.

Mrs D at 22 weeks of pregnancy was obsessed with the idea that she had acquired immunodeficiency syndrome (AIDS), and, despite tests, assurances, and reasoning, she could not be convinced. She avoided people and called her doctor continually. She was referred for psychological help and eventually her condition improved after brief psychotherapy.

Posttraumatic stress disorders are psychological symptoms occurring after a definable stressor, such as a personal tragedy or a major disaster. The symptoms include reexperiencing the trauma (flashbacks), recurrent intrusive thoughts or dreams, psychic numbing, and at least two of the following symptoms: hyperalertness, sleep disturbances, guilt, memory problems, avoidance of activities reminiscent of the event, and symptom exacerbation when in contact with specific activities or scenes.

In obstetrics, many events that patients have endured may be brought out again in a pregnancy. Childhood incest, rape or other sexual traumas, physical abuse, a very traumatic prior labor, and delivery or hospital experiences may be contributing to current difficulties. It is important for staff to inquire in a sensitive way about these events or the presence of anxiety disorders. They are treatable, and appropriate therapy affords patients considerable relief. The perception of anxiety is contagious. If the staff feel especially anxious around a certain patient, it may be because of that person's feelings and communications. Treatment of posttraumatic stress disorders consists primarily of psychotherapy in which patients are able to go over the details of the stressful events in their own time and gradually gain some mastery over them.

Atypical Psychological Reactions

Although most of the discussion so far has referred to psychological disturbance in the pregnant and postpartum woman, other important psychological reactions related to pregnancy alter a woman's life and/or family experiences. These include reactions manifested by the baby's father, the grandparents, and/or adoptive parents.[53]

Adoptive Parents

Adverse psychological reactions do occur among adoptive parents. In our service, Mrs B had proved infertile after the diagnosis and treatment of ovarian cancer. She became acutely depressed after the adoption of a much wanted baby. After treatment with antidepressant medications she recovered normally.

Infertility Patients

Patients who become pregnant after a long period of infertility or after the use of one or more of the new reproductive technologies can develop clinical depression. This is often a great disappointment to the professional staff, who cannot understand this response. Of interest, depressions occur with the same frequency in *successfully* treated infertility patients as in women who become pregnant without such assistance (see Chapter 16).

Grandparents

Grandparents can also develop a depressed state after the birth of a grandchild. This is especially likely to occur if they have had depressions after the birth of their own children.

Fathers and Pregnancy

The effect of pregnancy on fathers is a relatively neglected area.[64–67] The couvade syndrome (from the French word *couver* meaning to sit, eg, on eggs) refers to symptoms of pregnancy in men, and specifically to customs of childbirth in some societies in which the men develop certain types of behavior, such as going to bed at or about the time of birth for a definite number of days. In Western civilizations, men have more physical symptoms, usually gastrointestinal, during their partner's pregnancies. Up to 11% of fathers experience morning sickness, vomiting, or other abdominal distress during the peripartum period. Occasionally, in such cases if reassurance is ineffective and symptoms are distressing, supportive psychotherapy is necessary. Uncommonly, more severe psychological reactions are observed, usually in individuals with a preexisting neurotic personality style (see Chapter 15).

Pathophysiology

Psychopathology

Although the cause of the affective disorders in pregnancy and the postpartum period is not established, there are a number of hypotheses, some of them mutually exclusive. In general, these include biologic, cognitive, psychoanalytic, and sociocultural theories.[10,11,16,21,29,68,69]

Of all the peripartum affective disorders, there are features of the postpartum blues that strongly suggest a physiologic cause.[5,29] The condition is extremely common and it has a discrete time course. In the vast majority of cases, the blues generally resolves entirely or largely remits in less than 10 days. This alone strongly implies some type of maternal readjustment to the changes in the physiologic milieu of the puerperium. Further, the blues is generally unrelated to the circumstances of the delivery or to the condition of the newborn and occurs with a similar time scale in different societies.[29,33] The dysphoria of the blues is also quite similar to that observed in postoperative psychological reactions, suggesting a patterned response to an acute, stressful event.[70] Some investigators report a relationship between the occurrence of the blues and a history of premenstrual tension, but there is no consensus on this point.[13,38,69,71,72] Finally, the mood disturbances of the blues fluctuate, similar to those observed in other well-recognized disorders of cerebral dysfunction such as drug withdrawal states or thyrotoxicosis.[73,74]

Condon and Watson[69] are probably closest to the truth in describing the blues as a "hormonally induced emotional lability." Unfortunately, despite all of these observations, speculation, and research, no unifying physiologic explanation for the blues has been forthcoming. Further, it is unknown whether the maternity blues has a cause similar to that of the other puerperal affective disorders.

The role of maternal physiology in triggering peripartum depressions and/or psychoses is controversial and uncertain. There is general agreement that human depressive states are characterized by abnormalities in dopaminergic and noradrenergic activity in the central nervous system (CNS). It has been postulated that rapid hormonal changes in the puerperium and/or premenstrual period could influence psychotic relapses or breaks through effects on central dopamine neurotransmission.[59,71]

A brief review of the major theories of causes of these disorders is helpful to understand their complexity and clinical and physiologic associations.

The *biologic theories* for peripartum mood disturbances center around the major hormonal changes that occur with pregnancy and in the puerperium.[39,73,75–77] Mood and behavior changes associated with normal menses, administration of oral contraceptives, estrogen replacement therapy, and pregnancy have suggested to many a relationship between mood and sex steroid hormone levels, especially those of estrogen and progesterone.[18,59,78–85]

Sex Steroids

Estrogen and progesterone levels are extremely high during pregnancy and fall precipitously at delivery, reaching a baseline in 2 to 5 days.[12,82] The acute withdrawal of these hormones is considered a contributory factor to mental dysfunction. As estrogen and progesterone affect monoaminergic CNS neurotransmitters largely by reducing responses to dopamine, in theory it is reasonable to assume that such changes might modulate some aspects of mood.[22,78,82,86] Thus, when these steroids are abruptly withdrawn at delivery, vulnerable individuals could show evidence of acute mood changes and/or depression by exposing hypersensitive dopamine receptors in the limbic system.[39,87]

When *total* sex hormone concentrations are measured, a 100-fold drop in progesterone and a 10-fold decline in estrogen concentration postpartum are observed.[88] Data on the *active* concentrations of these hormones are less easily obtained. It is claimed that measurement of salivary sex steroid concentrations is an accurate reflection of the free hormone concentrations in the serum.[89–91] In a series of such studies, Harris and co-workers[91] report apparent differences in the concentration of both prolactin and progesterone in depressed versus normal women, modified by the presence or absence of breastfeeding. In these studies, an apparent progesterone "deficiency" and lower prolactin levels were found in depressed individuals.

When critically reviewed, the sex steroid hypothesis is less strong than it initially appears. Most circulating estrogen and progesterone is biologically inactive, bound to carrier globulins. Thus, despite apparent high total hormone concentrations during late pregnancy, the active or free levels are much lower, generally representing less than 3% of the total.[91,92]

Studies of treatment of depressed mood by administration of sex steroids are bedeviled by placebo responders and poor study design. Dalton[93] and Solthau and Taylor[94] have claimed success in treating postpartum depressions with natural progesterone, either intramuscularly or with vaginal or rectal suppositories. Dalton has also administered progesterone prophylactically in subsequent pregnancies for women with prior histories of postpartum depression and has claimed a significant increase in recurrence risk.[95] In a similar fashion, she had treated premenstrual syndromes (or late luteral phase dysphoria [LLPD]) with progesterone.[96] However, the efficacy of such treatment is poorly supported by prospective randomized trials and the role of progesterone in postpartum mood modulation is simply unclear. There are no scientifically valid and independently confirmed studies supporting the progesterone replacement therapy as effacious for either LLPD or peripartum depression. However, the salivary free hormone level studies as reported by Harris and co-workers[91] and others[62,90] and the available serum studies suggest that there are possibilities for treatment awaiting evaluation when studies with appropriate control groups and adequate numbers are designed.

These data are interesting but are not easy to interpret. Such studies are technically difficult to perform to isolate active hormone from bound and comparability of the various assays used is unclear.[92] Not surprisingly, the levels reported vary between investigators and the possible contribution of bound hormone entering the circulation from inactive stores after carrier protein dissociation is not established. At best, such data on sex steroid levels suggest that closer attention to the physiology of the major pregnancy sex steroids might tease out heretofore hidden complexities in hormonal milieu that are of consequence in tailoring therapy in individual cases.

Prolactin

Increased prolactin levels and active breast-feeding have been associated with postpartum depression and premenstrual tension.[12,97,98] It has been claimed that the administration of bromoergocryptine, an ergot polypeptide derivative that functions as a potent prolactin-inhibiting agent, is an effective treatment for depression. Such data tend to support the prolactin or at least to provide evidence that dopamine agonists are useful in the treatment of depression.[99] Unfortunately, results of studies of the relationship between prolactin and depression in nonpregnant patients are conflicting. The reported levels in depressed individuals have been stated to be lower, elevated, or the same as those for normal individuals.[100]

In sum, the situation for prolactin remains unsettled. This substance is known to be nonspecifically elevated in response to a number of unspecific stimuli, including major and minor surgery, routine exercise, and sexual intercourse.[101]

Thyroid Dysfunction

Hamilton[102] and others[62,78,103–106] have reported thyroid dysfunction as a contributory factor to postpartum depression. In fact, a well described, transitory postpartum thyroid dysfunction syndrome occurs in the first year post partum in 4% to 10% of women.[106–109] The majority of cases of documented postpartum thyroid dysfunction are without obvious clinical symptoms, at least insofar as directing medical attention to the possibility of thyroid disease.

This postpartum thyroid dysfunction syndrome is believed to be an autoimmune disease, precipitated by unknown postpartum alterations in the immune system.[105,106] Recurrences with repeated pregnancies have been described. This disorder is a destructive, lymphocytic inflammatory process strongly associated with the presence of serum antimicrosomal and antithyroglobulin antibodies.[104,106,108] The onset is commonly 6 weeks to 4 months post partum. In the initial, acute phase a nonpainful goiter may be present, accompanied by transient hyperthyroidism. In the subsequent 2- to 6-month healing phase that follows, hypothyroidism is common. Usually, thyroid function returns to normal within a year, but in some instances hypofunction persists.[110] In general, the antibody titers are lowest after delivery and then rise rapidly, reaching a maximum at 4 to 6 months, during the hypothyroid phase, then decline.[78,108,110]

In the best studied large population (N = 901), Fung and co-workers[103] found no association between postpartum thyroid dysfunction and sex or weight of the neonate, maternal age, parity, duration of breast-feeding, or presence of goiter at first presentation. Of interest in this study was an association between the presence of antimicrosomal antibodies and maternal smoking that warrants additional investigation.

A relationship between mood and thyroid function should not be rejected out of hand.[103,106] Independent of pregnancy or parturition, patients with thyroid dysfunction have been known for many years to display a variety of psychiatric symptoms.[111-114] Hypothyroid or hyperthyroid function can result in symptoms strikingly similar to clinical depression, anxiety/mania, or, rarely, frank psychosis.[115,116] Also, thyrotoxicosis can precipitate mania in predisposed patients with known bipolar disease.[89]

In animal models, thyroxine treatment increases noradrenaline and dopamine synthesis in the central nervous system, providing at least the framework for a plausible link between thyroid hormone and mood.[78,117,118] There are also data comparing clinically depressed patients to controls evaluating their responses to thyrotropin-releasing hormone (TRH) therapy.[117,119] Depressed individuals tend to have a blunted response to TRH and lower platelet serotonin (5-HT) uptake dynamics, again suggesting a possible link between thyroid function and the bioactive amines thought to be important in the central nervous system modulation of mood.

Despite these interesting associations, the importance of thyroid dysfunction in contributing to the incidence of postpartum depressions is not established. Certainly, the available data document that some women develop transitory and, uncommonly, permanent thyroid abnormalities in the first several months post partum. Further, in at least some of these individuals, there is an association between these thyroid abnormalities and depressed mood. However, most depressed women do not have demonstrable thyroid abnormalities, and by no means does clinical depression develop in all women with demonstrable thyroid abnormalities. Further, it is unclear whether the true psychoses have a different relationship to thyroid function than the less severe depressive states. For example, in a matched control study of 30 hospitalized patients with DSM-IIIR-defined psychoses (affective disorder with psychotic features N = 22; schizophrenia N = 4; atypical psychosis N = 4) with onset at least 4 weeks after delivery, no significant differences in either thyroid function or antibody pattern could be identified.[120] The use of routine postpartum antibody titers to screen for risk for depression cannot at present be supported except as a research tool. In individual cases of clinical depression it is reasonable to perform screens for thyroid function as an occasional case needing treatment may be identified.

Corticosteroids

There is considerable research interest in a possible link between abnormalities in corticosteroid metabolism and affective disorders.[121-124] Biologically active and total plasma cortisol levels are normally elevated during pregnancy.[125,126] Corticosteroid dynamics during pregnancy are characterized by dexamethasone resistance and increased responsiveness to adrenocorticotropin (ACTH), implying a relative tissue refractoriness to cortisol.[126] Serum cortisol levels typically increase slightly in the third trimester and peak about the time of delivery.[125] After parturition, cortisol levels drop rapidly.

There are limited data linking postpartum mood and serum cortisol levels.[77,127,128] For example, Ehlert and co-workers[129] studied salivary cortisol levels in 70 postpartum women and correlated elevated morning levels with the onset of blues symptoms. Unfortunately, in a very similar study of 40 primiparous women, Feksi and associates[90] could not establish any relationship between blues symptoms and cortisol concentrations. Similar data indicating no correlation were reported by Kuevi and co-workers.[127] Thus, the available data do not provide a consistent picture.

Both abnormalities in cortisol dexamethasone suppression as well as elevated serum levels of cortisol are common findings in nonpuerperal depression.[121,130,131] In recent years, special attention has focused on cortisol secretion and the response to the dexamethasone suppression test (DST) as biologic markers for depression. Although the majority of these studies were performed in nonpregnant individuals, the results have encouraged application of the DST challenge to recent parturients with mood disorders.[132-135] Unfortunately, although there is a high incidence of abnormal DST results post partum, there is also poor correlation between these results and affective mood disorders.[132,135] Apparently, transient DST test result abnormalities—specifically nonsuppression—occur normally in more than 50% of otherwise normal postpartum women. This high incidence of abnormal responders returns to normal levels within 6 weeks after delivery. Thus, the DST is unreliable during the puerperium as an indicator of depression.

Additional interesting data concern the relationship between corticotropin-releasing hormone (CRH) proopiomelanocortin-related peptides and peripartum mood.[62,73,136-138] For example, the levels of CRH, a potent ACTH-releasing hormone, rise from the second trimester to term with additional increases during labor.[73,125,139] At least some CRH is of placental origin, but the role of this placental secretion in regulating ACTH, β-endorphin (BEP), and cortisol secretion in normal human pregnancy is at best unclear.[139]

BEP levels similarly rise with labor and delivery, and thereafter decline rapidly postpartum.[74,137,138] In Smith and associates' study[73] combining a longitudinal investigation of BEP levels, CRH concentration, and maternal mood as judged by psychological testing, women with mood deterioration from 38 weeks to postpartum day 2 had statistically significant drops in plasma BEP levels, greater than those of women with stable or improving mood. They postulate that the acute stress-related withdrawal of endogenous opioids after delivery precipitate hypothalamic and limbic dysfunction akin to a drug withdrawal syndrome. The full implications of such interesting relationships await additional investigation in prospective, well-designed studies.[62,74,136]

Serotonin

Abnormalities in tryptophan metabolism are linked to depressive disease.[77,140,141] Tryptophan is a dietary amino acid that serves as a precursor for the neurotransmitter serotonin (5-hydroxytryptophan [5-HT]). Tryptophan is actively transported into the CNS. It is speculated that tryptophan transport is a rate-limiting step in 5-HT synthesis and thus that changing serum levels can alter CNS neurotransmitter availability.[12] A hypothalamic serotonin deficiency has long been felt to be part of the physiology of depression. As the hypothalamus is important in regulating temperature, sleep cycles, and libido and as such functions are commonly abnormal in depressed individuals, a connection between presynaptic deficiencies of neurotransmitters such as 5-HT and depression is a reasonable hypothesis.

An important line of research is investigation of platelet uptake of 5-HT as a model of synaptic function.[12,142–144] The theory is that platelet uptake dynamics and modulation by various drugs reflect presynaptic 5-HT uptake into CNS synaptosomes. Platelet models are also used to investigate α_2-adrenergic receptor (AAR) number and function, also thought to be involved in causing depression. In general, the number of AAR binding sites is greater in women with the maternity blues than normal postpartum and normal nonpregnant women. In theory at least, sex hormones might alter these monoamine receptor sites in the CNS, predisposing individuals to mood disturbances.

During normal pregnancy tryptophan levels are reduced. Postpartum, there is a biphasic rise over the first 5 days.[77,145] Individuals developing the blues are missing the early peak. Dietary replacement treatment with tryptophan is based on the theory that plasma unbound (ie, free) tryptophan modulates the central nervous system synthesis of 5-HT and thus mood.[77,145–150] Unfortunately for this interesting hypothesis, Harris's prospective trial of tryptophan was not successful in preventing the postpartum blues.[146] This indicates either that such disorders are not the result of low 5-HT levels or, minimally, that dietary replacement of tryptophan is ineffectual in elevating such levels and returning mood to normal.

The strength of the association between puerperal tryptophan concentrations and mood remains unsettled. In this regard, it is again important to differentiate between free and bound hormone. Albumin is the primary carrier protein for tryptophan, and albumin concentrations fall normally during gestation, largely by the normal expansion of intravascular volume. Further, there are significant seasonal as well as diurnal variations in tryptophan concentration and a close connection between tryptophan levels and patterns of nutrition—all of which must be accounted for in the critical review of any claimed association between specific levels and mood.[151,152,159] DeMyer and co-workers[151] have attempted to offset some of these methodologic problems by measuring the ratio of plasma tryptophan to five other amino acids, finding these values to correlate best with patients' clinical condition.

The situation for 5-HT remains unsettled. It may be that abnormalities in tryptophan levels in the blues are not etiologic but only serve as markers for another unknown mechanism. The recent discovery of potential adverse effects of orally administered l-tryptophan, even if they prove to be due to toxic contamination of the amino acid, is an additional reason for therapeutic caution in the use of this substance. In sum, the tryptophan story is one of more unanswered questions and interesting possibilities rather than firm data.

Despite these and other associations, the present data do not unequivocally establish a link between sex steroid levels, tryptophan levels, β-endorphin concentrations, or other "aberrant neuroendocrine secretory dynamics" and the common postpartum disorders of mood.[12,74,82,90,127,130,151] The thyroid function story is somewhat different. Substantial transient departures from normal values for thyroid tests appear to accompany parturition.[78] Some 4% to 8% of postpartum women have a condition of biochemically significant thyroid dysfunction, and, in unusual cases, frank hypothyroidism eventually results. Thus, there is suffcient evidence available to warrant performance of thyroid screens on women with serious puerperal mood disturbances. Unfortunately, it appears at present that this thyroid association will explain only a small percentage of the total cases of postpartum affective disorders—specifically the depressives—and, perhaps rarely, the psychotic disorders. Changes in thyroid function are probably not causative of the blues as the time course is wrong: the endocrinologic abnormalities are delayed in most cases to 3 to 4 weeks post partum. Further study of these and other hormonal substances is warranted. Yet, at present, a firm association between most of these reported abnormalities and the majority of peripartum mood disturbances is tenuous at best.

Other Causative Factors

Although the literature is riddled with inconsistencies and contradictions, there is evidence that the *level of depressive symptoms before pregnancy*,[153] *marital difficulties*,[154–156] *increased number of untoward life events*,[22] and a *high level of baseline symptoms*[31,70] are related to peripartum mood dysfunction. Further, friend and family support as well as other psychological stressors are thought by many authors to have an important role in affective states.[13,35,53,157–159] In critically reviewing these data, it remains unclear whether marital discord leads to depression or the converse.[22,160] The question of whether there are different types of depression with varying responses to life events or whether the differences between studies in the influence of these factors represent problems of sampling or perhaps interpretation remains moot.

The evidence that obstetric or perinatal complications necessarily increase the occurrence of postpartum mood disturbances is not compelling. However, throughout the literature, complications of gestation are suggested as associations with peripartum depressions, and this issue must be still regarded as unsettled.[29,161–163,167] Given the difficulties inherent in the data it is not surprising that the distinction between acute situational anxiety/depression and serious mood disturbances is difficult to establish. Further, social and demographic differences between populations affect results. Thus, there are honest differences in both observation and opinion among investigators as they report their clinical experience.

The general theory underlying our thinking concerning true peripartum depressive mood views this disorder in what O'Hara and associates call a diathesis-stress conceptualization.[42] In this formulation, a cognitive vulnerability to depression and/or a depression history combines with environmental events.[13,19,69] Thus, an individual who is potentially vulnerable either because of physiologic events, such as hormonal changes or the trauma of surgery, dysfunctional self-control attitudes, or a dysfunctional attributional style, can develop clinical depression in the face of sufficiently stressful events of life. In terms of postpartum depressions, the data supporting such a hypothesis are mixed. Perhaps this formulation is best considered as a reasonable working idea, tying together a great deal of otherwise incomprehensible data as we research for additional information.

Treatment

Treatment for peripartum depressions consists of the use of antidepressant drugs, psychotherapy, support groups (such as Depression after Delivery, a national group with local chapters), and family or personal counseling (see Chapters 21 and 22).

In serious cases, especially those with thought disorders, mania, or suicidal or homicidal ideation, referral to a psychiatrist or other mental health professional is necessary. Less severe cases can be managed by the non-psychiatrist after appropriate consultation, with careful attention to the effects of antidepressant drugs, if administered, and to the adequacy of the family and other social supports. Although occasional residual symptoms of the blues can persist for months, the condition is considered normal and treatment with psychotropic medications is not indicated.[165] However, as there is at least partial agreement in the literature that there is a link between the more severe forms of the blues and serious depressive disease, it is prudent to follow up on selected cases of the blues for several weeks to be certain that a clinical depression is not developing.[7,12,24,156,166] If such a disorder does occur after this period of observation, this attention will provide a ready source of contact for the patient and/or her family when additional assistance is needed.

As suggested by Chang and Renshaw,[44] the basics of therapy for more severe cases of depression and other psychiatric disorders during pregnancy include (1) close collaboration between the obstetrician and the psychiatric consultant, (2) daily visits by both clinicians during any antenatal admissions, (3) careful patient observation, (4) social support, (5) drug titration to achieve control with minimally effective dosages, and (6) a return to alternative treatments (behavioral, etc) when possible.

The use of psychotropic drugs, including lithium carbonate, the phenothiazides, and haloperidol, is effective in treating acute psychoses as well as in preventing their recurrence. When treating patients with mania, both lithium and probably the anticonvulsants should be avoided in the first trimester if possible. For these patients, the use of a benzodiazepine is preferable. If required, lithium can be administered after 12 weeks of gestational age. However, fetal hypotonia, cyanosis, and goiter have been reported as complications of lithium treatment and care is needed. Because lithium is renally excreted, the dosage needs to be decreased substantially or discontinued just before delivery. Maternal creatinine clearance declines post partum by approximately 50%, leading to possible acute lithium toxicity if the drug dosage is not decreased.

For individuals with clinical antepartum depression, supportative, cognitive, or behavioral therapy can be attempted in the first trimester. When drug treatment is necessary, the newer tricyclic agents such as nortriptyline hydrochloride or desipramine hydrochloride are better choices than imipramine hydrochloride or amitriptyline hydrochloride as they produce less orthostatic hypotension.

An antidepressant such as a tricyclic (amitriptyline hydrochloride or similar) 150 to 200 mg qhs frequently relieves depression, although therapy will be necessary for several weeks to achieve a full response. If psychotic symptoms are present, haloperidol to 100 mg/24 hours or chloropromazine 400 to 800 mg/24 hours will provide control.

As with all pharmacologic treatment during pregnancy, the lowest possible dose of medication should be administered for the shortest possible time, avoiding treatment in the first trimester, if possible. However, obvious clinical choices need to be made. If the clinical cost of tapering or discontinuing a drug is maternal disorganization, mania, or loss of ability to function socially or to take proper care of oneself, then the failure to treat causes more harm than good.

For patients having chronic treatment for anxiety, doses of benzodiazepines can be tapered in the first trimester or a tricyclic antidepressant attempted. Again, cognitive, behavioral, or supportive psychotherapy treatments can also be helpful, preventing the potential side effects of medications.

In selected cases, as in nonpuerperal depression, electroconvulsive treatment (ECT) is indicated, especially when drug therapy has not been successful.[165,167] With care, such treatment is safe during pregnancy, but it is uncommonly used because of concern for fetal well-being.

In terms of prognosis, more than 90% of women treated for a postpartum psychosis improve within 90 days or less.[168] Recovery may be delayed or incomplete in the subclass of women with schizophrenialike thought disorders, delusions, or hallucinations. Individuals with these conditions need long-term follow-up observation and the prognosis is more guarded.

After apparent clinical recovery from peripartum psychosis women should be followed closely for several months. Especially with schizophrenics, depressive reactions may follow improvement of the original psychosis.

It is prudent to counsel patients with psychoses carefully about future pregnancies as well as the likelihood of nonpuerperal recurrences. Chang and Renshaw[44] suggest a 2- to 3-year interval between pregnancies. We concur.

Conclusions

The affective disorders of pregnancy are an interesting and ultimately frustrating set of clinical conditions. The striking features of these conditions include their frequency, the variability of presentation in individual women, and the lack of a clear cause. The high incidence of the less severe form, the maternity blues; the lack of strong correlation with complications of pregnancy; the cross-cultural occurrence; and the discrete timing support the idea of a primary biologic cause, manifested in a variety of ways, as influenced by both cultural factors and individual personality. The blues are best viewed as a readjustment from the complex psychological and physiologic state of pregnancy to another in which the bioendocrinologic changes increase an individual woman's sensitivity to her personal circumstances. The cause of the true depressions and psychoses is less clear and remains highly controversial. Minimally, even if not directly causative in depressions and psychotic reactions, the biology of gestation probably exacerbates preexisting stresses, evoking symptoms in susceptible individuals.

References

1. Yalom ID, Lunde DT, Moos RH, et al: Post partum blues syndrome: A description and related variables. *Arch Gen Psychiatry* 1968:18;16–27.
2. Pitt B: Maternity blues. *Br J Psychiatry* 1973;133:431–433.
3. Hapgood CC, Elkind GS, Wright JJ: Maternity Blues: Phemonena and relationship to later postpartum depression. *Aust NZ J Psychiatry* 1988;22:299–306.
4. Hopkins J, Marcus M, Campbell SB: Postpartum depression: A critical review. *Psychol Bull* 1984;94:498–515.
5. Stein GS: The maternity blues, in Brockington IF, Kumar R (eds.): *Motherhood and Mental Illness*. London, Academic Press, 1982, pp 119–154.
6. Robin AA: The psychological changes of normal parturition. *Psychiatr Q* 1962;36:129–150.
7. Kendell RE, McGuire RJ, Connor Y, et al: Mood changes in the first three weeks after childbirth. *J Affect Disord* 1981;3:317–326.
8. Hamilton JA: The identity of postpartum psychosis, Brockington IF, Kumar R (eds.): *Motherhood and Mental Illness*. London, Academic Press, 1982, pp 1–20.
9. Herzog A, Detre T: Psychotic reactions associated with childbirth. *Dis Nerv Syst* 1971;37:229–235.
10. Brockington IF, Cox-Roper A: The nosology of puerperal mental illness, in Kumar R, Brockington IF (eds.): *Motherhood and Mental Illness: 2. Causes and Consequences*. London, Butterworth, 1988, pp 1–16.
11. Welner A: Childbirth-related psychiatric disease. *Comp Psychol* 1982;23:143–154.
12. Campbell J, Winokur G: Postpartum affective disorders: Selected biological aspects, in Wood D (ed.): *Recent Advances in Postpartum Psychiatric Disorders*. Washington DC, American Psychiatric Association Press, 1985, pp 20–35.
13. Thirkettle JA, Knight RG: The psychological precipitants of transient postpartum depression: A review. *Cur Psychol Res Rev* 1985;4:143–166.
14. Atkinson AK, Rickel AU: Depression in women: The postpartum experience. *Issues Ment Health Nurs* 1983;5:197–218.
15. Knight RG, Thikettle JA: Anxiety and depression in the immediate postpartum period: A controlled investigation of a primiparous sample. *Aust NZ J Psychiatry* 1986;20:430–436.

16. Brockington IF, Cernik KF, Schofield EM, et al: Puerperal psychosis: Phemonena and diagnosis. *Arch Gen Psychiatr* 1981;38:829–838.

17. Katona CLE: Puerperal mental illness: Comparison with non- puerperal controls. *Br J Psychiatry* 1982;141:447–452.

18. Paffenbarger RS: Epidemiological aspects of parapartum mental illness. *Br J Prev Soc Med* 1964;18:189–195.

19. Ryle A: The psychological disturbances associated with 345 pregnancies in 137 women. *J Ment Sci* 1961;107:279–286.

20. Brockington IF, Margison FR, Schofield E, et al: The clinical picture of the depressed form of puerperal psychosis. *J Affect Dis* 1988;15:29–37.

21. Cutrona CE: Nonpsychotic postpartum depression, a review of recent research. *Clin Psychol Rev* 1982;2:487–503.

22. O'Hara MW, Zekoski EM: Postpartum depression: A comprehensive review, in Kuman R, Brockington IF (eds.): *Motherhood and Mental Illness: 2. Causes and Consequences.* London, Butterworth, 1988, pp 17–63.

23. Harding JJ: Postpartum psychiatric disorders: A review. *Compr Psychiatry* 1989;30:109–112.

24. Cox JL: *Postnatal Depression: A Guide for Health Professionals.* Edinburgh, Churchill Livingstone, 1986.

25. Esquirol JED: *Mental Maladies: A Treatise on Insanities.* Hunt EK (trans): Philadephia, Les and Blanchard, 1845.

26. Marcé LV: *Traité de la Folie des Femmes Enceintes, des Nouvelles Accouchées et des Nourrices.* Paris, JB Baillière et Fils, 1858.

27. Zuckerman BS, Beardslee WR: Maternal depression: A concern for pediatricians. *Pediatrics* 1987;79:110–117.

28. Wrate RM, Rooney AC, Thomas PF, et al: Postnatal depression and child development—a three-year follow-up study. *Br J Psychiatry* 1985;146:622–627.

29. Kennerley H, Gath D: Maternity blues reassessed. *Psychiatr Dev* 1986;1:1–17.

30. Harris B: Maternity blues. *Br J Psychiatry* 1980;136:520–521.

31. Cox JC, Connor YM, Henderson I, et al: Prospective study of the psychiatric disorders of childbirth by self report questionnaire *J Affect Disord.* 1983;5:1–7.

32. Jarrahi-Zadeh A, Kane PJ, Van de Castle RL, et al: Emotional cognitive changes in pregnancy and early puerperium. *Br J Psychiatry* 1969;115:797–805.

33. Davidson JRT: Postpartum mood change in Jamaican women: A description and discussion of its significance. *Br J Psychiatry* 1972;121:659–663.

34. Harris B: "Maternity blues" in East African clinic attenders. *Arch Gen Psychiatry* 1981;38:1293–1295.

35. Cox JL: Childbirth as a life event: Sociocultural aspects of postnatal depression. *Acta Psychiatr Scand* 1988;(suppl):76–83.

36. Gard PR, Handley SL, Parsons AD, et al: A multivariate investigation of postpartum mood disturbance. *Br J Psychiatry* 1986;148:567–575.

37. Harris B, Huckle P, Thomas R, et al: The use of rating scales to identify post-natal depression. *Br J Psychiatry* 1989;154:813–817.

38. Pitt B: Atypical depression following childbirth. *Br J Psychiatry* 1968;144:1223–1225.

39. Nott PN, Franklin M, Armitage C, et al: Hormonal changes and mood in the early puerperium. *Br J Psychiatry* 1976;128:379–383.

40. Kumar R: Neurotic disorders in childbearing women, in Brockington IF, Kumar R (eds.): *Motherhood and Mental Illness,* London Academic Press, 1982, pp 71–118.

41. Jacobson L, Kaij L, Nilsson A: Postpartum mental disorders in an unselected sample: Frequency of symptoms and predisposing factors. *Br Med J* 1965;1:1640–1643.

42. O'Hara MW, Neunaber DJ, Zekoski ME: Prospective study of postpartum depression: Prevalence, course, and predictive factors. *J Abnorm Psychol* 1984;93:158–171.

43. Cutrona CE: Causal attributions and perinatal depression. *J Abnorm Psychol* 1983;92:161–172.

44. Chang SS, Renshaw DC: Psychoses and pregnancy. *Compr Ther* 1986;12:36–41.

45. O'Hara M, Zekoski E, Phillips L, et al: Controlled prospective study of postpartum mood disorders: Comparison of childbearing and non-childbearing women. *J Abnorm Psych* 1990;99:3–15.

46. Kaplan BJ: Causes and attributions of depression during pregnancy. *Women Health* 1983;8:23–32.

47. Nott PN: Psychiatric illness following childbirth in Southhampton: A case register study. *Psychol Med* 1982;12:557–561.

48. Padawer JA, Fagan C, Janoff-Bulman R, et al: Women's psychological adjustment following emergency cesarean versus vaginal delivery. *Psychol Women Q* 1988;12:25–34.

49. Davidson J, Robertson E: A follow up study of postpartum illness, 1946–1978. *Acta Psychiatr Scand* 1985;71:451–457.

50. Thuwe I: Genetic factors in puerperal psychosis. *Br J Psychiatry* 1974;125:378–385.

51. American Psychiatric Association: *Diagnostic and Statistical Manual of Mental Disorders* (ed. 3). Washington, DC, American Psychiatric Association Press, 1987.

52. McNeil TF: Women with nonorganic psychosis: Psychiatric and demographic characteristics of cases with versus without postpartum psychotic episodes. *Acta Psychiatr Scand* 1988;78:603–609.

53. Gise LH: Psychiatric implications of pregnancy, in Cherry SH, Berkowitz RL, Kase NG (eds.): *Rovinsky and Guttmacher's Medical, Surgical and Gynecologic Complications of Pregnancy* (ed. 3). Baltimore, Williams & Wilkins, 1988, pp 614–654.

54. Pugh TF, Jerath BK, Schmidt WM, et al: Rates of mental disease related to childbearing, *N Engl J Med* 1963;268:1224–1228.

55. Paffenbarger RS: Epidemiological aspects of mental illness associated with childbearing, in Brockington IF, Kumar R (eds.): *Motherhood and Mental Illness*, London, Academic Press, 1982, pp 19–36.

56. Dean C, Kendall RE: The symptomatology of puerperal illness. *Br J Psychiatry* 1981;139:128–133.

57. Brockington IF, Winokur G, Dean C: Puerperal psychosis, in Kumar R, Brockington IF (eds.): *Motherhood and Mental Illness.* London, Academic Press, 1982, pp. 37–70.

58. Kumar R, Robson KM: A prospective study of emotional disorders in childbearing women. *Br J Psychiatry* 1984;144:35–47.

59. Brockington IF, Kelly A, Hall P, et al: Premenstrual relapse of puerperal psychosis. *J Affect Dis* 1988;14:287–292.

60. Martin ME: Puerperal mental illness, a follow up study of 75 cases. *Br Med J* 1958;2:737–777.

61. Garvey MJ, Tuason VB, Lumry AE, et al: Occurrence of depression in the postpartum state. *J Affect Dis* 1985;5:97–101.

62. George A, Sardler M: Endocrine and biochemical studies in puerperal mental disorders, in Kumar R, Brockington IF (eds.): *Motherhood and Mental Illness: 2. Causes and Consequences.* London, Butterworth, 1988, pp 78–113.

63. Warks I, Lader M: Anxiety states (anxiety neurosis): A review. *J Nerv Ment Dis* 1973;150:3–18.

64. Wilson LG: Couvade syndrome. *Am Fam Physician* 1977;15:157–166.

65. Quill T, Lipkin M, Lamb GS: Health-care seeking by men in their spouse's pregnancy. *Psychosom Med* 1984;46:277–283.

66. Cavenar JO, Butts NT: Fatherhood and mental illness. *Am J Psychiatry* 1977;134:429–431.

67. Wainright WH: Fatherhood as a precipitant of mental illness. *Am J Psychiatry*

1966;123:40–44.

68. Treadway CR, Kane FJ, Jarrahi-Zadeh A, et al: A psychoendocrine study of pregnancy and puerperium. *Am J Psychiatry* 1969;125:1380–1386.

69. Condon JT, Watson TL: The maternity blues: Exploration of a psychological hypothesis. *Acta Psychiatr Scand* 1987;76:164–171.

70. Levy V: The maternity blues in postpartum and post-operative women. *Br J Psychiatry* 1987;151:368–372.

71. Dennerstein L, Lehert P, Riphagen F: Postpartum depression: Risk factors. *J Psychosom Obstet Gynecol* 1989;10(suppl):53–65.

72. O'Hara MW, Rehm LP, Campbell SB: Predicting depressive symptomatology: Cognitive-behavioral models and postpartum depression. *J Abnorm Psychol* 1982;91:457–461.

73. Smith R, Cubis J, Brinsmead M, et al: Mood changes, obstetric experience and alterations in plasma contisol, beta- endorphin and corticotrophin releasing hormone during pregnancy and the puerperium. *J Psychosom Res* 1990;34:53–69.

74. Brinsmead M, Smith R, Singh B, et al: Peripartum concentrations of beta endorphin and cortisol and maternal mood states. *Aust NZ J Obstet Gynaecol* 1985;25:194–197.

75. George AJ, Copeland JRM, Wilson KCM: Prolactin in the maternity blues. *Br J Pharmacol* 1980;70:102–103.

76. Steiner M: Psychobiology of mental disorders associated with childbearing. *Acta Psychiatr Scand* 1979;60:449–464.

77. Handley SL, Dunn TL, Waldron S, et al: Tryptophan, cortisol, and puerperal mood. *Br J Psychiatry* 1980;136:498–508.

78. Harris B, Fung H, Johns S, et al: Transient postpartum thyroid dysfunction and postnatal depression. *J Affect Dis* 1989;17:243–249.

79. Herzberg PN, Johnson AL, Brown S: Depression and oral contraceptives. *Br Med J* 1970;3:142–144.

80. Gyermark L, Genther S, Fleming N: Some effects of progesterone and related steroids in the nervous system. *Int J Neuropharmacol* 1967;6:191–193.

81. Nilsson A, Almgren PE: Psychiatric symptoms during the postpartum period as related to the use of oral contraceptives. *Br Med J* 1968;5:453–455.

82. Deakin JFW: Relevance of hormone-CNS interactions to psychological changes in the puerperium, in Kumar R, Brockington IF (eds.): *Motherhood and Mental Illness: 2. Causes and Consequences.* London, Butterworth, 1988, pp 113–132.

83. Kane FJ: Psychiatric reactions to oral contraceptives. *Am J Obstet Gynecol* 1968;103:1052–1063.

84. Denner Stein L, Judd F, Davies B: Psychosis and the menstrual cycle. *Med J Aust* 1983;1:524–526.

85. Dennerstein L, Burrows GD, Wood C, et al: Hormones and sexuality: Effect of estrogen and progesterone. *Obstet Gynecol* 1980;56:316–322.

86. Majewska MD, Harrison NL, Schwartz RD, et al: Steroid hormone metabolites are barbiturate-like modulators of the GABA receptor. *Science* 1986;232:1004–1007.

87. Cookson JC: The neurobiology of mania. *J Affect Dis* 1985;8:233–241.

88. Bulter J, Leonard BE: Postpartum depression and the effects of nomifensine treatment. *Int Clin Psychol Pharmacol* 1986;1:244–252.

89. Darue J, McGarrigle HHG, Lachelin GCC: Increased saliva oestriol to progesterone ratio before idiopathic preterm delivery: A possible predictor for preterm labour? *Br Med J* 1987;294:270–272.

90. Feksi A, Harris B, Walker RF, et al: "Maternity blues" and hormone levels in saliva. *J Affect Dis* 1984;6:351–355.

91. Harris B, Johns S, Fung H, et al: The hormonal environment of post-natal depression. *Br J Psychiatry* 1989;154:600–667.

92. Anderson PJB, Hancock KW, Oakey RE: Non-protein bound oestradial and progesterone in human peripherial plasma before labour and delivery. *J Endocrinol* 1985;104:7–15.

93. Dalton K: *Depression after Childbirth*. London, Oxford University Press, 1980.

94. Solthau A, Taylor R: Depression after childbirth. *Br Med J* 1982;284:980–981.

95. Dalton K: Prospective study into puerperal depression. *Br J Psychiatry* 1971;118:689–692.

96. Dalton K: *The Pre-menstrual Syndrome*. London, Heinemann, 1964.

97. Alder EM, Cox JL: Breast feeding and post-natal depression. *J Psychosom Res* 1983;27:139–144.

98. Alder E, Bancroft J: The relationship between breast feeding persistence, sexuality and mood in postpartum women. *Psychol Med* 1988;18:389–396.

99. Waehrens J, Gerlack J: Bromocriptine and imipramine in endogenous depression: A double-blind controlled trial in out-patient. *J Affect Dis* 1981;3:193–202.

100. Fava GA, Lisansky J, Buckman MT, et al: Prolactin, cortisol, and antidepressant treatment. *Am J Psychiatry* 1988;145:358–360.

101. Noel GL, Suh HJ, Stone JG, et al: Human prolactin and growth hormone release during surgery and other conditions of stress. *J Clin Endocrinol Metab* 1972;35:840–851.

102. Hamilton JA: *Postpartum Psychiatric Problems*. St. Louis, CV Mosby, 1962.

103. Fung HYM, Kologlu M, Collison K, et al: Postpartum thyroid dysfunction in mid Glamoragan. *Br Med J* 1988:296;241–244.

104. Hayslip CC, Fein HG, O'Donnell VM, et al: The value of serum antimicrosomal antibody testing in screening for symptomatic postpartum thyroid dysfunction. *Am J Obstet Gynecol* 1988;159:203–209.

105. Goldman JM: Postpartum thyroid dysfunction. *Arch Intern Med* 1986;146:1296–1299.

106. Amino BN, Hori H, Iwatahi Y, et al: High prevalence of transient post-partum thyrotoxicosis and hypothyroidism. *N Engl J Med* 1982;306:849–852.

107. Lowe TW, Cunningham FG: Thyroid disease in pregnancy. *Williams Obstetrics, Supplement No. 9*. Norwalk, CT, Appleton & Lange, 1990.

108. Jansson R, Bernarder S, Karlsson A, et al: Autoimmunethyroid dysfunction in the postpartum period. *J Clin Endocrinol Metab* 1984;58:681–687.

109. Gerstein H: How common is postpartum thyroiditis? *Arch Intern Med* 1990;150:1397–1400.

110. Fein HG, Goldman JM, Weintraub BD: Postpartum lymphocytic thyroiditis in American women: A spectrum of thyroid dysfunction. *Am J Obstet Gynecol* 1980;138:504–510.

111. Smith CK, Barish J, Correa J, et al: Psychiatric disturbance in endocrinologic disease. *Psychosom Med* 1972;34:69–86.

112. Young LD: Organic affective disorder associated with thyrotoxicosis. *Psychosomatics* 1984;25:490–492.

113. Josephson AM, Mackenzie TB: Thyroid-induced mania in hypothyroid patients. *Br J Psychiatry* 1980;137:222–228.

114. Cohen KL, Swigar ME: Thyroid function screenings in psychiatric patients. *JAMA* 1979;242:254–257.

115. Folks DG: Organic affective disorder and underlying thyrotoxicosis. *Psychosomatics* 1984;25:243–249.

116. Wilson WH, Jefferson JW: Thyroid disease, behavior, and psychopharmacology. *Psychosomatics* 1985;26:481–492.

117. Roy A, Karoum F, Linnoila M, et al: Thyrotropin releasing hormone test in unipolar depressed patients and controls: Relationship to clinical and biologic variables.

Acta Psychiatr Scand 1988;77:151–159.

118. Harris PE, Dieguez C, Lewis BH, et al: Effects of thyroid status on brain catecholamine biosynthesis in adult rats: Assessment by a steady-state method. *J Endocrinol* 1986;111:383–389.

119. Arato M, Rihmer Z, Banki CM, et al: The relationship of neuro endocrine tests in endogenous depression. *Prog Neuropsychopharmol Biol Psychiatr* 1983;7:715–718.

120. Stewart DE, Addison AM, Robinson GE, et al: Thyroid function in psychosis following childbirth. *Am J Psychiatry* 1988;145:1579–1581.

121. Dahl R, Puig-Antich J, Ryan N, et al: Cortisol secretion in adolescents with major depressive disorders. *Acta Psychiatr Scand* 1989;80:18–26.

122. Mason JW: A review of psychoendocrine research as the pituitary-adrenal cortical system. *Psychosom Med* 1968;30:576–607.

123. Railton IE: The use of corticoids in postpartum depression. *J Am Med Woman Assoc* 1961;16:450–452.

124. Rubin RT, Poland RE, Lesser IM, et al: Neuroendocrine aspects of primary endogenous depression: I. Cortisol secretary dynamics in patients and matched controls. *Arch Gen Psychiatry* 1987;44:328–336.

125. Campbell EA, Linton EA, Wolfe CDA, et al: Plasma corticotropin-releasing hormone concentrations during pregnancy and parturition. *J Clin Endocrinol Metab* 1987;64:1054–1059.

126. Nolten WE, Rueckert PA: Elevated free cortisol index in pregnancy: Possible regulatory mechanism. *Am J Obstet Gynecol* 1981;139:492–498.

127. Kuevi V, Causon R, Dixon AF, et al: Plasma immune and hormone changes in "postpartum blues". *Clin Endocrinol* 1983;19:39–46.

128. Cone BA: *Puerperal Depression*, in 3rd International Congress, Psychosomatic Medicine in Obstetric and Gynaecology, London, England, 1971. Basel, Kargen, 1972, pp 355–357.

129. Ehlert U, Patalla U, Kirschbaum C, et al: Postpartum blues: Salivary cortisol and psychological factors. *J Psychosom Res* 1990;34:319–325.

130. Christensen P, Lolk A, Gram LF, et al: Cortisol and treatment of depression: Predictive value of spontaneous and suppressed cortisol levels and course of spontaneous plasma cortisol. *Psychopharmacol* 1989;97:471–475.

131. Kitamura T, Kano S, Shima S, et al: Hormonal changes in major depressive disorder. *Keio J Med* 1989;38:40–52.

132. Greenwood J, Parker C: The dexamethasone suppression test in the puerperium. *Aust NZ J Psychiatry* 1984;18:282–284.

133. Kumar R, Alcser K, Grunhaus L, et al: Relationships of the dexamethasone suppression test to clinical severity and degree of melancholia. *Biol Psychiatry* 1986;21:436–444.

134. Mossman D, Somoza E: Maximizing diagnostic information from the dexamethasone suppression test. *Arch Gen Psychiatry* 1989;46:653–660.

135. Singh B, Gilhotra M, Smith R, et al: Postpartum psychoses and the dexamethansone supression text. *J Affect Dis* 1986;11:173–177.

136. Kimdball CD, Chang CM, Chapman MB: Endogenous opioid peptides in intrapartum uterine blood. *Am J Obstet Gynecol* 1984;149:79–82.

137. Newnham JP, Dennett PM, Ferron SA, et al: A study of the relationship between circulating β-endorphin-like immunoreactivity and postpartum "blues". *Clin Endocrinol* 1984;20:169–177.

138. Goland RS, Wandlaw SL, Stank RJ, et al: Human plasma beta-endorphin during pregnancy, labor, and delivery. *J Clin Endocrinol* 1981;52:74–78.

139. Sasaki A, Shinkawa O, Margioris AN, et al: Immunoreactive corticotropin-releasing hormone in human plasma during pregnancy, labor and delivery. *J Clin En-*

docrinol Metab 1987;64:224–229.

140. Young SN, Pihl RO, Ervin FR: The effect of altered tryptophan levels on mood and behavior in normal human males. *Clin Neuropharmacol* 1988;11:S207-S215.

141. Moller SE: Tryptophan to competing amino acids ratio in depressive disorder: Relation to efficacy of antidepressive treatments. *Acta Psychiatr Scand* 1985;72:9–31.

142. Snedden JM: Blood platelets as a model for monoamine containing neurones. *Prog Neurobiol* 1973;1:151–198.

143. Garcia-Sevilla JA, Zis AP, Hollingsworth PJ, et al: Platelet alpha-adrenergic receptors in major depressive disorder. *Arch Gen Psychiatry* 1981;38:1327–1333.

144. Metz A, Stump K, Cowan PJ, et al: Changes in platelet alpha 2 - adrenoceptor binding postpartum: Possible relation to maternity blues. *Lancet* 1983;1:495–498.

145. Gard PR, Handley SL: Human plasma amino acid changes at parturition. *Horm Metabol Res* 1985;17:112.

146. Harris B: Prospective trial of l-tryptophan in maternity blues. *Br J Psychiatry* 1980;137:233–235.

147. Nardini M, De Stefano R, Iannucelli M, et al: Treatment of depression with l-5-hydroxytryptophan combined with chlorimipramine, a double-blind study. *Int J Clin Pharmacol Res* 1983;3:239–250.

148. Schmid-Burgk W, Kim JS, Lischewski R, et al: Levels of total and free tryptophan in the plasma of endogenous and neurotic depressives. *Arch Psychiatr Nervenkr* 1981;231:35–39.

149. Young SN, Chouinard G, Annable L: Tryptophan in the treatment of depression. *Adv Exp Med Biol* 191;133:727–737.

150. von Lerber-Good WF: Neurotransmitter precursor therapies in affective disorders. *Int J Vitam Nutr Res* 1986;29(suppl):69–82.

151. DeMyer MK, Shea PA, Hendrie HC, et al: Plasma tryptophan and five other amino acids in depressed and normal subjects. *Arch Gen Psychiatry* 1981;38:642–646.

152. Dam H, Mellerup ET, Rafaelsen OJ: Diurnal variation of total plasma tryptophan in depressive patients. *Acta Psychiatr Scand* 1984;69:190–196.

153. Nilsson A, Kaij L, Jacobson L: Postpartum mental disorder in an unselected sample: The psychiatric history. *J Psychosom Res* 1967;10:327–339.

154. Kumar R, Robson K: Neurotic disturbance during pregnancy and the puerperium: Preliminary report of a prospective survey of 119 primiparae, in Sandler M (ed.): *Mental Illness in Pregnancy and the Puerperium.* London, Oxford Medical Publications, 1978, pp .

155. Watson JP, Elliot SA, Ruggit J, et al: Psychiatric disorder in pregnancy and the first postnatal year. *Br J Psychiatry* 1984;144:453–462.

156. Paykel ES, Emms EM, Fletcher J, et al: Life events and social support in puerperal depression. *Br J Psychiatry* 1980;136:339–346.

157. O'Hara MW: Social support, life events, and depression during pregnancy and the puerperium. *Arch Gen Psychiatry* 1986;43:569–573.

158. O'Hara MW, Rehm LP, Campbell SB: Postpartum depression: A role for social network and life stress variables. *J Nerv Ment Dis* 1983;171:336–341.

159. Meltzer ES, Kumar R: Puerperal mental illness, clinical features and classification: A study of 142 mother-and-baby admissions. *Br J Psychiatry* 1985;147:647–654.

160. Martell, LK: Postpartum depression as a family problem. *Matern Child Nurs J* 1990;15:90–93.

161. Nadelson CC: "Normal" and "special" aspects of pregnancy: A psychological approach, in Nadelson CC, Notman MT (eds.): *The Woman Patient, Medical and Psychological Interfaces,* vol. 1. New York, Plenum Books, 1978, pp .

162 Gennaro S: Postpartal anxiety and depression in mothers of term and preterm

infants. *Nurs Res* 1988;37:82–85.

163. Entwisle DR, Doering SG, Reilly TW: Sociophysiological determinants of women's breast feeding behavior: A replication and extension. *Am J Orthopsychiatry* 1982;52:244–260.

164. Powers PS: Psychiatric disorders in pregnant women. *Med Aspects Hum Sex* 1989;23:47–54.

165. Oates MR: The treatment of psychiatric disorders in pregnancy and the puerperium. *Clin Obstet Gynecol* 1986;13:385–395.

166. Pleshette N, Asch S, Chase J: A study of anxieties during pregnancy, labor, the early and late puerperium. *Bull NY Acad Med* 1956;32:436–433.

167. Kramer BA: Electroconvulsive therapy use during pregnancy. *West J Med* 1990;152:77– .

Chapter 9

Chronic Mental Illness

William H. Miller, Jr., MD

Canst thou not minister to a mind diseas'd,
Pluck from the memory a rooted sorrow,
Raze out the written troubles of the brain,
And with some sweet oblivious antidote
Cleanse the stuff'd bosom of that perilous stuff
Which weighs upon the heart?
  —*Macbeth* IV, iii, 24
  William Shakespeare (1564–1616)

The treatment of the pregnant chronic mentally ill woman often creates a feeling of apprehension among obstetrical clinicians. The treatment of such patients is commonly based more on folklore and anecdote than empirical evidence—an approach that this chapter will critique. Included in this review is: (1) a survey of the current literature, focusing on the effect of pregnancy on mental health, as well as the impact of mental illness on the outcome of a pregnancy, and (2) a discussion of various issues important to the development of a reasonable treatment in these often difficult individuals.

Clinical Presentation and Differential Diagnosis

Background Studies

Much of the literature concerning mental illness during pregnancy is from Scandinavia, where standardized systems of health care exist. For example, Nielsen and Kaij, from Sweden, studied the effect of pregnancy on mental health in an unselected population of women.[1] Fifty percent of the women reported worsened mental health with pregnancy, 5% reported improved mental health, and 45% reported no change. Not surprisingly the occurrence of psychiatric symptoms during pregnancy was strongly related to a history of prior psychiatric problems (see Chapter 6).

McNeil and Kaij, also from Sweden, studied women with previous psychotic illnesses.[2] They found that 45% of these women experienced their mental health as a problem during their pregnancy, compared to only 13% of a control population. When psychiatric interviews were performed on these patients, assessing the effects of pregnancy on their mental health, evidence of worsening mental disturbance was found in 39% of previously psychotic women, compared to 4% of controls. As a clinical observation, only 35% of these previously psychotic women had a notation in their medical records relevant to their mental status! Fifty-eight percent of those with no such mental status notation were found to have significant increased mental disturbances.

Mental illness has important effects on the outcome of pregnancy. For example, in 1961, Sobel reported a 2.2 times increase in the deaths of infants of schizophrenic women.[3] In both 1972 and 1977, Sameroff and Zax observed an increase in obstetric complications among women diagnosed with a mental illness.[4,5] In these studies, women with depression had infants with lower Apgar scores and required more resuscitation. Women with a diagnosis of schizophrenia had significantly more low-birth-weight infants. In contrast, McNeil and co-workers in 1974 found no relation between obstetrical complications and the degree of mental disturbance.[6] In 1975, Reider et al, in a study from the United States, reported an increase in fetal and neonatal deaths in offspring of schizophrenics—7.5% versus 3.8% compared to a control group.[7] As a reflection of the difficulty of the literature in this field, Cohler and co-workers in 1975 were unable to find a significant relationship between maternal mental illness and the development of pregnancy and/or birth complications.[8] The latter authors did note that when obstetrical complications occurred during pregnancy and childbirth in mothers with a mental illness, this led to a worsening of the mother's mental condition.

In one of the largest available studies, Wrede and co-workers followed 171 schizophrenic women matched with 171 controls.[9] Of these women, 54 were diagnosed as chronic schizophrenic and 117 as mildly schizophrenic. In comparing chronic schizophrenic women versus controls, there were significant increases in various medical and pregnancy complications. Obstetric complications consisted of nausea, heartburn, and bleeding in the first trimester and proteinuria and hypertension in the third. In addition, significant increases in labor and delivery complications were also reported—22% in the schizophrenic group as a whole, compared to 9% in the control group. These complications included long labors (greater than 36 hours), abnormalities of fetal heart rate pattern, abnormal presentations, an increased incidence of instrumental delivery, and low Apgar scores (less than 3), as well as an increased likelihood of postpartum hemorrhage. In addition, nurses assessed the offspring of the schizophrenic women, and they reported that they were less healthy than those of the control group. The pediatric assessments took into account vital signs, episodes of cyanosis, irritability, and various neurological abnormalities. Not surprisingly, compliance with prenatal care was poor among these disorganized individuals. Among the control patients, 1.8% were not compliant with prenatal care, as compared to 9.6% in the chronic schizophrenic group.

The data from a recent study from the Oregon Health Sciences University involving 84 women admitted for inpatient psychiatric treatment is helpful in putting this issue into perspective. Eighty-eight percent of these women were unemployed, with 36% claiming no address, most of whom were living on the street. This was a group of severely ill women (Table 9.1). Fully 62% were involuntarily admitted, 32% had a history of more than five previous psychiatric admissions, and 60% had experienced more than 5 years of diagnosed mental illness. Sixty-seven percent had previously used psychotropic medication, but only 20% were on psychotropic medication at admission. Although these

Table 9.1 Oregon Sample of Pregnant Hospitalized
Psychiatric Patients

Diagnosis	n	Percent
Schizophrenia	37	44
Adjustment disorder	16	19
Substance abuse/dependence	9	11
Bipolar disorder	9	11
Depressive disorder	3	4
Conduct disorder	4	5
Schizoaffective disorder	3	4
Atypical psychosis	2	2
Dementia	1	1
Total	84	

women were admitted at varying times during pregnancy and 45% had at least one prenatal visit, only 15% had adequate prenatal care. Fifty-seven percent ended up receiving psychiatric medications during their hospitalization, with an average stay of approximately 44 days. Only 19% of these women had planned to become pregnant, but 65% had a positive attitude toward their gestation.

This population of chronic mentally ill pregnant women was clearly at high risk for obstetrical and social complications. Over 60% of these women were actively abusing alcohol or illicit psychoactive substances while pregnant, a substantially higher percentage than other urban populations.[10] The adverse impact of substance abuse on pregnancy and neonatal outcome is substantial and well documented[11,12] (see Chapter 10). The related issue of homelessness, with its associated hazard of exposure, added to poor nutrition, inadequate medical care, and frequent exposure to trauma were serious contributing factors.

By reviewing birth certificates, the perinatal outcome of 43 of these patients was obtained. Twenty-one of the patients were from a long-term state facility with an average stay of 77 days, and 22 patients were from an acute care university hospital psychiatric unit, with an average stay of 7 days. The demographic characteristics between these two groups did not differ to any significant degree. Their psychiatric history and obstetrical history were also similar.

It was originally hypothesized that the group of patients from the state hospital would have better perinatal outcome than patients from the university psychiatric unit because of better access to prenatal care. However, when the groups were compared in terms of the incidence of small-for-gestational-age infants, adequate versus no prenatal care, pregnancy complications, and congenital anomalies, no significant differences were found. Several other variables were studied: greater than 30-day stay versus less than 30-day stay, greater than 60-day stay versus less than 60-day stay, psychotic diagnosis versus nonpsychotic diagnosis, greater than five previous admissions and invol-

Table 9.2 Comparison of Patients Who Kept Follow-up Obstetrical Prenatal Appointment vs. Those Who Did Not

	Kept appointment (%)	Did not keep appointment (%)	
Number of patients	12	14	
Average age (years)	24.5	31.35	1*
Married	7 (58)	3 (21)	
Single	4 (33)	11 (79)	
Unemployed	7 (58)	14 (100)	2*
Living situation			
Husband/family	9 (75)	3 (21)	
Apartment alone	2 (17)	2 (14)	
No address	1 (8)	9 (64)	3*
Voluntary admission	10 (83)	7 (50)	
Involuntary admission	2 (17)	7 (50)	
Psychiatric history			
Previous admissions			
0	5 (42)	6 (43)	
5 or less	4 (33)	3 (21)	
More than 5	3 (25)	5 (36)	
Substance use	6 (50)	10 (71)	
Previous psychiatric medications	6 (50)	8 (57)	
Obstetrical history			
Previous prenatal visit	10 (83)	4 (29)	4*
Adequate prenatal care	8 (67)	1 (7)	5*
Attitudes			
Pregnancy planned	8 (67)	1 (7)	6*
Positive attitude	10 (83)	10 (71)	
Negative attitude	0	0	
Ambivalent	2 (17)	4 (29)	
Discharge diagnosis			
Schizophrenia	2 (17)	8 (57)	
Adjustment disorder	7 (58)	1 (7)	
Substance abuse	1 (8)	2 (14)	
Depression	1 (8)	1 (7)	
Conduct disorder	1 (8)	0	
Bipolar disorder	0	1 (7)	
Atypical psychosis	0	1 (7)	
Psychotic	2 (17)	10 (71)	

* Statistical significance: 1, $T = 3.17$, $df = 23.85$, p < 0.0042;
2, $\chi^2_2 = 4.7888$, $df = 1$, $p < 0.0286$;
3, $\chi^2_2 = 6.3462$, $df = 1$, $p < 0.0118$;
4, $\chi^2_2 = 5.7492$, $df = 1$, $p < 0.0165$;
5, $\chi^2_2 = 7.6562$, $df = 1$, $p < 0.0057$;
6, $\chi^2_2 = 7.6562$, $df = 1$, $p < 0.0057$;
7, $\chi^2_2 = 5.7492$, $df = 1$, $p < 0.0165$ (psychotic vs all other diagnoses).

From Miller et al,[18] with permission.

untary versus voluntary admissions status. Again, no significant differences were found in regard to perinatal outcome. It was assumed longer hospitalization meant better prenatal care, hence improved perinatal outcome. Yet there were no differences in the number of obstetrical consultations between the two groups. Twenty-nine percent of patients received an obstetrical consultation when admitted in the first trimester, 77% were admitted in the second trimester, and 80% were admitted in the third trimester. The average number of days prior to an obstetrical consult was 34 days in the state hospital. This indicates that the amount of prenatal contact received in this state hospital was minimal and not much different from that in the acute care facility.

It is important to recognize that these patients were *not* a normal population of obstetric cases. In comparing these 43 mentally ill patients to outcomes recorded in the state of Oregon's statistics, there are several significant differences. These include an increased incidence of intrauterine growth retardation, inadequate prenatal care, and pregnancy complications in the mentally ill group. Low birth weight is considered to be an important predictor of developmental problems.[13] Among the known risk factors for low-birth-weight infants, inadequate prenatal care—defined as fewer than five visits or not seen until the third trimester—plays an significant role.[13] Based on national statistics, the incidence of inadequate care is 87.2 per 1000 births, strikingly different from the incidence of 409 per 1000 births in this group of hospitalized psychiatric patients.[14]

Recently, several review articles looking at long-term inpatient management of pregnant psychiatric patients have shown improved perinatal outcome as a result of close prenatal observation permitting appropriate obstetrical intervention.[15–17] If adequate obstetrical care could be provided in a long-term setting, it would be important to identify which factors lead to lack of outpatient compliance with prenatal care. Noncompliant patients could then be referred to a long-term facility where continued psychiatric treatment *and* prenatal care could be provided.

A study of patients admitted to an acute care psychiatric unit in a university hospital, with an average stay of 7 days, found 52% of the patients kept their outpatient follow-up prenatal care appointment.[18] There were several important differences between the group who kept their follow-up prenatal care appointment versus those who did not (Table 9.2). The group that did not keep the prenatal care appointment tended to be experiencing an unplanned pregnancy, to be older, unemployed, living on the street, with no previous prenatal care, and with a psychotic presentation. No difference was noted in the psychiatric history or incidence of admitted substance abuse. Also, no specific hospital interventions during the short stay were noted to have significantly improved the ability of the patient to keep the follow-up prenatal care appointment.

Pathophysiology

Table 9.1 shows that the majority of inpatient pregnant patients (61%) had disorders involving psychosis. Psychosis is defined as a gross distortion of reality, including hallucinations, paranoid ideation, and/or delusions. Psychosis can be a symptom for a number of diagnoses, such as schizophrenia and affective disorders (including depression and bipolar disorder), as well as drug-induced states.

Schizophrenia includes psychotic symptoms and behavior changes. There are disturbances in functioning at work or socially, or problems related to self-care. By definition these difficulties need to have been below levels of previous functioning and to have been present for a period of greater than 6 months. Schizophrenia occurs at a rate of approximately 12% if a parent has a diagnosis of schizophrenia and up to 40% if both parents have the disorder. These data and twin studies support a genetic component in the etiology of this illness. Nongenetic factors in etiology may include birth trauma, family environment, and stressful life events. It appears that there is a polygenic predisposition which, with exposure to specific polyvariant environmental insults, may move an individual toward a clinical illness.

Affective disorders include both depression and bipolar illness (see Chapter 6). These illnesses can include psychotic symptoms. The major feature of the affective disorders is mood alteration. Depression is characterized by chronic low dysphoric mood changes, while bipolar disorders involve mood cycling—manic or elevated moods alternating with varying episodes of depressed mood.

Depression is the most frequent of the affective disorders, occurring in 10% to 20% of women. Specific biological factors, including changes in neurotransmitters (norepinephrine and serotonin) and neuroreceptors, as well as neuroendocrine changes in the limbic-hypothalamic-pituitary-adrenal axis, are important in the pathophysiology of depression. In addition, psychosocial factors such as stressful life events and maladaptive coping mechanisms are generally believed to play a major role in provoking specific depressive episodes.

Bipolar illness has a more specific genetic background, as reflected in pedigree studies. Fifty percent of bipolar patients have a family history of an affective disorder, and the concordance rate for monozygotic twins is 67%. The specific psychological and environmental factors are balanced to play a minimal role in bipolar illnesses. The classical course of this illness is characterized by episodic mood changes occurring as frequently as monthly or as rarely as every 2 to 4 years.

Treatment

Treatment decisions in mentally ill pregnant women are affected by illness characteristics, including the specific diagnosis, the severity of symptoms, and the usual time course of the illness in the individual person. Other issues that need consideration include the history of previous response to pharmacological and nonpharmacological treatments, and the availability of a support system. Further, placement of the woman in the least restrictive environment, consistent with appropriate evaluation and treatment, is critical. If the woman is hospitalized, the length of stay is important, as well as her history of previous compliance with treatment. As always, practical choices need to be made. For example, it is difficult to justify treating a patient for only a few days in the hospital with any type of psychotropic medication unless unusual circumstances exist.

There are distinct risks to be considered in *failing* to treat. As has been suggested, neglect of the prenatal care, followed perhaps by infant neglect, is a problem especially in these chronically mentally ill women (see Chapter 11). Also of importance is the high incidence of the abuse of drugs and alcohol, perhaps used as self-medication. Denial of the pregnancy and the risks of infanticide in a patient who has psychotic or manic symptoms is a serious, but fortunately rare occurrence.[19] The lack of treatment also contributes to homelessness, with its increased risk of exposure and trauma, the risk of suicide, impaired attachment to the child, and related difficulties in parenting.

Drug Therapy

Sixty-five percent of all patients receiving psychotropic drugs are women, of whom 50% are of childbearing age.[20] Ten percent to 20% of women of childbearing age are taking an antidepressant.[20] In considering drug therapy during pregnancy it is best to assume that *all* psychotropic drugs have some effect on the fetus.[21-23]

There are distinct limitations in our knowledge concerning the risk and benefits to drug use during pregnancy (see Chapter 19). The critical research on how psychotropic medication effects developing pregnancy cannot be performed for both practical and ethical reasons. Not surprisingly, many problems exist with the available data. Much of the literature consists of anecdotal case reports involving relatively small numbers of patients. This means that risk-benefit ratios are unclear, and present practice may either underestimate or overestimate the risks involved. The best that can be done is to use drugs cautiously, be aware of the limitations of the available literature, and choose agents with the best track record and lowest theoretical risk.

In individuals on chronic medication, preconceptual counseling is important. In such discussions, if possible, the effects of the individual's illness on pregnancy, the genetic risks, and the potential medication effects on the developing pregnancy need to be reviewed. An important issue is the possibility of stopping or decreasing doses of medicine prior to conception or changing to less potentially toxic compounds.

The stage of pregnancy also influences decisions regarding interventions with medications. In the first trimester, there is the concern of a possible increase in fetal loss or anomaly secondary to drug exposure during the period of early organogenesis.[24,25] Concerns during the second and third trimester focus more on long-term neurobehavioral effects from fetal exposure to psychotropic medications.

Maternal concerns related to effects of drugs on the maternal-fetal circulatory system, such as orthostatic hypotension or fetal withdrawal,[26] need to be considered. Specifically, at the time of delivery, it is important to consider metabolic and hormonal changes occurring in the mother and their impact on maternal and fetal blood levels of medication. In regard to lactation, most psychotropic medications cross into the breast milk.[27] Other concerns include postpartum psychiatric disorders, as in bipolar patients, where the incidence of a postpartum psychosis/depression is increased. In this setting, the prophylactic administration of psychotropic medication has been tried and bears consideration.[28]

Other Treatments

In unusual and acute situations, restraints may be needed in order to temporarily control an agitated or aggressive patient and allow time for assessment. When using restraints in pregnancy, it is important to avoid placing the woman in supine position in order to decrease the chance of supine hypotension. Restraining a person on their side with a cross-leg technique or simply putting a pillow underneath their hip to tilt them to the left can be helpful in avoiding supine hypotension. The only studies on the potential long-term effects of restraints in pregnancy were performed in animal models. These studies indicate that restraints reduce the liter size in rats and resulted in growth retardation in monkeys.[31,32] The clinical implications of such data for human medicine are at best unclear but serve to remind the clinician that the use of restraints is a *potential* fetal threat. Chemical control of unacceptable behavior is best.

Electroconvulsive therapy is valuable in certain situations and with attention to detail can be a safe method of treatment during pregnancy.[32] In the acutely catatonic, manic, or suicidal patient with a depressive disorder, especially if medications have not been successful, electroconvulsive therapy (ECT) may be the treatment of choice. Attention to oxygenation, relaxation, and adequate fetal monitoring is important. One must not forget that this procedure also entails the giving of an anesthetic. Several case reports document the dramatic effectiveness and safety of ECT during pregnancy when there is close attention to maternal and fetal condition.[33] With care, ECT retains a role in clinical management (see Chapter 20).

Obstetrical Surveillance

Most important in the obstetrical management of women with chronic psychiatric disease is ongoing, regular prenatal care. Routine examinations and serial ultrasonic studies allow the detection of most of the important problems that may arise during a woman's pregnancy. Problems are evaluated and treated in the usual manner. Early ultrasound is valuable in the chronic mentally ill patient. Often, there are questionable dates or date-size discrepancies, and an ultrasound is critical in establishing the true estimated date of confinement. It is important to emphasize that appropriate ongoing prenatal care with the usual attention to detail and usual studies of fetal growth is the most important obstetrical surveillance that we can provide for this group of patients.

Intrapartum management is the same as that for normal patients. It is prudent to inform the pediatrician of the labor and provide a reliable support person. Issues of operative delivery and anesthesia, ideally, should have been discussed long before the onset of labor. During labor it is certainly reasonable to administer epidural anesthesia, if possible, to reduce maternal distress.

Several types of medications are useful in pregnant women for sedation in acute agitation. One is haloperidol (Haldol), 2.5–5 mg IM, q 30 minutes, not to exceed 20–30 mg in a 24-hour period. Another neuroleptic medication that can be very effective is droperidol (Fentanyl), 1–2 cc IM q 1–2 hours, not to exceed 6 cc in a 24-hour period. When using neuroleptics, one must be cognizant of the possibility of a dystonic reaction, which should be treated with small parenteral doses of either diphen- hydramine (Benadryl) or benzotropine. Also effective in controlling acute agitated or aggressive behavior is lorazepam

(Ativan), administered as 1–2 mg po IM q 1–3 hours, not to exceed 10–12 mg in a 24-hour period. If given to a laboring woman, all of these drugs will cross the placenta and affect the neonate and likely alter the fetal heart rate pattern on the electronic fetal monitoring strip. The pediatrician must be informed that such medications have been given so that proper support will be available when the child is born.

Conclusions

Pregnancy is a period of emotional stress and, for some women, a time of high potential for psychiatric breakdown. This is particularly true for women with a history of mental disturbance.

The preponderance of evidence indicates that there is a relationship between chronic mental illness and increased pregnancy/birth complications. Ongoing prenatal care improves the outcome of pregnancy, particularly among this high-risk, indigent, and/or substance-abusing population. The sometimes complicated process required to link with various health care providers is difficult for this group of patients. Their misperceptions and bizarre behavior often prevent them from appropriate use of available services. This is a setting in which the impact of the clinician is critical. It should be emphasized that it is the lack of consistent, competent obstetrical care that is the major factor in the increase of pregnancy and birth complications characteristic of this population of the chronically mentally ill.

Identification of this problem and responding to it are different issues. Special strategies are often required to cajole these individuals into care programs. For example, community mental health centers assume great importance for psychiatric patients identified as noncompliant with routine prenatal care follow-up. Close case management is helpful in treating the chronically mentally ill, by improving psychiatric and medical care.[34] Providing obstetrical information and training to mental health care providers increases awareness of the importance of ongoing prenatal care, which improves obstetrical follow-up for this group of patients.

The group of pregnant women noncompliant with their arranged prenatal follow-up contains a large proportion (50%) of involuntary patients. In a study done in the state of Oregon, the patient's pregnancy did not appear to affect the process of commitment.[13] The legal issues in these cases are particularly difficult. In the courtroom, a woman's individual rights can conflict with those of the fetus. Forced treatment versus the rights of the mother to determine her own care is a difficult ethical question[35,36] (see Chapters 2 and 3). Involuntary intervention with pregnant women, even with clear medical indications and a firm belief in moral ascendency, is at best controversial. However, in selected cases, involuntary commitment needs reexamination if adequate prenatal care cannot be provided in other ways.

Unfortunately, under most circumstances it is difficult to obtain long-term inpatient care for these women. The developing concept of outpatient commitment has recently emerged in some states and may provide a partial solution.[37] This permits monitoring of the patient's follow-up with psychiatric and obstetrical care, using the alternative of involuntary inpatient care when necessary. If legal and ethical issues can be clarified, such outpatient commitment could provide some leverage in encouraging outpatient prenatal follow-up for otherwise poorly compliant women.

In selected cases, brief psychiatric hospitalization of these pregnant mentally ill women provides an opportunity to influence the outcome of their pregnancy. This allows physicians and staff to get information about the pregnant patient, including past and current pregnancy histories. This information can help identify those patients at risk for compliance with ongoing prenatal care. Early in pregnancy is an ideal time to get prenatal laboratory tests and information for dating pregnancy, as well as for performing fetal surveillance. All of these influence the woman's prenatal care needs and, eventually, the outcome of the pregnancy. Obstetrical consultations during a patient's hospitalization should be obtained. This may provide an opportunity to develop an ongoing relationship with prenatal care providers and/or mental health care providers, leading to improved follow-up care after discharge.

One of the most difficult problems a psychiatric unit faces is admitting a poorly compliant pregnant patient. One of the most difficult situations in a labor/delivery and postpartum unit is an acutely ill psychiatric patient. Education and consultation/liaison between these two specialties cannot be overemphasized for improving the outcome for these challenging pregnancies.

References

1. Nielson, Kaij L: Women with non-organic psychosis: Mental disturbance during pregnancy. *Acta Psychiatr Scand* 1984;70:127–139.
2. McNeil TF, Kaij L: Women with non-organic psychosis: Pregnancy's effect on mental health during pregnancy. *Acta Psychiatr Scand* 1984;70:140–148.
3. Sobel DE: Infant mortality and malformations in children of schizophrenic women. *Psychiatr Q* 1961;35:60–64.
4. Sameroff A, Zax M: Perinatal characteristics in the offspring of schizophrenic women. *J Nerv Ment Dis* 1973;157:191–199.
5. Zax M, Sameroff A, Babigian H: Birth outcomes in the offspring of mentally disordered women. *Am J Orthopsychiatry* 1977;47:218–230.
6. McNeil TF, Persson-Blennow I, Kaij L: Reproduction in female psychiatric patients: Severity of mental disturbance near reproduction and rates of obstetric complications. *Acta Psychiatr Scand* 1974;50:23–32.
7. Rieder RO, Rosenthal D, Wender P, Blumenthal H: The offspring of schizophrenics: Fetal and neonatal deaths. *Arch Gen Psychiatry* 1975;32:200–211.
8. Cohler BJ, Gallant DH, Grunebaum HU, et al: Pregnancy and birth complications among mentally ill and well mothers and their children. *Soc Biol* 1975;22:269–278.
9. Wrede G, Mednick SA, Huttunen MO, Nilsson CG: Pregnancy and delivery complications in the births of an unselected series of Finnish children with schizophrenic mothers. *Acta Psychiatr Scand* 1980;62:369–381.
10. Chasnoff IJ: Drugs and women: Establishing a standard of care. *Ann NY Acad Sci* 1989;562:208–210.
11. MacGregor S, Keith LG, Chasnoff IJ, et al: Cocaine use during pregnancy: Adverse perinatal outcome. *Am J Obstet Gynecol* 1987;157:686–690.
12. Cherukuri R, Minkoff H, Feldman J, et al: A cohort study of alkaloidal cocaine ("crack") in pregnancy. *Obstet Gynecol* 1988;72:147–151.
13. Center for Health Statistics: *Medicaid Support and Birth Outcome*. Portland, Oregon Department of Human Resources, 1986.

14. Center for Health Statistics: *Oregon Vital Statistics*. Portland, Oregon Department of Human Resources, 1987.

15. Chang SS, Renshaw DC: Psychosis and Pregnancy. *Compr Ther* 1986;12:36–41.

16. Mugtader S, Hamann MW, Molnar G: Management of psychotic pregnant patients in a medical-psychiatric unit. *Psychosomatics* 1986;27:31–33.

17. Spielvogel A, Wele J: Treatment of the psychotic pregnant patient. *Psychosomatics* 1986;27:487–492.

18. Miller WH, Resnick MP, Williams MH, Bloom JD: The pregnant psychiatric inpatient: A missed opportunity. *Gen Hosp Psychiatry* 1990;12:373–378.

19. Slayton RI, Soloff PH: Psychiatric denial of third-trimester pregnancy. *Clin Psychiatry* 1981;42:471–473.

20. Carmen E: Inequality and women's mental health: An overview. *Am J Psychiatry* 1981;138:1319–1330.

21. Kerns L: Treatment of mental disorders in pregnancy: A review of neuroleptics, antidepressants, and lithium carbonate. *Jeff J Psychiatry* 1986;4(2):22–36.

22. Nurnberg GH, Prudic J: Guidelines for treatment of psychosis during pregnancy. *Hosp Community Psychiatry* 1984;35:67–71.

23. Guze BH, Guze PA: Psychotropic medication use during pregnancy. *West J Med* 151:296–298.

24. Weber LW: Benzodiazepines in pregnancy—an academic debate or teratogenic risk? *Biol Res Pregnancy Perinatol* 1985;6:151–167.

25. Jones KL, Lauo Ru, Johnson BA, Adams J: Pattern of malformation in the children of women treated with carbamazine during pregnancy. *N Engl J Med* 1989;320:1661–1666.

26. Eggermont E: Withdrawal symptoms in neonate associated with maternal imipramine therapy. *Lancet* 1973;2:680–686.

27. American Academy of Pediatrics Committee on Drugs: Psychotropic drugs in pregnancy and lactation. *Pediatrics* 1982;69:241–244.

28. Inwood DG (ed.): *Recent Advances in Postpartum Psychiatric Disorders*. Washington, DC, American Psychiatric Association Press, 1985.

29. Cohen LS, Heller UL, Rosenbaum JF: Treatment guidelines for psychotropic drug use in pregnancy. *Psychosomatics* 1989;30:25–33.

30. Wiebold JL, et al: The effect of restraint stress in early pregnancy in mice. *J Reprod Fertil* 1986;78:185–192.

31. Golub M, Anderson J: Adaptation of pregnant Rhesus monkeys to short-term chair restraint. *Lab Anim Sci* 1986;36:507–511.

32. Remick R, Maruice W: ECT in pregnancy. *Am J Psychiatry* 1978;135:761–762.

33. Varan LR, Gillieson MS, Skane DS, et al: ECT in acutely psychotic pregnant women with actively aggressive homicidal impulses. *Can J Psychiatry* 1985;30:363–367.

34. Bond GR, Miller LD, Krumweed RD, Ward RS: Assertive case management in three CMHCs: A controlled study. *Hosp Community Psychiatry* 1988;39:411–418.

35. Soloff PH, Jewell S, Roth LH: Civil commitment and the rights of the unborn. *Am J Psychiatry* 1979;136:114–115.

36. Kolder VE, Gallagher J, Parons MT: Court-ordered obstetrical interventions. *N Engl J Med* 1987;316:1192–1196.

37. APA Task Force Report No. 26: New outpatient commitment guidelines stress clinician's role in assuring appropriate care. *Hosp Community Psychiatry* 1987;38:1343–1344.

Chapter 10

Anorexia and Bulimia

Leon Speroff, MD

> Women who are very lean, have miscarriages when
> they prove with child, until they get into better
> condition.
> > *Aphorisms*
> > —Hippocrates (c 460–375 BC)

St. Wilgefortis was the seventh daughter of the king of Portugal, living around the year 1000.[1] When confronted with an arranged marriage (she had made a vow of virginity to become a nun), she turned to intense prayer. The intensity of the prayer was marked by anorexia and the growth of body hair. Confronted with this new appearance, the king of Sicily changed his mind about the marriage, and Wilgefortis's father had her crucified. Around 1200, the legend of Wilgefortis spread throughout Europe. The fact that the cult that developed centered around women with different names has suggested that many girls underwent an experience similar to that of Wilgefortis.

St. Wilgefortis became a symbol of a woman who liberated herself of female problems. She became a protectress of women with sexual problems, including difficulties associated with childbirth. Indeed, women who wished to rid themselves of their husbands prayed to her, since she had successfully resisted both a father and a potential husband. In England, she was known as St. Uncumber because women believed that with her intervention they could be "uncumbered" of their husbands.

Thus emerged the medieval dark ages explanation (with ascendancy to sainthood) of a girl's response (anorexia nervosa) to her fears of marriage and sexuality. Our understanding of the reason for this extraordinary behavior today continues to focus on an inability to cope with the onset of adult sexuality, with a return to the prepubertal state. Both anorexia nervosa and bulimia nervosa (binge eating) are distinguished by a morbid fear of fatness.

Clinical Presentation

Anorexia Nervosa

It is a common experience for a physician to be the first to recognize anorexia nervosa in a woman with the complaint of amenorrhea. It is also not infrequent that a physician will evaluate and manage an infertility problem due to hypogonadotropism and not be aware of a developing case of anorexia. Because the mortality rate associated with this syndrome is significant (5%–15%), and because the obstetrical consequences are potentially serious, it is important that clinicians be alerted to the importance of this condition.

Anorexia nervosa occurs almost exclusively in young white middle- to-upper-class females under age 25 (Table 10.1). Although eating disorders do occur in other races, recognition is hampered by the stereotype of the patient as white and middle class.[2] The families of anorectics are success-achievement-appearance oriented. Serious problems may be present within the family, but the parents make every effort to maintain an apparent marital harmony, glossing over or denying conflicts. Anorexia can be considered to be a condition that identifies a genuinely disturbed family.[3]

At puberty, normal weight gain may be interpreted as excessive, and this can trip the teenager over into true anorexia nervosa. Excessive physical activity can be the earliest sign of incipient anorexia nervosa. Such children are characteristically overachievers and strivers. They seldom give any trouble, but are judgmental and then demand that others live up to their rigid value system, often resulting in social isolation.

The cultural value our society places on thinness definitely plays a role in eating disorders. Both occupational and recreational environments that stress

Table 10.1 Diagnosis of Anorexia Nervosa

1. Onset between ages 10 and 30 years

2. Weight loss of 25%, or weight 15% below normal for age and height

3. Special attitudes:

    Denial

    Distorted body image

    Unusual hoarding or handling of food

4. At least one of the following:

    Lanugo

    Bradycardia

    Overactivity

    Episodes of overeating (bulimia)

    Vomiting, which may be self-induced

5. Amenorrhea

6. No known medical illness

7. No other psychiatric disorder

8. Other characteristics:

    Constipation

    Low blood pressure

    Hypercarotenemia

    Diabetes insipidus

thinness put women at greater risk for anorexia nervosa and bulimia. Basically, an eating disorder progressively becomes a method of solving a psychological dilemma.

It is uncertain whether the incidence of eating disorders is increasing or whether a perceived increase is due to greater recognition and a growing population. A survey of schoolgirls in the United Kingdom discovered a prevalence of 1 in 20.[4] The serious case of anorexia nervosa is seen more often by an internist. However, the borderline anorectic frequently presents to a gynecologist, pediatrician, or family physician. Such a patient is often a teenager who has low body weight, amenorrhea, and hyperactivity (excellent grades and many extracurricular activities). The amenorrhea can precede, follow, or appear coincidentally with the weight loss.

Besides amenorrhea, constipation is a common symptom, often severe and accompanied by abdominal pain. The preoccupation with food may manifest itself by large intakes of lettuce, raw vegetables, and low-calorie foods. Hypotension, hypothermia, rough dry skin, soft lanugo-type hair on the back and buttocks, bradycardia, and peripheral edema are the most commonly encountered clinical signs. Long-term diuretic and laxative abuse may produce significant hypokalemia and occasionally muscular weakness. An elevation of the serum carotene is not always associated with a large intake of yellow vegetables, suggesting that a defect in vitamin A utilization is present. The characteristic yellowish coloration of the skin is usually seen on the palms.

Pathophysiology
Hypothalamic Dysfunction

The various problems associated with anorexia represent dysfunction of the body mechanisms regulated by the hypothalamus: appetite, thirst and water conservation, temperature, sleep, autonomic balance, and endocrine secretion.[5] Endocrine studies can be summarized as follows: follicle-stimulating hormone (FSH) and luteinizing hormone (LH) levels are low, cortisol levels are elevated due to decreased clearance in the face of a normal production rate, prolactin levels are normal, thyroid-stimulating hormone (TSH) and hypothalamic (T_4) levels are normal, but the 3,5,3'-triiodothyronine (T_3) level is low and reverse T_3 is high. Indeed, many of the symptoms can be explained by relative hypothyroidism (constipation, cold intolerance, bradycardia, hypotension, dry skin, low metabolic rates, hypercarotenemia). This appears to be a compensation to the state of undernourishment, with a change from formation of the active T_3 form of thyroid hormone to the inactive metabolite, reverse T_3. With weight gain, all of the metabolic changes revert to normal. Even though normal gonadotropin secretion may be restored with weight gain, 30% of patients remain amenorrheic.[5]

The central origin for the amenorrhea is suggested by the demonstration that the response to gonadotropin-releasing hormone (Gn-RH) is regained at approximately 15% below the ideal weight, and this return to normal responsiveness occurs before the resumption of menses.[6] Patients with anorexia nervosa have persistent low levels of gonadotropins similar to prepubertal children. With weight gain, sleep-associated episodic secretion of LH appears, similar to the early pubertal child. With full recovery, the 24-hour pattern is similar to that of an adult, marked by fluctuating peaks. This sequence of changes with increasing and decreasing weight is explained by increasing and decreasing pulsatile secretion of Gn-RH.

Exercise and Amenorrhea

Competitive female athletes, as well as women engaged in strenuous recreational exercise or in other forms of demanding activity such as ballet and modern dance, have a significant incidence of menstrual irregularity and amenorrhea. There appear to be two critical influences: the level of body fat and the effect of stress itself. The critical weight hypothesis states that the onset and regularity of menstrual function necessitate maintaining weight above a critical level and, therefore, above a critical amount of body fat.[7]

In addition to the role of body fat, stress and energy expenditure play an independent role. Warren has pointed out that dancers will have a return of menses during intervals of rest, despite no change in body weight or percent body fat.[8] High energy output and stress, therefore, may act independently, in addition to low body fat, in suppressing reproductive function. It is not surprising that a woman with low body weight who is engaged in competitive activity (athletic or aesthetic) is highly susceptible to anovulation and amenorrhea.

The site of Gn-RH secretion, the arcuate nucleus area in the hypothalamus, is rich in opioid receptors and endorphin production. There is considerable evidence indicating that endogenous opiates inhibit gonadotropin secretion by suppressing hypothalamic Gn-RH. Women studied during a period of endurance conditioning demonstrate a steadily increasing endorphin output after exercise.[9–11] This link of endorphins to the menstrual suppression associated with exercise is plausible, but yet unproven. How this suppression is further intensified or activated by a state of low body fat is unknown.

In the subculture of exercise and amenorrhea, the characteristics strikingly remind one of anorexia nervosa: significant physical exercise, a necessity for control of the body, striving for artistic and technical proficiency, and the consequent preoccupation with the body, together with the stressful pressures of performing and competition. Individuals in this lifestyle are prone to develop what can be called the anorectic reaction. Fries[12] has described four stages of dieting behavior which can form a continuum:

1. Dieting for cosmetic reasons
2. Dieting due to neurotic fixation on food intake and weight
3. The anorectic reaction
4. True anorexia nervosa

Differential Diagnosis

There are important distinctions between the *anorectic reaction* and true *anorexia nervosa*. Women with established anorexia have a misconception of reality and a lack of insight into the disease and their problem. They do not consider themselves underweight and display an impressive lack of concern over their dreadful physical condition and appearance. The doctor- patient relationship is difficult. There is often no visible emotional involvement and a great deal of mistrust. On the other hand, women with the anorectic reaction have the capability for self-criticism. They can see the problem and describe it with insight and an absence of denial. As the exercising woman deliberately makes an effort to decrease body weight, the individual with the anorectic reaction develops her syndrome consciously and voluntarily just as in anorexia nervosa. A clinician may be the first to be aware of the problem, having encountered the patient because of the present complaint of either amenorrhea or now uncontrolled weight loss. Early recognition, concentrated counseling, and confidential support may intercept and prevent a worsening of the problem.

Bulimia Nervosa

Bulimia is a syndrome marked by episodic and secretive binge eating followed by self-induced vomiting, fasting, or the use of laxatives and diuretics.[3] It appears to be a growing problem among young women (up to 4% in some estimates); however, careful study indicates that while bulimic behaviors may be relatively common, clinically significant bulimia is not (approximately 1.0% of female students and 0.1% of male students in a college sample, and 1.1% of females and 0.5% of males in a general practice population).[13-15] Bulimic behavior is frequently seen in patients with anorexia nervosa, but not in all. Patients with bulimia tend to be older and married. The binge eating is followed by some excessive behavior to avoid getting fat.[16] Although this is usually self-induced vomiting, it can also result from excessive exercise or an outrageously strict diet. Patients with bulimia have a high incidence of depressive symptoms, and a problem with shoplifting (usually food). They also are often dependent upon drugs and alcohol. A woman with bulimia is anxious, lonely, and frustrated. Her habitual binging and purging soon interfere with normal social activity, increasing her isolation. The most common complication of bulimia is due to the frequent vomiting: electrolyte imbalance with metabolic sequelae. Various pharmacotherapeutic interventions have yielded good short-term, but poor long-term results, with a high rate of relapse.

There is a growing tendency to divide patients with anorexia nervosa into bulimic anorectics and dieters. Bulimic anorectics are older, less isolated socially, and have a higher incidence of family problems. Body weight in a "pure" bulimic fluctuates but it does not fall to the low levels seen in anorectics.

Treatment

Despite remarkable endocrine changes, extensive laboratory testing in these patients is not necessary. The changes seen are simply secondary to undernourishment. The clinician's attention is better directed to the psychosocial origin of the problem. Continued weight loss in an adult weighing less than 100 pounds requires psychiatric consultation. Some would argue that any patient with an eating disorder requires psychiatric intervention. However, it is disappointing that despite the impressive studies on anorexia, there is no specific or new therapy available. This only serves to emphasize the need for early recognition in order to allow psychological intervention *before* the syndrome is entrenched in its full severity. Physicians (and parents) should pay particular attention to weight and diet in young women with amenorrhea.

Prognosis is excellent with early recognition, and simple weight gain may reverse the state of amenorrhea. The degree of reversibility is unknown, although general experience indicates that the majority of women regain ovulation when stress and exercise diminish or cease.[17,18] However, these patients are often unwilling to give up their routines of exercise, and a sensitive clinician can perceive that the exercise is an important means for coping with daily life. Hormone replacement therapy is therefore encouraged for these hypoestrogenic patients. It is now apparent that the exercise is not sufficient to balance the loss of estrogen protection against osteoporosis.

Clinical Issues

Eating Disorders and Pregnancy

It has been estimated that a typical pregnancy requires approximately 300 extra calories per day above that needed in the nonpregnant state.[19] With sufficient caloric intake, weight gain during pregnancy averages 10 to 12 kg. Women who are underweight prior to pregnancy need to increase their energy intake and gain 12 to 15 kg. Imagine the reaction of a patient with an eating disorder when confronted with these facts. This is fuel for the fire (the morbid fear of fatness).

Prior to the 1970s, obstetricians vigorously advised their patients to limit weight gain during pregnancy. This sadly misplaced advice could be traced to the false belief that excessive weight gain was the cause or a major contributor to preeclampsia, made labor more difficult, and had a permanently detrimental impact on a woman's figure. More appropriate recommendations emerged in the 1970s, based upon a growing body of information derived from scientific studies. These studies documented the importance of prepregnancy weight as well as weight gain during pregnancy as two very important determinants for infant birth weight.

The critical issue is the relationship between the diet of the mother and the well-being of the fetus. There are three classic studies of acute famine during the dark days of World War II in Leningrad, Holland, and Wuppertal.[20–22] The mean birth weight during the siege of Leningrad declined 550 g to 2789 g. During the Dutch famine, mean birth weight decreased by 300 g; there was no decrease in infants conceived during the famine whose mothers received adequate rations during the third trimester. In Wuppertal, mean birth weight was depressed by 170 to 227 g. These differences are proportional to the level of official rations, the conditions being the worst in Leningrad.

Studies of restriction of calories during pregnancy indicated ready achievement of lesser maternal weight gain, at the expense of lighter birth weights.[23] Women who gain less than 20 pounds compared to those who gain more than 20 pounds are 2.3 times more likely to deliver infants of low birth weight and 1.5 times more likely to have a fetal death.[24] These studies finally led to the abandonment of strict caloric limitations for pregnant women.

In general, studies of dietary supplementation have indicated increases in mean birth weights.[24] The Special Supplemental Food Program for Women, Infants, and Children (WIC) was begun in the United States in 1973. A review of this program finds a significant impact of less preterm labor and delivery, an increase in mean birth weight, and a reduction in late fetal death.[25] These improvements are attributed to an improved maternal physiological status, not upgraded health care. The head circumferences of infants of mothers who participated in WIC were significantly larger, presumably reflecting accelerated brain growth.

Gradually, it came to be appreciated that there is a linear relationship between birth weight and maternal weight gain at all levels of prepregnancy weight.[26-30] However, as prepregnancy weight increases, the importance of maternal weight gain diminishes.[31] Thus, in underweight women, the importance of both prepregnancy weight and weight gain during pregnancy is magnified.

Now that the many circumstances that influence infant birth weight are better recognized, a modern look at this subject is especially helpful. After adjusting for maternal age, race, parity, weight gain, socioeconomic status, cigarette consumption, and gestational age, there is a statistically significant linear relationship between prepregnancy body mass and birth weight, as well as between prenatal weight gain and birth weight.[32,33] Furthermore, the fetal death rate increases exponentially as birth weight decreases at each gestational age.[34] Most importantly, a low prepregnancy weight can be overcome; weight gain during pregnancy (beginning in the first trimester) in underweight women can bring an infant into the normal range for birth weight.[35]

Low birth weight in an infant can be directly attributed to two main influencing factors: prematurity and fetal growth retardation. In developing countries, the major factor is intrauterine growth retardation, while in developed countries, prematurity is the predominant influence.[36] In patients with eating disorders, the outcome of pregnancy is significantly influenced by both factors. This reflects a pregnancy in a subculture struggling with the nutritional risks usually encountered in a developing country in addition to the threat of preterm labor and delivery.

In view of the well-recognized correlation between maternal weight (prepregnancy weight and pregnancy weight gain) and infant size, it is logical to expect a problem with pregnancy outcome in patients with eating disorders. Older reports were anecdotal in nature and usually failed to provide birth weights, since our awareness of the importance of body weight to pregnancy outcome is a relatively recent development.[37-43]

Complications of Pregnancy

More recent reports have documented problems with intrauterine growth retardation and preterm labor. The average maternal weight gain in seven pregnancies in patients with anorexia nervosa was 8 kg; all infants demonstrated retarded growth in the third trimester, followed by accelerated growth after birth.[44] A review of 23 pregnancies in 74 women treated for anorexia or bulimia documented the importance of the severity of the disorder.[45] Women in remission gained more weight and had higher birth weights and 5-minute Apgar scores. Women with active disease had worsening symptoms and psychological problems during pregnancy. The smallest birth weights were born to those with anorexia and bulimia. All the women who were ill at conception continued to be ill. Of the women who successfully breast-fed for 6 months, 9 of the 10 were in remission. The rate of preterm labor and delivery in patients with eating disorders is twice the normal incidence, and in a study of 50 Danish women, the perinatal mortality rate was six times the normal rate.[46]

While some patients with eating disorders do well during pregnancy, the clinician should not be misled.[47] After the pregnancy rapid deterioration usually takes place. Expert help during the pregnancy is highly recommended. Some useful warning signs are the following:

1. Unusual concern regarding body shape
2. Aversion to being weighed
3. Lack of weight gain

Because underweight women frequently are anovulatory, it is not surprising that they represent a significant population in whom ovulation is induced. About 25% of patients with amenorrhea are underweight because of self-imposed dietary restriction.[48] Comparing the outcome of pregnancy in underweight women after spontaneous and induced ovulation, it is apparent that inadequate weight has serious consequences.[49] The underweight women who underwent induction of ovulation failed to gain weight adequately during pregnancy despite care and counseling. As expected, fetal growth retardation and preterm labor were significant problems (Table 10.2).

The seriousness of the problem is heightened because of its presence at conception and during the first trimester. A study of adolescent pregnancy concluded that inadequate weight gain before 24 weeks gestation was associated with a significantly increased risk of having a small-for-gestational-age infant, even when later weight gains brought the cumulative weight gain to within normal adult standards.[50] Later inadequate weight gain was associated with an increased risk of preterm delivery. These results suggest that prevention of preterm delivery and of intrauterine growth retardation requires an effort encompassing the entire pregnancy, best begun prior to conception. A rise in weight of more than 6 kg by the 28th week of pregnancy has predictive value, indicating with a high degree of probability that the rest of pregnancy will progress normally.[51]

An issue requiring further study is the impact of an eating disorder on parenting after delivery. The obstetrician can contribute to this situation with the potential, albeit currently unproven, for positive long-term consequences.

Table 10.2 Intrauterine Growth Retardation (IUGR), Induced Ovulation, and Maternal Weight.

Category	Incidence of IUGR (%)
Normal weight, induced ovulation	2.5
Underweight, spontaneous ovulation	18.0
Underweight, induced ovulation	54.0

Treatment

Dietary restriction decreases birth weight. Dietary manipulation can have as great an impact as a serious famine. The impact on perinatal morbidity and/or mortality has been poorly assessed, but there is reason to believe that preterm labor is increased and that children with impaired intrauterine growth have more problems later in life.

Because growth retardation before the third trimester is associated with potentially serious long-term morbidity, physicians treating amenorrhea associated with weight loss should consider solving the dietary problem before subjecting a fetus to a struggle during intrauterine life. Patients with an active eating disorder should wait for remission before attempting pregnancy. These messages, therefore, apply especially to two groups of physicians: obstetricians and reproductive endocrinologists.

Conclusions

When encountering a pregnant patient with an eating disorder, the obstetrician should seek expert consultation to achieve and maintain remission of the disorder during the pregnancy. Careful serial monitoring of maternal weight gain and of fetal growth is essential. Ultrasonic evaluation of fetal growth every 2 to 3 weeks in the third trimester is best. Consideration should be given to special dietary supplementation, especially when delayed fetal growth is demonstrated. Full exploitation of the pregnancy is warranted to provide motivation for effective resolution of this psychodynamic disorder.

The best results are achieved with stabilization of the eating disorder prior to pregnancy. The reproductive endocrinologist should hesitate before embarking on a program of ovulation induction in such women. The reward of pregnancy should be offered as an inducement to reach a normal prepregnancy weight. Patients with an eating disorder who are considering pregnancy must be made aware of the potential adverse impact of their condition on fetal growth and development.

The timing of psychiatric intervention is important. The prospect of pregnancy should stimulate a preconceptual effort by the patient's physicians. At no other time will the patient's physicians have such a strong ally, the motivating force behind the desire for pregnancy.

References

1. Lacey JH: Anorexia nervosa and a bearded female saint. *Br Med J* 1982;285:1816–1817.
2. Robinson P, Andersen A: Anorexia nervosa in American blacks. *J Psychiatr Res* 1986;19:14–36.
3. Herzog DB, Copeland PM: Eating disorders. *N Engl J Med* 1985;313:295–303.
4. Szmukler GI: The epidemiology of anorexia nervosa and bulimia. *J Psychiatr Res* 1985;19:143–153.
5. Warren MP, Vande Wiele RL: Clinical and metabolic features of anorexia nervosa. *Am J Obstet Gynecol* 1973;117:435–455.
6. Warren MP: The effects of undernutrition on reproductive function in the human.

Endocr Rev 1983;4:363–377.

7. Frisch RE: Body fat, menarche, and reproductive ability. *Semin Reprod Endocrinol* 1985;3:45–54.

8. Warren MP: Effect of exercise and physical training on menarche. *Semin Reprod Endocrinol* 1985;3:17–26.

9. Howlett TA, Tomlin S, Hgahfoong L, et al: Release of beta- endorphin and met-enkephalin during exercise in normal women: Response to training. *Br Med J* 1984;288:1950–1956.

10. Russell JB, Mitchell DE, Musey PI, Collins DC: The role of beta-endorphins and catechol estrogens on the hypothalamic- pituitary axis in female athletes. *Fertil Steril* 1984;42:690–698.

11. Laatikainen T, Virtanen T, Apter D: Plasma immunoreactive beta-endorphin in exercise-associated amenorrhea. *Am J Obstet Gynecol* 1986;154:94–100.

12. Fries H: Secondary amenorrhea, self-induced weight reduction and anorexia nervosa. *Acta Psychiatr Scand* [Suppl] 1984;248.

13. Schotte DE, Stunkard AJ: Bulimia vs bulimic behaviors on a college campus. *JAMA* 1987;258:1213–1218.

14. Herzog DB, Copeland PM: Bulimia nervosa—psyche and satiety. *N Engl J Med* 1988;319:716–717.

15. Kins MB: Eating disorders in a general practice population. Prevalence, characteristics and follow-up at 12 to 18 months. *Psychiatr Med* 1989;14(suppl):1–34.

16. Fairburn CG, Cooper PJ: The clinical features of bulimia nervosa. *Br J Psychiatry* 1984;144:238–246.

17. Bullen BA, Skriinar GS, Beitins IZ, et al: Induction of menstrual disorders by strenuous exercise in untrained women. *N Engl J Med* 1985;312:1349–1355.

18. Stager JM, Ritchie-Flanagan RB, Robertshaw D: Reversibility of amenorrhea in athletes. *N Engl J Med* 1984;310:351–352.

19. Hytten FE, Chamberlain G (eds.): *Clinical Physiology in Obstetrics*. Oxford, Blackwell, 1980.

20. Antonov AN: Children born during the siege of Leningrad in 1942. *J Pediatr* 1947;30:250–259.

21. Smith CA: The effect of wartime starvation in Holland upon pregnancy and its product. *Am J Obstet Gynecol* 1947;53:599–608.

22. Dean RFA: The size of the baby at birth and the yield of breast milk, in *Studies of Under-nutrition. Wuppertal 1946–49*. London, Medical Research Council: Special Report Series, No. 275, Her Majesty's Stationery Office, 1951, pp 346–378.

23. Campbell DM, MacGillivray I: The effect of a low calorie diet or a thiazide diuretic on the incidence of pre-eclampsia and on birthweight. *Br J Obstet Gynaecol* 1975;82:572–577.

24. Rush D: Effects of changes in protein and calorie intake during pregnancy on the growth of the human fetus, in Calmers I, Enkin M, Keirse MJNC (eds.): *Effective Care in Pregnancy and Childbirth*. Oxford, Oxford University Press, 1989, pp 255–280.

25. Taffel SM: *Maternal Weight Gain and the Outcome of Pregnancy: United States, 1980*. Washington, DC, National Center for Health Statistics, Series 21, no. 44, DHHS (PHS) 86, Public Health Service, U.S. Government Printing Office, 1986.

26. Peckham CH, Christianson RE: The relationship between prepregnancy weight and certain obstetric factors. *Am J Obstet Gynecol* 1971;111:1–7.

27. Simpson JW, Lawless RW, Mitchell CA: Responsibility of the obstetrician to the fetus. II. Influence of prepregnancy weight gain on birthweight. *Obstet Gynecol* 1975;45:481–487.

28. Harrison GG, Udall JN, Morrow G: Maternal obesity, weight gain in pregnancy, and infant birth weight. *Am J Obstet Gynecol* 1980;136:411–412.

29. Gormican A, Valentine J, Satter E: Relationships of maternal weight gain, prepregnancy weight, and infant birth weight. *J Am Diet Assoc* 1980;77:662–667.

30. Arbuckle TE, Sherman GJ: Comparison of the risk factors for pre-term delivery and intrauterine growth retardation. *Paediatr Perinat Epidemiol* 1989;3:115–129.

31. Winikoff B, Debrovner CH: Anthropometric determinants of birth weight. *Obstet Gynecol* 1981;58:678–684.

32. Abrams BF, Laros RK: Prepregnancy weight, weight gain, and birth weight. *Am J Obstet Gynecol* 1986;154:503–509.

33. Seidman DS, Ever-Hadani P, Gale R: The effect of maternal weight gain in pregnancy on birth weight. *Obstet Gynecol* 1989;74:240–246.

34. Myers SA, Ferguson R: A population study of the relationship between fetal death and altered fetal growth. *Obstet Gynecol* 1989;74:325–331.

35. Bruce L, Tchabo JG: Nutrition intervention program in a prenatal clinic. *Obstet Gynecol* 1989;74:310–312.

36. Villar J, Belilzan JM: The relative contribution of prematurity and fetal growth retardation to low birth weight in developing and developed societies. *Am J Obstet Gynecol* 1982;143:793–798.

37. Kay DWK, Leigh D: The natural history, treatment and prognosis of anorexia based on a study of 38 patients. *J Ment Sci* 1954;100:411–431.

38. Beck JC, Brockner-Mortensen K: Observation on the prognosis in anorexia nervosa. *Acta Med Scand* 1954;149:409–430.

39. Dally P, Sargant W: Treatment and outcome of anorexia nervosa. *Br Med J* 1966;2:793–795.

40. Farquharson RF, Hyland H: Anorexia nervosa: The course of 15 patients treated from 20 to 30 years previously. *J Can Med Assoc* 1969;94:411–419.

41. Theander S: Anorexia nervosa: A psychiatric investigation of 94 female patients. *Acta Psychiatr Scand* 1970;214(suppl):1–194.

42. Hart T, Kase N, Kimball CP: Induction of ovulation and pregnancy in patients with anorexia nervosa. *Am J Obstet Gynecol* 1970;108:880–884.

43. Willi J, Hagemann R: Langzeitverlaufe von anorexia nervosa. *Schweiz Med Wochenschr* 1976;106:1459–1465.

44. Treasure JL, Russell GFM: Intrauterine growth and neonatal weight gain in babies of women with anorexia nervosa. *Br Med J* 1988;296:1036–1038.

45. Stewart DE, Rasking J, Garfinkel PE, MacDonald OL, Robinson GE: Anorexia nervosa, bulimia, and pregnancy. *Am J Obstet Gynecol* 1987;157:1194–1198.

46. Brinch M, Isager T, Telstrup K: Anorexia nervosa and motherhood: Reproduction pattern and mothering behaviour of 50 women. *Acta Psychiatr Scand* 1988;77:611–617.

47. Lacey JH, Smith G: Bulimia nervosa. The impact of pregnancy on mother and baby. *Br J Psychiatry* 1987;150:777–781.

48. Knuth UA, Hull MGR, Jacobs HS: Amenorrhea and loss of weight. *Br J Obstet Gynaecol* 1977;84:801–807.

49. van der Spuy ZM, Steer PJ, McCusker M, Steele SJ, Jacobs HS: Outcome of pregnancy in underweight women after spontaneous and induced ovulation. *Br Med J* 1988;296:962–965.

50. Hediger ML, Scholl TO, Belsky DH, Ances IG, Salmon RW: Patterns of weight gain in adolescent pregnancy: Effects on birth weight and preterm delivery. *Obstet Gynecol* 1989;74:6–12.

51. Lauckner A, Lauckner W: Significance of initial weight and weight development for the course and outcome of pregnancy. *Zentralbl Gynakol* 1988;110:1018–1029.

Chapter 11

Perinatal Substance Abuse

William H. Miller, Jr., MD and M. Gayle Doucette, MSSA

> They are drunken
> but not with wine
> —Isaiah 29:9

Substance abuse is a serious, cyclic, and self-perpetuating social and medical problem. Addictive behavior has a deleterious impact on the mental and physical health of individuals and major social and legal ramifications. In some communities, substance abuse is already intergenerational. Further, at present, we are barely keeping pace with the problem as it relates to pregnant women. It is increasingly apparent that no segment of our society is free of drug exposure. All of us share in the expense of treatment for drug-related complications and those in clinical medicine now share some of the dangers.

The problems of substance abuse are both complex and frustrating. There are substantial barriers to the adequate identification and treatment of pregnant women who abuse drugs. These difficulties are beyond the simple technical issues of population screening and evaluating fetal or neonatal effects. Chemical dependency is a "soft" and often illusive diagnosis compared to other conditions in obstetrics and gynecology. Also, clinicians commonly perceive pregnant drug abusers as undesirable and difficult patients. Many health care providers feel uncomfortable and undereducated when assessing or treating pregnant women for alcohol and drug use. There are also limitations in our training. For most clinicians, their medical or nursing school experience included little in-depth education about chemical dependency. Thus, many practitioners are ill prepared for this type of history taking as well as medical management for this patient population. Due to the inexperience of many practitioners and their reluctance to become involved in such matters, the diagnosis of substance abuse promotes feelings of helplessness leading at times to the denial that any problem exists. Other perceptions interfere with complete evaluation. In private practice especially, there is a peculiar fear of offending an individual and driving them away if "difficult" or unacceptable questions are asked.

This chapter provides an overview of substance abuse in pregnancy. There are five important objectives: (1) to review the epidemiology of perinatal substance abuse; (2) to detail the medical, obstetrical, and neonatal complications from such abuse; (3) to discuss some psychosocial issues facing the substance-exposed patient; (4) to discuss methods of obtaining a substance-abuse history; and (5) to explore the needs for development of multidiscipline treatment programs targeted at substance-exposed pregnancies.

Ideally, a greater understanding of this complex and unfortunate situation will lead to improved identification and treatment of these problem pregnancies and an increased willingness among practitioners to be more involved in their care.

Epidemiology

Chemical dependency is a disease affecting at least 8 million women between the ages of 15 and 44. This disorder is one of the most commonly missed and potentially dangerous of all obstetric and neonatal diagnoses.[1] However, this omission is not limited to those providing obstetrical care, as 78% of women with substance-abuse problems have never talked with any physician about their problem.[2] Further, many clinicians still believe "nice women" and "good mothers" should not and do not drink to excess or abuse drugs. Consequently, there are a series of major barriers against a woman bringing substance-abuse problems to her doctor's attention, including the shame she feels about her disease, her fear that the physician will think she is "bad" or will be angry with her, and the realistic fear that exposure will lead to legal or social service entanglements.

Unfortunately, in the last several years the substance-abuse problem for pregnant women appears to have become worse and not better. Smith, in a review of the epidemiology of cocaine and alcohol abuse, reports several disturbing trends.[3] For instance, the city of San Francisco reported that cocaine-related cases from coroner's and emergency room data from 1984 to 1985 increased 55% and 47%, respectively. Similar increases have been reported from other major urban areas such as Denver, Los Angeles, and Miami. In 1985, these cities reported cocaine overdose as their number one cause of death. A parallel increase is seen in the number of patients seeking treatment for cocaine abuse. Pharmacologic manipulation of cocaine has changed the pattern of drug use. Since 1986, crack, a crystalline form of cocaine, has become readily available and accessible in all geographic locations and to virtually everyone. Crack is also inexpensive, costing as little as $10 per "hit." People of all ages have been seduced into the business of selling crack cocaine, and the result has been devastating to the health and well-being of many. Recent changes in the sex ratio for cocaine abuse are also of major importance. Increasing numbers of women of the childbearing age are now involved with cocaine addiction. In addition, there has been an increase in polysubstance abuse, with cocaine, opiates, marijuana, tobacco, and alcohol used in various complex combinations.[3]

The National Association for Perinatal Addiction Research and Education (NAPARE) performed a hospital incidence study in 1987, surveying 36 hospitals with over 150,000 deliveries. Overall, the average incidence of illicit psychoactive drug use during pregnancy was 11%.[4] This study found no difference in incidence when comparing hospitals with less than 25% indigent patients to hospitals with greater than 50% indigent patients. The screening protocol used to determine if a woman was a substance abuser was a major factor influencing the actual reported incidence. When clinical suspicion was the only factor leading to drug screening, an incidence of 3% was noted. This compares to an incidence of 16% when all patients were screened by protocol independent of clinical presentation or social standing.[4,5] If these percentages are extrapolated to national birth statistics, then there are more than 350,000 pregnancies exposed to illicit psychoactive substances every year in the United States and the actual number could be considerably higher.

There are other equally disturbing data. In a recent study from Pinellas County, Florida, blinded urine drug screens were performed on women enrolling for prenatal care. Over a 6-month period 380 women from the public health care system and 335 women receiving private health care were studied. There was an overall incidence of 14.8% positive urine screens for alcohol, marijuana, cocaine, and opiates. Of great interest, there were no significant differences in the rates of positive testing in the public versus the private sector or white versus black populations. However, the study workers did find that black substance abusers were 10 times as likely to be reported to social service agencies compared to white substance abusers, despite this apparently equal incidence of documented abuse.[5] These data emphasize the high incidence and widespread social impact of abuse as well as the unequal response of clinicians and social service agencies to such problem pregnancies.

Other substances continue to be abused during pregnancy, including marijuana. Marijuana is relatively easy to obtain and with a reputation of being "harmless" it holds tenaciously to its widespread popularity begun in the mid-1960s. In 1985, about 5,640,000 women 18 years old and over used marijuana—an increase from the number 5,590,000 in 1982.[1] Marijuana is also a popular second drug among those who use cocaine. Babies born to mothers who smoke marijuana are likely to be small for gestational age and to show neurological distress such as abnormal startle reflex, tremors, and inability to shut out disturbing stimuli.

Although our focus is on illicit psychoactive substances, much of what will be discussed also applies to alcohol abuse. Abuse of alcohol is still a major problem and more than 18 million Americans drink alcohol to excess.[6] In women, both the rate of heavy drinking and the incidence of alcohol problems have increased during the past generation. The prevalence of alcoholism in female relatives of alcoholic individuals rose from 6%–7% in 1969 to nearly 21% in 1983.[6,7] Latest estimates show fetal alcohol syndrome (FAS), the third leading cause of birth defects, affects one in every 500 babies born in the United States.[6,8] The effects of alcohol go beyond FAS to include more subtle abnormalities including increased rates of spontaneous abortion, intrauterine growth retardation, and various nonspecific anomalies.[9]

Figure 11.1 presents a paradigm which will be used as a model for discussing the various aspects of substance abuse and its effect on pregnancy, mother, infant, and family.

Patient Profile

Experience has identified three different but overlapping groups of women identified as substance abusers. First is a group of older women, usually over 25 years of age. They are often poorly educated, unemployed, and have other children. This group commonly shows up in an emergency room with an obstetrical complication such as bleeding or preterm labor. After intensive med-

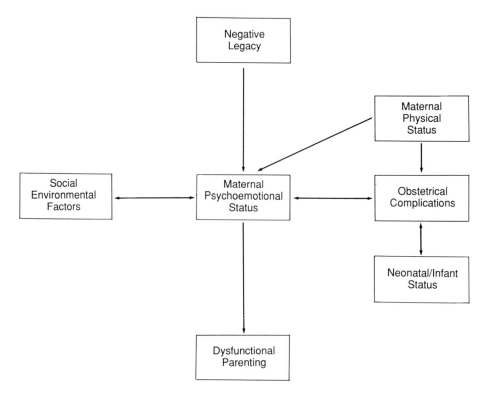

Figure 11.1 A paradigm for perinatal substance abuse.

ical and social intervention, the patient is discharged with a well-thought-out discharge plan. All too often, they fail to show up for any follow- up care, only to be seen when the next crisis occurs. An important initial intervention for this group is obtaining regular prenatal care.

The second group frequently presents to a prenatal clinic in midgestation. After persistent questioning, the patient admits to some type of substance use. This group is usually very concerned about the pregnancy and is seeking prenatal care. They are often younger, unmarried, and with their first pregnancy. These women frequently come from a background of substance abuse in their family of origin and/or in their current peer group. They are usually easier to engage in treatment, but will most likely drop out of treatment if not provided with adequate social support.

The third group is commonly the most unrecognized. These women are usually better educated and employed and/or living with someone employed. They are often older and could be placed in the middle or higher socioeconomic income class. This group is frequently seen by the private prenatal care providers and is often not evaluated for substance abuse for various reasons.

Diagnosis

One need not be an expert in treating chemical dependency in order to identify the problem. A physician can learn much about a patient's drinking and substance-use habits by asking a few simple questions. It is important that the clinician have a nonjudgmental, honest, concerned approach to the history taking. Focusing on the amount of substance used seldom elicits a truthful answer. This may be more true for women than men because of the cultural stigma applied to women using alcohol or drugs. Therefore, questions such as "You don't drink, do you?" or "How much do you drink?" may communicate the clinician's desire to avoid the issue, as well as increasing the guilt, denial, and resistance the patient already feels. The patient and clinician begin to work together to cover up the issue of psychoactive substance use.

General guidelines are available which suggest appropriate introductions to the subject of substance abuse. The natural flow of questions permits such queries to be easily posed within the context of routine history taking.[10] Although these questions were developed primarily for the evaluation of alcohol abuse, the approach is equally valid for other types of substance abuse. The question "Has anyone in your family had a drinking (or drug) problem?" can be incorporated with other questions about family history relating to diabetes, twins, cancer, etc. This indicates substance use is important to the care provider. "Do you ever drink any wine, beer, or mixed drinks?" can be asked when discussing the patient's other habits. If they sometimes do drink, then try to define the drinking behavior by focusing on past behavior, which is less threatening. An example would be "When did you first start drinking?" followed by "How often did you drink at that time?" then "How old were you when you first got drunk?" and "How much were you drinking at the time?" The severity of the problem can be estimated by the patient's reported behaviors when she uses psychoactive substances. Questions such as "Did you get into any trouble because of drinking?" followed by "How much could you drink then?" are helpful.

One can then move to the present after discussing past behaviors, which are less threatening than present behaviors. Questions such as "How much can you hold now?" or "How much can you drink at one time?" are better than "How much do you drink now?" The answers may be more than the interviewer anticipates. Different people have varying perspectives and tolerances, and abusers commonly hold more than others. It can be helpful to suggest a range of ingestion, usually specifying high amounts. If the individual does not drink, they will usually laugh and say "Certainly not."

Although these questions focus on alcohol, it is important to ask about other drug use in the same manner. If one suspects substance abuse, it is helpful to ask about the circumstances, such as amounts used and patterns of use, as well as focusing on psychosocial disruptions that the ingestions produce (see Appendix 11.1).

Clinical Presentation and Differential Diagnosis

Several behavioral indicators should raise the clinician's suspicion regarding the possibility of substance use during pregnancy including:

1. Women who admit to substance abuse prior to pregnancy, but state they have stopped using upon learning of the pregnancy
2. Women who present for labor and delivery without prior prenatal care

3. Women who enter prenatal care late in pregnancy
4. Women who receive only sporadic prenatal care, frequently missing appointments
5. Women who present with premature labor, delivery, or abruptio placentae
6. Women who deliver an unexplained stillborn infant or an infant with anomalies

Clinical identification is closely tied to the complex issue of drug screening. This is usually performed by urinary studies. For patients who match the criteria for suspected use, knowledge that there will be random screening for drugs at prenatal visits can be the motivation needed to remain drug-free during pregnancy. Screening at the time of labor and delivery is also important since even infrequent drug users will sometimes use a stimulant like cocaine to precipitate labor.

Some hospitals practice screening the urine of newborns born to suspected drug abusers with or without informing the parent or obtaining parental consent. Justification for not notifying the parent has been under the guise of child protection, although this practice is generally not condoned and is legally controversial. Because both false-positive and false-negative test results can be due to degrees of operator proficiency, storage of kits, and other factors, at least two tests are usually performed when screening urine for drugs: an initial screen and a confirmation test.

When they can be combined, urinary screening as well as an appropriate history assist in the accurate identification of "at-risk" pregnancies. Frank and co-workers,[11] studying a known cocaine-using population in Boston, found that if a substance-abuse history alone was used without a screen, 26% of the cocaine abusers were not correctly identified. Perhaps more important, 50% of abusing individuals would have been missed if only urine screens were used without a good substance abuse history. This reinforces the importance of *both* an interview directly inquiring about psychoactive substance use *as well as* performance of urinary drug testing if the extent of drug use in a population is to be accurately estimated.

Thus, in clinical application, neither the many testing techniques nor interview techniques are free from problems. The denial, fear, and guilt felt by the pregnant substance user inhibits her discussion of substance use. Urine drug screening, which at first blush appears to be an ideal method for evaluation, does not accurately identify all cases and is potentially subject to laboratory error. Urinary testing is also irregularly applied and bedeviled by ethical and legal controversies.

Pathophysiology

Medical Complications

The list of potential medical complications from substance abuse is extensive (Table 11.1).[12] These problems are either the direct result of substance abuse or are related to the lifestyle of abusing individuals. Illnesses such as diabetes, hepatitis, and hypertension can have dramatic influence on the outcome of

Table 11.1 Potential Medical Complications of Substance Abuse

Anemia	Phlebitis
Bacteremia	Pneumonia
Cardiac disease,	Septicemia
especially endocarditis	Urinary tract infections
Cellulitis	Cystitis
Cerebrovascular accidents	Urethritis
Poor dental hygiene	Pyelonephritis
Diabetes mellitus	Condyloma acuminatum
Gastritis/pancreatitis	Gonorrhea
Hepatitis—acute or chronic	Herpes
Hypertension	Syphilis
Myocardial infarction	AIDS
Pelvic inflammatory disease	Insomnia
Trauma	Menstrual dysfunction

the pregnancy by increasing perinatal morbidity.[13] Urinary tract and venereal infections are important risk factors for preterm labor and delivery.[13] Acquired immunodeficiency syndrome (AIDS), of course, is a major concern in all aspects of medicine, including its effect on the newborn infant, for whom there is a 30% or greater human immunodeficiency virus (HIV) transmission rate.[14] Chronic menstrual irregularities make dating the pregnancy uncertain, creating management difficulties in complicated pregnancies, especially when the mother appears late in gestation.

Obstetrical Complications

Table 11.2 lists most of the frequent obstetrical complications of substance abusers.[12] There are two major groups of problems. The first is *infection*, ie, chorioamnionitis, septic thrombophlebitis, premature rupture of membranes, and preterm labor. This may be related to increased exposure to pathogens or perhaps to a decrease in immune response associated with substance abuse or the abusing lifestyle. The second is *vasospasm*, or constriction of the blood vessels, ie, abruptio placentae, preterm labor, premature rupture of membranes, and intrauterine growth retardation. These complications are particularly relevant to cocaine abuse. It is theorized that vasospasm leads to chronic or possibly recurrent episodes of ischemia of the uterus, placenta, and fetus. Again, a past or current history of such complications should lead the clinician to consider the possibility of substance abuse.

Several studies have found increases in the incidence of specific obstetric complications in substance-exposed pregnancies compared to the incidence in the general obstetric population. For example, dramatic increases are found in premature rupture of membranes (21.1% for cocaine users versus 3.9% for controls), pregnancy-induced hypertension (12.7% versus 4.5%), abruptio placentae (4.2% versus 0.9%), and stillbirth (7.1% versus 1.4%).[10,11] Using matched controls, MacGregor and co-workers performed a prospective study of the effects of cocaine use in pregnancy. He found statistically significant increases

Table 11.2 Potential Obstetrical Complications of
Substance Abuse

Abortion	Intrauterine death
Abruptio placentae	Intrauterine growth retardation
Amnionitis	Placental insufficiency
Breech presentation	Postpartum hemorrhage
Cesarean section	Preeclampsia (PIH)
Chorioamnionitis	Premature labor
Eclampsia	Premature rupture of membranes
Gestational diabetes	Septic thrombophlebitis

in obstetrical complications, including premature labor (24% versus 3.4%), premature delivery (22% versus 2%), abruptio placentae (9% versus 1%), and intrauterine growth retardation (22% versus 2.5%).[17] These increases are dramatic and have been confirmed elsewhere, which causes great concern among obstetrical clinicians.[18]

A follow-up study compared a group of cocaine abusers who stopped using the drug by the second trimester of pregnancy to a group who continued use throughout pregnancy. In the group stopping cocaine use during the second trimester, the incidence of premature delivery and intrauterine growth retardation returned to normal.[19] This information reinforces the benefits of efforts to curb drug use in pregnancy.

Neonatal Complications of Substance Abuse

There are three major areas in which the neonatal effects of substance abuse in pregnancy are manifested: *congenital anomalies, neonatal and infant medical complications,* and *neurobehavioral changes.* Recent studies have revealed some major congenital anomalies associated with substance abuse, specifically cocaine. Binghol et al,[20] Chasnoff et al,[21] and Chavez et al,[22] in separate studies reported statistically significant increases in various anomalies, including genitourinary, gastrointestinal, cardiovascular, and central nervous system defects. These anomalies are thought to have a vasospastic etiology presumably related to the pharmacologic effect of the drug. Constriction of the blood flow in the fetus leads to decreases in circulation. Ischemia then develops in specific organ systems at various critical stages of development. This could result in the specific anomalies seen such as ileal atresia, hypospadias, cerebral vascular accidents, etc.

Many neonatal and infant medical complications are linked to maternal substance abuse (Table 11.3).[12] In a recent study, Biagas and co-workers reported an incidence of 20% positive urine drug screens from infants with medical complications resulting in the need for treatment in a neonatal intensive care unit.[23] The incidence of sudden infant death syndrome (SIDS) is found to increase from an expected rate of 0.5% in the general population to 15% in infants whose mothers used cocaine during pregnancy.[24] Although there is some dispute over the validity of certain of these data, nonetheless there is sufficient information to generate major concern.

Table 11.3 Potential Neonatal Complications of Substance Abuse

Sudden infant death syndrome	Intracranial hemorrhage
Respiratory distress syndrome	Meconium aspiration
Intrauterine growth retardation	Pneumonia
Autoimmune deficiency syndrome	Septicemia
Neonatal abstinence syndrome	Hypoglycemia
Hypocalcemia	Hyperbilirubinemia

The neurobehavioral effects in infants from pregnancies exposed to substance abuse are among the most difficult to assess. These effects may have a long-term impact on child development. Various investigators have tested infants with intrauterine exposure to different drugs, including opiates and cocaine. Using the Brazelton Neonatal Behavioral Assessment Scale shortly after birth, several statistically significant changes have been noted among drug-exposed infants. These abnormalities include a decrease in the infant's ability to interact with its environment, an increase in motor reflex deficits, and an increase in difficulties with irritability and inconsolability.[25,26] With these deficits, it is not hard to imagine the difficulties facing the new mother in parenting an affected infant.

The Movement Assessment Infants Scale (MAI), originally developed to assess the risk for cerebral palsy, provides an assessment of reflex and motor dysfunction in an infant at 3 to 4 months of age. The MAI places the infant in one of these risk categories for developing motor developmental dysfunction at 1 to 2 years of age: no risk, questionable risk, or high risk. Using the MAI, 27% of cocaine-exposed infants were placed in the no-risk category, compared to 1.3% of the control group.[27]

In contrast, 43% of the cocaine-exposed infants were placed in the high-risk category, compared to 1.3% of the control group. This indicates the cocaine-exposed infant could be at approximately 40 times greater risk for developmental problems than those not exposed to cocaine in utero. These developmental problems may include difficulties with concentration and group interaction, cognitive impairment, and motor problems affecting coordination and balance. Fortunately, recent studies involving early physical therapy and parenting intervention have shown promise in the treatment of such developmental problems.[27] The long-term neurobehavioral outcome for these infants remains uncertain and further longitudinal study is needed.

Psychosocial Pathology

It is important to remember that substance abuse is not a problem confined to the lower socioeconomic groups, but the specific needs of this particular group may be greater because of the lack of social and economic support available to them. Such individuals frequently have poor family and social support networks.

Noncompetitive peer relationships with other women are also commonly lacking. Often isolated and associating with unreliable, abusive men, such women are vulnerable to physical and sexual abuse.[26]

Self-esteem influences one's ability to mother an infant. These women often come from families where they did not experience their mother as a supportive, nurturing figure. This negative legacy often results in a lack of exposure to appropriate mothering. This can lead to concerns regarding their own ability to mother.[3] These concerns can result in ambivalent feelings toward the pregnancy, labor, and delivery, as well as their own self-worth. Events such as the perception of fetal movement and the performance of ultrasonic scans are often dreaded rather than anticipated. These events unmistakably validate the reality of the pregnancy, demanding a major change in how the pregnant woman relates to the world. These ambivalent feelings can lead to a delay in the pursuit of prenatal care, which impedes optimal obstetrical intervention.

Issues of *body image* are of great importance to this population. On one hand, there is poor attention to their physical needs, leading to deterioration in their physical health, as discussed earlier. On the other hand, their bodies are often their leverage in life, being a mediator for attachments and human interactions. The physical changes the women go through can therefore be viewed as dangerous and threatening to their way of life.[29] This is in contrast to most women, who anticipate these physical changes as positive and exciting, despite the normal discomforts and concerns regarding the changes from pregnancy.

The ability to maintain trusting *relationships* is often a recurring problem for these women. These difficulties may extend back to the woman's childhood. It often starts with an inconsistent relationship with her parents. Again, this negative legacy is reinforced by problems in other relationships. This can affect the development of a trusting relationship with providers of medical and substance-abuse treatment. The lack of trusting relationships can lead to inconsistent compliance with substance-abuse treatment and follow-up prenatal care. The bonding—or forming a relationship with the baby—that starts early in the pregnancy is often delayed or does not occur. The woman, therefore, may not be emotionally prepared for the realities of childbirth and the dependency needs of her newborn child.[29] These problems would be amplified by a difficult pregnancy and/or infant.

Using the Beck's Depression Index, several studies show an incidence of depression in 75% of substance-abusing pregnant women.[30,31] Some older populations have an incidence as high as 90%.[27] Even without the influence of substance abuse, depression can greatly influence one's ability to parent. For example, Weismann and co-workers found less involvement with their children, impaired communication, increased friction, lack of affection, and an increase in the guilt and resentment toward the child in non-substance-abusing depressed women.[32] Substance- abuse treatment in women with a diagnosis of depression seems to have a better outcome with concurrent treatment of the depression.[33]

A substance-abusing mother is likely to be a *dysfunctional parent.* Such women may deliver an unstable, irritable infant who interacts poorly with its environment. The infant may also have physical problems resulting from birth complications, making it more susceptible to fatigue and illness. This is further complicated by a lack of maternal support stemming from living in an unstable, drug-infested environment. Often these women are also victims of poverty, with its lack of the basic necessities for survival. The woman may have ambivalence regarding her own parenting skills. Emotional scars from her childhood, as well as feelings of guilt over any maternal or neonatal problems resulting from the substance abuse, will play a role in her ability to parent. She may be depressed or have other psychiatric disorders. The added burden of substance abuse only increases the difficulties.

This problematic triad of an unstable infant, environment, and mother sets up a vicious cycle, reinforces dysfunctional parenting, and encourages *child abuse*. Several studies have confirmed the relationship of past and future violence in the home to substance abuse in pregnancy.[34,35] An unsupported parent, who is using her child to fulfill her own personal needs, is coupled with an infant attempting to communicate its own urgent needs. The infant's attempts to communicate are viewed as inappropriate and are in competition with the mother's needs. This can result in the rejection of the infant's efforts. The mother, out of frustration, may neglect or punish the child abusively. Such abusive families are commonly involved with substance abuse. In New York City, 50% of child abuse and neglect cases involve the use of psychoactive substances by the offending care giver. If alcohol abuse is included, the figure reaches 64%.[36]

Treatment

In the 1970s methadone clinics were developed for pregnant women. This experience gave us our first glimpse of the pregnant substance-abusing population and taught us an extremely important lesson. The use of the drug methadone in and of itself did not decrease perinatal morbidity. The dramatic decreases in morbidity associated with these programs were due to improved compliance with prenatal care, a prerequisite to receiving the drug.[37] This confirms research looking at the positive impact of prenatal care on perinatal morbidity in non-substance-abusing populations and is important in the development of treatment programs for pregnant substance abusers.[38,39] That is, while a woman is pregnant, a high priority needs to be placed on the *continuity of prenatal care*, perhaps even above the priority of abstinence. This can be a difficult concept for individuals trained in substance-abuse treatment, where abstinence is commonly a prerequisite for program entry. No woman should be denied access to competent prenatal care, regardless of her current substance-abuse history.

If a specific program for substance-exposed pregnant women is not available in the community, several options are still available. It is important to discuss with the woman the impact of her drug or alcohol use, being careful to avoid a judgmental approach. Recommendations should be specific. The use of drugs and alcohol should be limited as much as possible, if the patient is unable to totally stop. She should also be advised to avoid intermittent or binge use. The clinician should refer her to a substance-abuse treatment program by providing specific names and phone numbers, and by making an appointment. The prenatal care provider should not lose contact with the patient. If a woman refuses the referral, continue to see the patient and re-question her about her substance use at each visit. Continue to make the referral and praise her if she eventually does follow up on your suggestion.

The diagnosis, the referral, and the mother's response must be documented in the medical record, as it is helpful for others caring for the mother and her child. It is also legally prudent to make a chart notation to the effect that possible adverse effects of drug and alcohol use in pregnancy for both the woman and her unborn child were discussed. The chart entry should also include a statement to the effect that the woman has been informed that there are limits to the accuracy of diagnosis for any adverse fetal effects and that treatment may not be possible if such adverse effects do occur.

Substance-abuse treatment programs fall into several categories: long-term residential rehabilitation (6–18 months), short-term inpatient rehabilitation (4 weeks), inpatient detoxification (5–7 days), intensive outpatient (4 days/week for 4 or more weeks), and outpatient after-care treatment (weekly meetings). Some programs require the woman to be drug-free before acceptance, others will accept patients at the height of addiction. Many have admission restriction related to third-party reimbursement. There are few programs exclusively for women, even though it has been recognized that chemically dependent women have emotional and social needs that are different from those of men[8]; almost none have child care available.[11]

Unfortunately, a major barrier to comprehensive intervention with pregnant substance abusers is the difficulty, if not impossibility, of locating substance-abuse treatment programs that will accept pregnant women. A national survey in 1989 reported two thirds of hospitals had nowhere to refer pregnant substance users for chemical dependency treatment. There is a particular lack of residential treatment programs specific for pregnant patients. Frequently, staff is not available to provide medical treatment in the event of spontaneous abortion or other obstetrical complications. Even physicians experienced in treating chemically dependent patients with medication to counteract withdrawal symptoms are reluctant to become responsible for monitoring of withdrawal when a fetus is also involved. Obstetricians and neonatologists must both advocate for treatment programs and be able to identify themselves as available for education and consultation to treatment staff in the programs that do exist.

It is important to strive to develop both medical and behavioral interventions during the antepartum and postpartum period for substance-exposed infants, mothers, and families. The interplay of the many factors described earlier may result in the loss of benefits gained by interventions focused only on an individual aspect of the problem. Programs should include services from prenatal care providers, infant/child health care providers, mental health care providers, social services, substance-abuse counselors, family counselors, and other medical and social care providers in our communities. Practical concerns, such as child care and transportation, are often not addressed in substance-abuse treatment programs and need to be considered. Women's health issues, including contraception and family planning, are also relevant. Issues of co-dependency and violence require special attention in treatment programs designed for this population. Parenting intervention will play a vital role in improving the outcomes of these families, breaking the cycle of intergenerational substance abuse.

In developing such programs, it is important to maintain a nonjudgmental approach to this group of patients, showing respect, empathy, and honest concern for the individual. The attempt is to create an atmosphere that encourages participation in treatment programs and prenatal care. Consistent support and continuing education is extremely valuable in creating a work environment that prevents burnout and maintains enthusiasm among the various participants.

The Perinatal Center for Chemical Dependency in Chicago has functioned for over 13 years, pioneering the treatment of substance-abusing pregnant women. In a personal communication, they report that approximately 50% of their clients stop using substances while pregnant. Unfortunately, these women were found to have a 70% relapse rate postpartum; a large part of this is due to their environment. A few hours a week of contact with a treatment program, compared to substantially more hours exposed to drugs, crime, poverty, and violence, has questionable long-term benefit. Long-term residential treatment could improve the effectiveness of substance-abuse treatment by removing these individuals from this harsh environment. The lifestyle changes and retraining necessary to prevent recidivism may be more successfully obtained in a residential setting.

One of the easiest yet most effective interventions a physician can provide pregnant substance users is education about the effects of alcohol, drugs, and smoking on both mother and child. Educational materials such as posters, brochures, and videotapes are readily available from local chapters of national organizations like the American Lung Association (effects of alcohol and drugs), March of Dimes (information on most teratogenic substances), and the Children's Defense Fund, which markets and produces many effective posters. Materials that focus specifically on drug and alcohol problems as they relate to women in general or pregnant women specifically are available and are written in easy-to-understand language. Ross laboratories distributes a flyer on the effects of cocaine on fetal development free of charge. These might well be displayed in a doctor's waiting room, with enough for distribution for patients and/or families. Physicians can also consider developing their own fact sheets on drug abuse during pregnancy which could be included with material given to each patient who comes to the office/clinic for treatment (pregnant or not).

Other valuable information includes posters and/or flyers with telephone numbers and addresses to community resources such as drug treatment programs, and support groups like Alcoholics Anonymous, Narcotics Anonymous, and Cocaine Anonymous. The telephone number to the National Drug Abuse treatment referral hot line is 1-800-662- HELP and is open 24 hours a day. In addition, the National Association for Perinatal Addiction Research and Education (NAPARE) has a hot line specifically oriented to pregnant women (1-800-638-BABY). They provide education and treatment referral to programs focusing on obstetrical care and substance-abuse treatment. This is a valuable service for patients and prenatal care providers.

Conclusions

All the areas shown in the paradigm in Figure 11.1 are interrelated. One could draw an arrow from "dysfunctional parenting" to "negative legacy," creating the self-perpetuating cycle of dysfunction. This increasing family dysfunction will result in the need for more mental health and substance-abuse treatment programs. The long-term learning and developmental disabilities affecting the children exposed to psychoactive substances during pregnancy will require extensive intervention at many different levels. This could result in far-reaching long-term socioeconomic consequences secondary to the increased demands on public and mental health systems and educational systems, as well as unemployment, crime, and homelessness.

Although the substance-abuse problem seems overwhelming, there are positive aspects that need emphasis: (1) participation in prenatal care alone can have a dramatic influence on the outcome of the pregnancy, (2) stopping substance use during the pregnancy can further decrease perinatal morbidity, (3) not all babies exposed to drugs in utero have bad outcome, (4) proper early physical therapy intervention can ameliorate some of the developmental problems these babies encounter, and (5) there is a population of women who do not relapse postpartum after treatment.

Pregnancy and parenthood are times of introspection for both men and women. These can often provide the impetus to seek and participate in treatment for oneself, significant other, or one's children. Chemically dependent women frequently perceive a pregnancy as a "second chance in life" and are motivated to become drug-free and enter a treatment program.[42] Pregnancy may provide a window of opportunity, allowing one to break this pathological cycle. More research is needed to develop creative treatment programs focusing on the specific needs of women and families in their respective communities. Ongoing measurements of outcome are needed to continually improve our treatment of this difficult population.

References

1. Silver S: Scope, specifics of maternal drug use, effect on fetus are beginning to emerge from studies. *JAMA* 1989;261:1688–1689.
2. Trost C: Born to lose, babies of crack users crowd hospitals, break everybody's heart. *Wall Street Journal*, July 1989;70(192).
3. Smith DE: Cocaine-alcohol abuse: Epidemiological, diagnostic and treatment considerations. *J Psychoactive Drugs* 1986;18:117–129.
4. Chasnoff IJ: Drugs and women: Establishing a standard of care. *Ann NY Acad Sci* 1989;562:208–210.
5. Chasnoff IJ, Landress HJ, Barrett ME: The prevalence of illicit drug or alcohol use during pregnancy and discrepancies in mandatory reporting in Pinellas County, Florida. *N Engl J Med* 1990;332:1202–1206.
6. Blume S: Women and alcohol: A review. *JAMA* 1986;256:1467–1470.
7. Altman LK: Scientists say a specific gene may foreshadow alcoholism. *New York Times*, April 18, 1990;139:A1.
8. Wright JM: Fetal alcohol syndrome: The social work connection. *Health Soc Work* 1981;607:5–10.
9. Ouellette EM, Rosett HL, Rosman NP, et al: The adverse effects on offspring of maternal alcohol abuse during pregnancy. *N Engl J Med* 1977;297:528–530.
10. U.S. Department of Health and Human Services: *Preventing Fetal Alcohol Effects: A Practical Guide for OB/GYN Physicians and Nurses*. DHHS publication 83–1163, 1983.
11. Frank DA, Zuckerman BS, Amano H: Cocaine use during pregnancy: Prevalence and correlates. *Pediatrics* 1988;82:888–895.
12. National Institute on Drug Abuse: *Drug Dependence in Pregnancy: Clinical Manage-*

ment of Mother and Child. Washington, DC, Services Research Monograph Series, U.S. Department of Health, Education, and Welfare, 1979.

13. Burrows GN, Ferris TF (eds.): *Medical Complications of Pregnancy* (ed. 3). Philadelphia, WB Saunders, 1988.

14. Feinkind L, Minkoff HL: HIV in pregnancy. *Clin Perinatol* 1988;15:189–202.

15. Pelosi M, Frattarola M, Apuzzio J, et al: Pregnancy complicated by heroin addiction. *Obstet Gynecol* 1975;45:512–515.

16. Rementria JL, Nunaj NN: Narcotic withdrawal in pregnancy: Stillbirth incidence with case report. *Am J Obstet Gynecol* 1973;116:1152–1156.

17. MacGregor S, Keith LG, Chasnoff IJ, et al: Cocaine use during pregnancy: Adverse perinatal outcome. *Am J Obstet Gynecol* 1987;157:686–690.

18. Cherukuri R, Minkoff H, Feldman J, et al: A cohort study of alkaloidal cocaine ("crack") in pregnancy. *Obstet Gynecol* 1988;72:147–151.

19. Chasnoff IJ, Griffith DR, MacGregor SN, et al: Temporal patterns of cocaine use in pregnancy: Perinatal outcome. *JAMA* 1989;261:1741–1744.

20. Binghol N, Fuch M, Diaz V: Teratogenicity of cocaine in humans. *J Pediatr* 1987;110:93–96.

21. Chasnoff IJ, Chisun GM, Kaplan W: Maternal cocaine use and genitourinary tract malformations. *Teratology* 1988;37:201–204.

22. Chavez GF, Mulinare J, Cordero J: Maternal cocaine use during early pregnancy as a risk factor for congenital urogenital anomalies. *JAMA* 1989;262:795–798.

23. Biagas KV, Chasnoff IJ, Davis CL, et al: Urine toxicology: Testing in newborns admitted to neonatal intensive care. *Pediatr Res* 1989;25, Part 2, Abstract No. 1234.

24. Word SL, Schutz S, Kirshna V: Abnormal sleeping ventilatory patterns in infants of substance-abusing mothers. *Am J Dis Child* 1986;140:1015–1019.

25. Griffith D, Chasnoff IJ, Dirkes K: Neurobehavioral development of cocaine-exposed infants in the first month of life. *Pediatr Res* 1988;23:55–57.

26. Schneider JW, Chasnoff IJ: Cocaine abuse in pregnancy: Its effects on infant motor development—A clinical perspective. *Top Acute Care Trauma Rehab* 1987;2:59–69.

27. Schneider JW: Motor assessment and parent education beyond the newborn period, in Chasnoff IJ (ed.): *Drugs, Alcohol, Pregnancy and Parenting*. Boston, Kluwer Academic Publishers, 1988, pp 115–125.

28. Mondanaro-Escamilla J: Women: Pregnancy, children and addiction. *J Psychoactive Drugs* 1977;9:59–68.

29. Burn WJ, Burns KA: Parenting dysfunction in chemically dependent women, in Chasnoff IJ (ed.): *Drugs, Alcohol, Pregnancy and Parenting*, Boston, Kluwer Academic Publishers, 1988, pp 159–172.

30. Regan DO, Leifer B, Finnegan LP: Depressive self-concept and violent experience in drug-abusing women and their influence upon parenting effectiveness. *Natl Inst Drug Abuse Res Monogr Ser* 1985;54:332.

31. Burns K, Malamed J, Burns W: Chemical dependence and clinical depression in pregnancy. *J Clin Psychol* 1985;41:851–854.

32. Weissman M, Paykel E, Kleiman G: The depressed woman as a mother. *Soc Psychiatry* 1972;7:98–108.

33. Rounsaville BJ, Dolinsky ZS, Babor TF, Meyer RE: Psychopathology as a predictor of treatment outcome in alcoholics. *Arch Gen Psychiatry* 1987;44:505–513.

34. Oehlberg SM, Regan DO, Rudrauff ME, Finnegan LP: A preliminary evaluation of parenting, depression and violence profiles in methadone-maintained women. *Natl Inst Drug Abuse Res Monogr Ser* 1980;34:380–386.

35. Regan DO, Leifer B, Finnegan LP: The incidence of violence in the lives of pregnant drug-dependent women. *Natl Inst Drug Abuse Res Monogr Ser* 1984;54:330.

36. Corrigan EM: *Alcoholic Women in Treatment*. New York, Oxford Press, 1980.

37. Lee M, Stryker JC, Sokol RJ: Perinatal care for narcotic- dependent gravidas. *Perinatol Neonatol* 1985;9:35–40.
38. Rosner MA, Keith L, Chasnoff I: The Northwestern University Drug Dependence Program: The impact of intensive prenatal care on labor and delivery outcomes. *Am J Obstet Gynecol* 1982;144:23–27.
39. Niswander K, Henson G, Elbourne D: Adverse outcome of pregnancy and quality of obstetric care. *Lancet* 1984;2:827–831.
40. American Academy of Pediatrics and American College of Obstetricians and Gynecologists: *Guidelines for Perinatal Care*. Elk Grove Village, IL, American Academy of Pediatrics Press, 1983.
41. Millman RB: Evaluation and clinical management of cocaine abusers. *J Clin Psychiatry* 1988;49:27–32.
42. Smith J, Deitch K: Cocaine: A maternal, fetal and neonatal risk. *J Pediatr Health Care* 1987;1:120–124.

Appendix 11.1

The following are recommended as baseline questions which can easily be added to any medical history protocol. If the physician or nurse feels a need to justify these questions to the patient, they might begin this section by stating, "I'm now going to ask a few simple questions that may seem irrelevant or surprise you, but your honest answers are important so that I can help you and your baby experience the easiest and safest pregnancy possible."

Alcohol

1. How often do you drink wine, liquor, or beer?
2. How many drinks would you say you had last week?
3. Do you drink every day? How many glasses or cans?
4. How much is the maximum you might drink in any one evening?
5. Have you ever passed out from drinking? How many times?

Depending on the patient's responses to these questions, the physician might be interested in pursuing a more extensive history. If so, the Michigan Alcoholism Screening Test is a useful guide. This assessment tool includes questions such as: Does your husband (boyfriend, mother, etc) ever worry or complain about your drinking? Do you ever drink before noon? Are you always able to stop drinking when you want to?

Other Substance Abuse

When assessing for drug use, a physician again need only ask simple questions, beginning with the least threatening.
1. Do you smoke cigarettes? How many each day?
2. What prescription drugs have you taken during the past 6 months? How frequently and for how long did you take this medication?
3. Have you ever used diet pills? Medication to help you sleep? Medication to calm your nerves or relax?
4. Do you smoke marijuana? How many joints would you say you had last week?
5. What other drugs have you tried: cocaine, "crack," heroin, others?
6. How much and how frequently do you take these drugs now?
7. Who do you use drugs with?

Drinking and drug-use habits of the patient's family, spouse, and peers reflect both the environment in which a woman lives and the pressures to which she is exposed. These questions should be asked even if assessment of patient's drinking and/or drug habits is negative.

1. Was anyone in your family ever hospitalized for a drug- related illness? Or, in your opinion, should have been treated?
2. Does anyone in your family have a history of your opinion, should have been treated? (or, in your opinion, should have been treated?)
3. Does your husband (boyfriend, mate) drink? Use drugs?
4. Do you ever worry about your husband's (boyfriend's, mate's) drinking habits or drug use?

Chapter 12

Disorders of Mother-Infant Attachment

Ronald Davidoff, MD and John P. O'Grady, MD

You see her eyes are open
Ay, but their sense is shut
   —*Macbeth* V, i, 27
   William Shakespeare (1564–1616)

Attachment is a classic term used to describe the bond between mother and child necessary for the survival of the infant and ensuring that they will be in close proximity to one another. However, this definition does not include the fact that there may be caretakers other than the mother and that the short time span that is implied in this definition may be much longer.[1] Attachments are psychobiologically adaptive and assist the organization, equilibrium, and growth of the individual. When such attachments never develop or are disrupted by separations, serious sequelae may ensue.

Disorders of mother-infant attachment include delayed attachment (the most common disturbance), some instances of child abuse and neglect, and a rare but severe group of disorders including denial of pregnancy, rejection of the infant, and infanticide.[2] Most of these problems can, and generally do, occur in the absence of major mental illness. All are complexly influenced by factors that include frank maternal psychopathology or limitations of cognitive development, physical illness in the infant, and social pressures. The present chapter discusses the character, recognition, and management of these and other disturbances of the mother-infant bond and their importance in influencing perinatal events.

Clinical Presentation

Delay in attachment has several roots. This issue derives much of its power from the cultural expectations that are popularly assumed about the immediate bond thought to be normally present between a mother and her child. Deviations from that standard are potential sources of self-doubt and recrimination.

Although disenchantment with the newborn does occur in otherwise normal women, this reaction is transitory and is most often linked to an unpleasant birth experience.[5,6] Other women may speak of the disappointment of not replicating the attachment experience with one child (typically the first-born child) with another. Again, this is generally a transient event.

Some mild disturbances can be seen as expressions of the disappointment felt by some mothers at certain physical characteristics of the newborn.[7] The most common of these is disappointment with the sex of the child. This occurs in those for whom there was a strong preference for either a boy or girl or those who had developed a compelling fantasy about the sex of the child during gestation. Likewise, if another family member had expressed a strong preference, the delivery of a child of the "wrong" sex might be felt as a failure by the mother and this sense of failure become an obstacle to attachment. Examples of this include the father who wishes for a son or the widowed grandparent who hopes for a child to carry the name (or the cathected energy, to use a psychoanalytic vocabulary) of a departed spouse.

The birth of an ill or deformed child is a potentially more serious obstacle to normal attachment.[8] The more severe the illness in the newborn, the more likely there may be delay in attachment or even eventual abandonment of the child.

Technical requirements of the sick child, eg, catheters, monitors, and respirators, can become obstacles that limit the physical access of parents to the child for holding and cuddling as well as sustained, private time between mother and child.[9] It can also create the impression in the mother that she is not first in importance in her child's life compared to the doctors and nurses.[10] The very fact of the illness of the child can foster a sense of guilt and responsibility that may overwhelm the mother. In the more severely ill or handicapped child, parents may judge that the child's needs exceed their capabilities. This may become a cause of emotional detachment.[11] Similarly, the mother who has scant social support (or outright stigma and condemnation) may feel taxed beyond her abilities with even a healthy baby, have trouble with attachment, or even abandon custody of the infant. The problem for the socially unsupported mother of a sickly child is even worse.

In neonatal intensive care units, sensitivity to such issues has resulted in the encouragement of participation by the parents in the caring for the child.[12] But abandonment remains a problem. This may be understood as an extreme form of disturbed attachment in a setting of severe newborn illness.

Child Abuse and Neglect

Child abuse is a serious societal problem that generally is not a manifestation of a mental disorder.[3] Injuries to children by abusive adults commonly occur as random manifestations of annoyance or anger in family settings in which violence is common. Such violent responses to undesirable events have strong cultural patterning.[13,14] Although abuse occurs at all levels of society, it is more common when families are at or near the poverty level.[13,15,16] Also, abusive families are usually dysfunctional, and frequently have poor social supports. Other characteristics common to families practicing child abuse include a history of abuse during a parent's childhood, marital dysfunction, early parenthood, low self-esteem, a parent's using the child for emotional support, and absence of supportive personal relationships by the abuser.[15,17] There is also evidence that childhood abuse experiences increase the probability of development of chronic problems with aggressive behavior in such individuals. This emphasizes the potential long-term deleterious effects of early neglect. An extensive discussion of this subject is beyond the scope of this chapter, and interested readers are referred to the papers cited.

Denial of Pregnancy and Infanticide

Occasionally, especially in primigravidas, the perception of pregnancy is delayed until the second trimester but only rarely later. Similar events are encountered from time to time in massively obese women with long-standing histories of amenorrhea or oligomenorrhea. Uncommonly, such women seek treatment only during labor, apparently mystified about the sudden onset of colicky abdominal pain. To their apparent surprise they go on to deliver an "unanticipated" infant. In the authors' experience these women are usually delighted by the pregnancy and there is no associated psychopathology. However, in the majority of women, the changes in menses, breast size and sensations, and abdominal girth, and quickening are difficult even for the most blasé or inexperienced to ignore. In contrast, *denial of pregnancy* is a specific psychological problem, different from this occasionally encountered, unusual condition of simple delayed recognition, which is virtually restricted to the morbidly obese.

In true denial of pregnancy the woman unconsciously refuses to recognize that she is pregnant, ignores the signs and symptoms of advancing gestation, and does not seek prenatal care.[19-22] What is more remarkable than the apparent inattention of such women to their own bodily changes is the fact that occasionally family and even physicians experience this process, failing to recognize the true state of affairs.[23,24] The infants born of such denied pregnancies have generally survived but are at high risk caused by the absence of prenatal care and the possibility of maternal inattention at delivery as a disproportionate number are "toilet births."[25] Unfortunately, some of these neonates are also lost because of impulsive action by their mothers, usually suffocation. Although some of these individuals are clearly psychotic, most are not.[19,20,26-28]

Pathophysiology

Psychopathology: Denial of Pregnancy

How the process of denial suppresses the awareness of the physical symptoms of pregnancy is of practical interest for several reasons. Early diagnosis of pregnancy not only gives women the opportunity for choices concerning abortion or continuation but allows for prenatal care. Further, successful denial of the major physical signs and symptoms of pregnancy is a particularly striking form of negation of reality that seems incomprehensible to most nonphysicians and physicians alike. Such denial is usually seen only among children, the psychotic or individuals with certain neurologic disorders and intellectual limitations.[24]

Denial can be used as a psychodynamic mechanism for the avoiding of

Table 12.1 Summary: Cases of Denial of Pregnancy

Author	Age	Marital Status	Gravidity/ Parity	Denial Lifted	Comments
Bascom[81]	NS	S	1/0	At 39 weeks (time when patient presented at ER for jogging injury and pregnancy diagnosed)	Infant custody relinquished
Brozovsky and Falit[24]	15	S	1/0	At home birth	Neonaticide (neonate thrown from window)
	14	S	1/0	At home birth	Neonaticide with neonate thrown from window, patient claimed amnesia(?) for the event
Finnegan and co-workers[33]	24	S	1/0	At home birth	Neonaticide/?still-birth (events around neonatal death unclear, legal charges dropped)
	39	S	2/1	At home toilet birth	Custody relinquished; patient had prior, similar episode
	20	S	1/0	Never (persistent denial of pregnancy, labor, hospital birth)	Rapid neonatal death of premature infant after hospital delivery
Milstein and Milstein[19]	18	S	1/0	At home birth	Custody relinquished
Slayton and Soloff[20]	26	S	2/0	At hospital birth (psychiatric hospital at 38 weeks, but denial persisted despite staff interventions)	Custody relinquished
Soloff and co-workers[82]	20	S	2/1	At hospital birth (psychiatric hospital at 38 weeks, but denial persisted despite staff interventions)	Custody battle (custody relinquished, then sought)
Green and Manohar[22,23]		S	1/0	2 Weeks after delivery, while hospitalized	Neonaticide/probation

pain and objective dangers.[23,29] Anna Freud viewed it as a part of normal development in children.[30] For the child, dangerous or unpleasant or unwanted parts of external reality or certain sensory impressions can be blocked from awareness, usually unconsciously, by use of fantasy or special behavior. Although it is normal in children, Freud considered denial a pathologic condition in adults. Other writers disagree and have described denial as a common adult defense mechanism that is at times adaptive.[29,31]

Denial of Pregnancy: Selected Cases

The complexity of denial of pregnancy and its association with infanticide are reflected in the selected cases included in Table 12.1. Their dramatic presentation in the emergency room, to the family at home, or elsewhere was the stimulus for the original case publication, although the quality of the clinical description varies greatly. Although broad generalizations are not possible, given such a limited number of cases, certain clinical observations are in order supplementing the analyses previously presented.

Three categories of patients were encountered. One group was clearly psychotic.[6,32] These women had lost contact with reality despite interventions by family and their care givers. They believed that their abdominal distention meant they were filled with "gas." They were convinced that the labor contractions that they felt were either the onset of menses or simple dyspepsia. The patient described by Slayton and Soloff[20] hallucinated noises she believed were machines in the basement grinding up products of a previous second-trimester miscarriage. In this fantasy these machines were controlled by the physicians who had treated her for her prior pregnancy loss. These women were so profoundly disorganized that their mental dysfunction would have been immediately apparent to any experienced observer.

The second group of patients had limited cognitive abilities and major ego deficits that suggested a borderline or inadequate personality disorder and passivity.[24,28,33] Both of Brozovsky and Falit's[25] patients murdered their babies. These women had gone to the bathroom with an urge to move their bowels and then delivered an "unanticipated" infant. The authors described these women as experiencing maternal deprivation during their own upbringing and having limited capacity to care for themselves or others. With these patients, as with others, family and physicians did not recognize their pregnancy. Brozovsky and Falit[24] believed their patients experienced psychotic breaks at the time of delivery leading to varying forms of amnesia and impulsive murderous behavior.

The third group included women with the highest level of functioning. These patients had performed well in school or work, had friends, and were considered capable. They were from very rigid, religious homes, with enormous pressures to be "good" and not give in to sexual impulses.[22] Milstein and Milstein[19] wrote that with their patient, the "denial served to allay anxiety by disavowing thoughts, intolerable." They believed that their patient not only denied an awareness of body changes but also experienced "suppression of actual changes"!

Silverblatt[23] has also briefly described six cases from the University of New Mexico: four teenagers and two multigravidas. One patient was psychotic, the others not. In one of their cases, incest was part of the denial process. Incest may be a more common link in cases of child murder than is commonly recognized, but little reliable data is available.[34]

Rejection of the Newborn

The condition of *rejection of the newborn* has classically been closely linked to postpartum mental disorders (especially affective psychosis) although there is controversy on this point.[2–4]

Extreme forms of newborn rejection are uncommon, and it is fair to say all are poorly studied. This partially explains the inconsistency in the literature. Most reports involve only small numbers of individuals, and little systematic research has been possible. Much in the field remains uncertain. For example, the relationships between severe forms of newborn rejection to the less intense "bonding disorders"[32] or the transitory episodes of rejection in otherwise normal women are unknown.[6,13]

Infanticide

There is no more dramatic expression of the mother's denial of the neonate's right to exist than her killing the baby soon after delivery. Such cases capture public and professional attention and usually evoke intense interest.

Much in the literature of infanticide consists of case reports, and no systemic studies have been possible. Further, the interests and approach of psychological/psychiatric authors who review or comment on cases differ from those of students of forensic and legal medicine. Terminology is also inconsistent from article to article. Not surprisingly, the literature contains much that is contradictory, frankly speculative, or simply anecdotal.

As mentioned, readers of the infanticide literature are cautioned that terminology is not consistent among the various writers.[35] *Neonaticide* is usually defined as child killing within the first 24 hours of life or at least within the first week.[15,28,36,37] *Infanticide* is variously described but is most consistently interpreted to designate infant murders occurring within the first year of life, usually not including those cases defined as neonaticides.[15,37,38] Delay and associates,[39] however, use a broader definition for infanticide, accepting simply murder of an infant "par un de ses parents," and remark on the differences between the legal and psychiatric definitions of this entity. *Filicide* commonly refers to childhood homicides (less than 18 years of age) perpetuated by the victim's parents or stepparents.[15,38] Resnick[28] defines filicide as the murder of a "son or daughter" older than 24 hours; Montag and Montag[40] use the terms for similar killings of victims older than 1 year of age.

As Krugman[41] points out from a review of Jason's[38] data, there are two major categories of child killing. One is *intrafamilial*, usually associated with the use of bodily force. These victims are usually less than 3 years of age, the reasons for the killing are often unclear, and the setting usually characterized by familial or parental violence. In contrast, *extrafamilial* murders commonly involve older children involved in altercations or criminal acts. In such later killings, the use of weapons is common and most of these victims are above 12 years of age. Childhood murders between 3 and 12 years present a mixed pattern. The preponderance of the psychiatric literature and the thrust of the current review concerning child killing are focused on the youngest group.

Approximately 5% of all deaths between 1 and 17 years of age are due to murder.[15] In the United States, killings of children primarily involve deaths of individuals older than 1 year of age. Overall statistics of child killing reveal a slight male predominance in both offenders and victims. The best summed American data, admitting problems of underreporting, reports an incidence of neonaticide (deaths less than 1 week of age) of 1.3/100,000 live births and infanticide (deaths between 1 week and 1 year of age) of 4.3/100,000 infants.[15]

In the particular case of infanticide, not surprisingly, the mother is commonly but not invariably the offender.[39,42,43] For these early murders, the means of killing is usually strangulation or other application of force.[44] Such killings rarely involve the use of weapons such as guns or knives. More than 90% of cases of infanticide involve only the victim and the offender and such killings are more frequent in rural than in urban settings.

Later homicides within the first year of life have a different overall pattern. In these later killings, males become the principal offenders. Again, the large majority of these killings occur at the hands of parents or stepparents without the use of weapons.

For older children (older than 1 year, less than 18 years), killing of males is substantially more common (male/female ratio 62%/38%), weapons are likely to be used (55%), and only about one third are perpetrated by parents or stepparents. With increasing age of the victim, the pattern of killing becomes progressively similar to that for adult primary homicide. Thus, as the victim's age rises, the causes of murder begin to include social altercations and purely criminal behavior.[15] The overall problem of childhood homicide, particularly among older children, cannot be separated from the larger issues of child abuse and general societal violence.

It is suspected that some cases of real or attempted infanticide are concealed within the statistics for sudden infant death syndrome or are otherwise unreported, but the incidence of such incorrect attribution is unclear.[27,41,45-50] There are other rare causes for childhood killing. For example, bizarre neurologic disorders such as epileptic automatism may be associated with violent behavior leading to murder.[51]

The volitional destruction of the newborn is a serious legal issue and potential criminal charges against the mother and/or male partner if he is involved are certainly possible[52] (see Chapter 2). In terms of the current literature, the modern controversies about the active or passive killing of deformed or severely ill neonates are *not* the subject of this review; interested readers are referred elsewhere.[53-58]

History

Infanticide and child abandonment have a long history and in the past were practiced by many groups for economic and/or social reasons.[28,40,44,50,53,58-60] A number of societies living in settings of great environmental pressure such as the !Kung Bushmen of the Kalahari desert or certain Arctic Inuit societies (eg, the Netsilik) periodically killed normal newborns. Newborn killing as a form of population control was also once common in Japan.[46,53,61] Such killings occurred to permit or enhance the possibility of survival of the other members of the group by reducing food pressure and the distractions of child care.[53,62] In Greek, Roman, and Chinese civilizations normal and abnormal newborns were put to death or abandoned under specific circumstances.[54,63] For example, in Sparta, infanticide was practiced against weak or deformed neonates for the good of the state. Roman law permitted infanticide in instances of newborn malformation if five neighbors of the affected family would give their assent. In Rome otherwise unwanted children were also abandoned in established locales with the expectation that at least some of these children would be adopted by others.[53] Historically, in a number of societies, infanticide was also practiced selectively against certain sexes—usually, but not invariably, against female children, or against twins.[28,59] In cross-cultural studies such twin infanticide has been correlated with an inferior societal position for women.[64] At times children were also sacrificed in religious ceremonials as offerings to propitiate one or another of the gods.[61,65] Such sacrificial practices occurred in MesoAmerican and South American Precolumbian societies as well as among other social groups. Illegitimacy, expecially in societies in which there were strong prohibitions against illicit sexual activity, has also been a major social factor in infanticide.[28,66]

Historically, although the newborn's risk of death was higher if it proved to be anomalous, the mother giving birth to a malformed infant could also be at risk if the preternatural birth was interpreted as a sign of the gods' displeasure, as evidence of witchcraft, or as the result of intercourse with animals.[54] The true historic incidence of infanticide in Western societies is controversial, and child abandonment perhaps more common.[67,68] In Europe in the 18th century, infanticide and child desertion or abandonment to public or religious institutions were the subject of much discussion among the socially minded, leading to the founding of institutions for foundlings and various legislative remedies.[54,61,64,69] Such methods of control of family size were not replaced until the following century, when there was a rapid expansion of the practice of induced abortion.[60]

Differential Diagnosis

Despite the limitations of a retrospective literature review, a discussion of Resnick's studies of 200 years of infanticide reports is nonetheless valuable.[28,34] He makes an important clinical differentiation between killing of the newborn within the first 24 hours of life, which he terms *neonaticide*, and murder more than 24 hours after delivery, termed *filicide*.[24,28] Most subsequent writers have reported that there is a real clinical distinction between early and late forms of child homicide. In Resnick's study, neonaticide involved young (less than or equal to 25 years) unmarried women without strong evidence of accompanying psychosis or depression. The killings were not associated with maternal suicide attempts, and the primary reason for the killing was simply unwanted pregnancy. As noted by other workers, repetition of infanticide is believed to be rare, but the exact incidence is unknown.[21,27,70]

Women performing neonaticide display a fairly consistent set of characteristics, reflected in the experience of the current authors as well as noted in other case reports (Table 12.2).

In contrast to the circumstances surrounding early childhood killings, in Resnick's study filicide was much more likely to be performed by a deranged individual. Such murders were often associated with an attempted (or successful) suicide effort.

Scott,[71] d'Orban,[72] Wilkey and associates,[37] Bourget and Bradford,[42] and Resnick[34] provide a more extensive classification of child murder cases based on the source of the impulse to kill. In general, these authors identify *battering mothers* whose killing results from aggressive or impulsive acts; murder by *mentally ill mothers*; killings by *retaliating women* whose aggression was displaced from partner to child (Stern's "Medea complex");[73] cases involving *unwanted children*; *euthanasia*, the killing of abnormal children for altruistic reasons; and finally *neonaticide*.

Mental illness accompanies many later childhood homicides. In d'Orban's[72] review of 89 cases of child murder in England, 41% of the involved women had a history of prior psychiatric illness requiring treatment. Echoing Resnick's findings about the low level of mental disease in women killing newborns, those individuals with a prior psychiatric treatment history included 89% of retaliating women, 56% of those mentally ill, and 31% of the battering women but only 10% of the neonaticidal women. In this study and in the report of Lesnik-Oberstein[74] several social factors were importantly associated with child killers. These included a history of marital disorder and violence, housing and financial difficulties, and youthful parenthood. Again, in d'Orban's study as in Resnick's, the neonaticide group was distinct and notable for the lowest rating for family, social, and psychiatric stress in comparison to the other categories. These data emphasize the differences in the women involved in neonaticide as compared to other groups of child killers.

d'Orban also noted that sucessful or attempted maternal suicide was most frequent among mentally ill mothers (54%). In the majority of cases, the intention of the would-be suicide was self-destruction and the infant's murder became an extension of the mother's suicide or suicide attempt. In most instances, when mental dysfunction is associated with childhood killing, the primary disease is either schizophrenia or a major affective disorder, usually depression.[75]

In child murders involving parents with psychiatric disturbances a fre-

Table 12.2 Clinical Findings Characteristic of Neonaticide

Young mother

Unmarried mother

No prior psychiatric history

Rarely a history of clinical depression

Passive personality

Either maternal efforts to conceal pregnancy or denial of pregnancy

No special preparations for birth or killing of the baby

No accompanying suicide attempt

From Refs. 27,28,32,34,44

quent pattern is "altruistic" killing, commonly associated with depressive illness. The motivation appears to arise from a psychotic belief that killing the child spares the infant from some type of suffering that the parent finds intolerable.[29]

A further observation in cases involving neonaticide is that of maternal passivity.[26] As we have observed, most of these women are young, are immature, and lack criminal records. Among married women who kill newborns, extramarital paternity is common and the murder is often performed to prevent detection. Most of these women outwardly deny pregnancy to friends and family, and make no specific preparations for labor/delivery or for the killing of the baby. In general, either the neonatal murder results from an impulsive act or the child is lost because of inattention or abandonment. Thus, the majority of these killings appear to occur simply because the child is not wanted.[28]

In instances of child abuse or battering, true homicidal intent is usually lacking. The infant is commonly killed under circumstances of acute or unusual stress without specific premeditation.[29]

The unfortunate trends of modern society add an additional category to those of d'Orban/Scott and Resnick, that is, murder or attempted child murder related to substance abuse or drug reaction.[76,77] Foster and Narasimhachari[77] describe a "near-miss" filicide after a psychotic break in a woman with a prior history of mental illness. An acute ingestion of phencyclidine hydrochloride was apparently the precipitating stimulus, resulting in a violent, aggressive, and acutely agitated state only controlled with physical restraints and major antipsychotic medications. Sensitive serum and cerebrospinal fluid (CSF) assays documented the presence of phencyclidine hydrochloride. Eventual recovery to normal of the mother was observed.

Treatment

Prevention of infanticide is likely possible only in a minority of cases in which serious maternal mental disease can be diagnosed or recurrent child abuse identified. The clear identification of the families at risk has eluded clinicians in the past and doubtless will do so in the future.

Unfortunately, although it is difficult if not impossible to identify at-risk pregnancies for infanticide, some features may prove helpful to the clinician. At least some cases of filicide are performed by suicidal women and/or individuals with serious mental disturbances, especially involving fantasies of possession.[34,72,78-80] Margison[78] suggests particular attention to individuals with a prior history of violence and those with delusions of nihilism, possession, or unusual powers. Other signs to note are psychotic symptoms combined with excessive attention to the child's condition, maternal hypochondriasis, or delusions of guilt.[70] Many but not all of these women have a previously established psychiatric diagnosis, such as schizophrenia, mania, or depression with suicidal ideation.[72,79,80]

In individual cases, attention to maternal disorganization and threats or gestures of self-destruction can help identify such women and result in their referral to a psychiatrist and/or psychiatric social worker. However, if the past is a reliable guide, it is extraordinarily difficult to identify such women accurately.

In some instances of apparent sudden infant death syndrome (SIDS) or "near-miss" SIDS, child abuse or real or attempted infanticide may have occurred.[15,45,46,48-50] Although most of these instances are seen in emergency services or by pediatricians, obstetrical clinicians should remain alert if such cases or family histories come to their attention.

The situation for classic neonaticide is no better. In many instances the pregnancy has been concealed and prenatal care has been minimal or nonexistent. Some cases involve the syndrome of denial of pregnancy in which the woman is not consciously aware of her gestation and has not sought prenatal care. If so, medical personnel have little or no opportunity to interact with her.

The central problem for the clinician in all these individuals is that of unacceptable behavior. In denial of pregnancy, the individual suppresses maternal signs and symptoms of pregnancy, makes no birth preparations, and may be unable to act appropriately once the delivery occurs. Here the neonate may be lost from lack of attention to the simplist details such as an open airway. This condition is not necessarily restricted to psychotic women or those of limited mentation.[26,28,33] Various forms of aggression against the neonate occur. These commonly involve strangulation/suffocation with some subsequent attempts at concealment. Rarely such acts are performed with the assistance of others. Truly psychotic women represent a special group in which thought disorders, hallucinations, and bizarre behavior coexist and infant killing is possible, albeit uncommon.

Unfortunately, in most cases prevention is a fond hope. This leaves the clinician in the position of damage control when cases involving possible infanticide are seen in emergency services, offices, or clinics. The best course is to record carefully what the woman, her friends, family, or accompanying persons say and to list objective data concerning the condition of the child and the mother. As obstetricians are most likely to become involved in such cases involving out-of-hospital deliveries, most of the initial concerns are technical, related to assuring maternal and/or neonatal stability after an unattended birth. The woman should be carefully examined for retention of placental fragments, lacerations, and uterine tonus. Oxytocin (Pitocin) or ergonovine maleate (Ergotrate) is administered and any necessary repairs performed. Thereafter, the mental status and level of organization of the woman need assessment. Obviously bizarre activity and disorganized or delusional thinking should lead to prompt referral to a psychiatrist or appropriate drug exposure testing, if the clinical picture suggests ingestion. The rare possibility of an organic lesion or medication reaction should also be considered.

If there is any suspicion of active or passive infanticide or child abuse, the local authorities must be notified as the case involves a possible felony. If the circumstances are unclear, the clinician is still mandated by the laws concerning the reporting of possible child abuse to notify the appropriate authorities. This is another instance in which failure to document the clinical situation adequately is of no benefit to either the patient or the clinician. If child abuse or infanticide is suspected or possible, the practitioner becomes minimally a witness of fact—a responsibility that cannot be eluded. If the syndrome of denial of pregnancy is thought to be a possibility, the woman should minimally be admitted for observation and not simply discharged to home.

Conclusions

In nonpsychotic women the deliberate killing of the newborn is a dramatic, albeit rare event. The patterns of child killing are different, depending on the age of the infant. Prevention is unlikely except among individuals with known mental disorders who may come to the attention of clinicians. Among women killing newborns, denial and rationalization are common defense mechanisms. Youth, inexperience, and illegitimacy characterize such pregnancies. Maternal desperation, desire for concealment, and, infrequently, overt or covert assistance of others commonly accompany the act of neonaticide. Murders of older infants have a more complex pattern. Floridly psychotic or delusional women who kill their children are also rarely encountered.

Obstetric clinicians may become involved in such cases either by interaction in delivery settings with women experiencing denial of pregnancy or by family encounters in which psychiatric disease or child abuse is suspected. Practitioners may well encounter personal, professional, and legal difficulties when they become entangled in such complex and emotionally charged events.

References

1. Hunter R, Kilstrom N, Kraybill EN, Loda F: Antecedents of child abuse and neglect in premature infants: A prospective study in a newborn ICU. *J Pediatr* 1978;61:629–635.

2. Melhuish EC, Grambles C, Kumar R: Maternal mental illness and the mother-infant relationship, in Kumar R, Brockington IF (eds.): *Motherhood and Mental Illness: 2. Causes and Consequences*. London, Butterworth, 1988, pp 191–211.

3. Brockington IF, Cox-Roper A: The nosology of puerperal mental illness, in Kumar R, Brockington IF (eds.): *Motherhood and Mental Illness: 2. Causes and Consequences*. London, Butterworth, 1988, pp 1–16.

4. Tetlow C: Psychosis of childbearing. *J Ment Sci* 1955;101:629–639.

5. Robson K, Kumar R: Delayed onset of maternal affection after childbirth. *Br J Psychiatry* 1980;135:347–353.

6. Kumar R, Robson K: A prospective study of emotional disorders in childbearing women. *Br J Psychiatry* 1984;144:35–47.

7. Herman M: Psychiatry in the neonatal ICU. *Clin Perinatol* 1980;7:33–46.

8. Ross G: Parental responses to infants in intensive care. *Clin Perinatol* 1980;7:47–60.

9. Klaus M, Kennel J: *Parent-Infant Bonding* (ed. 2). St. Louis, CV Mosby, 1976.

10. Jacques NC, Hawthorne-Amick JT, Richards MP: Parents and the support they need, in Davis JA, Richards MP, Robertson NR (eds.): *Parent-Baby Attachment in Premature Infants*. New York, St. Martin's Press, 1983.

11. Beskwith L, Cohen SE: Preterm birth: Hazardous obstetrical and postnatal events as related to caregiver-infant behavior. *Infant Behav Devel* 1978;1:403–410.

12. Gemaro S: Maternal anxiety, problem solving ability and adaptation to the premature infant. *Pediatr Nurs* 1985;11:343–348.

13. Anselmo S: *Early Childhood Development: Prenatal through Age Eight*. Columbus, Merrill, 1987.

14. Parke RD, Lewis NG: The family in context: A multilevel interactional analysis of child abuse, in Henderson RW (ed.): *Parent-Child Interaction: Theory, Research, and Prospects*. New York: Academic Press, 1981.

15. Jason J, Gilliland JC, Tyler CW: Homicide as a cause of pediatric mortality in the United States. *Pediatrics* 1983;72:191–197.

16. Jason J, Andereck ND: Fatal child abuse in Georgia: The epidemiology of severe physical child abuse. *Child Abuse Negl* 1983;7:1–9.

17. Helfer R: The relationship between lack of bonding and child abuse and neglect, in Klaus MH, Leger T, Trause MA (eds.): *Maternal Attachment and Mothering Disorders: A Round Table* (ed. 2). Skillman, NJ, Johnson & Johnson, 1982.

18. Dodge KD, Bates JE, Pettit GS: Mechanism in the cycle of violence. *Science* 1990;250:1678–1683.

19. Milstein KK, Milstein PS: Psychophysiologic aspects of denial in pregnancy: Case report. *J Clin Psychiatry* 1983;44:189–190.

20. Slayton RI, Soloff PH: Psychotic denial of third trimester pregnancy. *J Clin Psychiatry* 1981;44:471–473.

21. Wilkins AJ: Attempted infanticide. *Br J Psychiatry* 1985;146:206–208.

22. Green CM, Manohar SV: Neonaticide and hysterical denial of pregnancy. *Br J Psychiatry* 1990;156:121–123.

23. Silverblatt H: Denial of pregnancies extended to physicians. *Psychiatr News*, Nov. 20, 1981, pp 23, 30.

24. Brozovsky M, Falit H: Neonaticide: Clinical and psychodynamic considerations. *J Am Acad Child Psychiatry* 1971;10:673–683.

25. Mitchell EK, Davis JH: Spontaneous births into toilets. *J Forensic Sci* 1984;29:591–596.

26. Saunders E: Neonaticides following "secret" pregnancies: Seven case reports. *Public Health Rep* 1989;104:368–373.

27. Bartholomew AA: Repeated infanticide. *Aust NZ J Psychiatry* 1989;23:440–442.

28. Resnick PJ: Murder of the newborn: A psychiatric review of neonaticide. *Am J Psychiatry* 1970;126:1414–1420.

29. Dorpat T: *Denial and Defense in the Therapeutic Situation*. New York, Jason Aronson, 1985.

30. Freud, A. *Normality and Pathology in Childhood*. New York, International Universities Press, 1965.

31. Hackett TP, Casem NH: Development of a quantitative rating scale to assess denial. *J Psychosom Res* 1974;18:93–100.

32. Brockington IF, Winokur G, Dean C: Puerperal psychosis, in Brockington IF, Kumar R (eds.): *Motherhood and Mental Illness*. London, Academic Press, 1982, pp 31–69.

33. Finnegan P, McKinstry E, Robinson GE: Denial of pregnancy and childbirth. *Can J Psychiatry* 1982;27:672–674.

34. Resnick PJ: Child murder by parents: A psychiatric review of filicide. *Am J Psychiatry* 1969;126:325–334.

35. Rodenburg M: Child murder by depressed parents. *Can Psychiatr Assoc J* 1971;16:41–48.

36. Arboleda-Florez J: Neonaticide. *Can Psychiatr Assoc J* 1976;21:31–34.

37. Wilkey I, Pearn J, Petrie G, et al: Neonaticide, infanticide and child homicide. *Med Sci Law* 1982;22:31–34.

38. Jason J: Child homicide spectrum. *Am J Dis Child* 1983;137:578–581.

39. Delay J, Lampérière T, Escourolle R, et al: Contribution à l'étude de l'infanticide pathologique. *Sem Hop Paris* 1957;69:4069–4080.

40. Montag BA, Montag TW: Infanticide: A historical perspective. *Minn Med* 1979;62;368–372.

41. Krugman RD: Fatal child abuse: Analysis of 24 cases. *Pediatrician* 1983–85;12:68–72.

42. Bourget D, Bradford JMW: Homicidal parents. *Can J Psychiatry* 1990;35:233–238.

43. Scott PD: Fatal battered baby cases. *Med Sci Law* 1973;13:197–206.

44. Kaye NS, Borenstein NM, Donnelly SM: Families, murder, and insanity: A psychiatric review of paternal neonaticide. *J Forensic Sci* 1990;35:133–139.

45. Bass M, Krarath RE, Glass L: Death-scene investigation in sudden infant death. *N Engl J Med* 1986;315:100–105.

46. Emery JL: Families in which two or more cot deaths have occurred. *Lancet* 1986;1:313–315.

47. Emery JL, GIlbert EF, Zugibe F: Three crib deaths, a baby minder and probable infanticide. *Med Sci Law* 1988;28:205–211.

48. Minford AMB: Child abuse presenting as apparent "near-miss" sudden infant death syndrome. *Br Med J* 1981;282:521.

49. Meadow R: Recurrent cot death and suffocation. *Arch Dis Child* 1989;64:179–180.

50. Cashell AW: Homicide as a cause of the sudden infant death syndrome. *Am J Forensic Med Pathol* 1987;8:256–258.

51. Hindler CG: Epilepsy and violence. *Br J Psychiatry* 1989;155:246–249.

52. Damme C: Infanticide: The worth of an infant under law. *Med Hist* 1978;22:1–24.

53. Post SG: History, infanticide, and imperiled newborns. *Hastings Cent Rep* 1988;18:14–17.

54. Moseley KL: The history of infanticide in Western society. *Issues Law Med* 1986;1:344–361.

55. Duff R, Campbell AGM: Normal and ethical dilemmas in the special-care nursery. *N Engl J Med* 1973;289:890–894.

56. Turnbull HR: Incidence of infanticide in America: Public and professional attitudes. *Issues Law Med* 1986;1:363–389.

57. Keyerlingk EW: Against infanticide. *Law Med Health Care* 1986;14:154–157.

58. Lomis MJ: Maternal filicide: A preliminary examination of culture and victim sex. *Int J Law Psychiatry* 1986;9:503–506.

59. Hunton RB: Maori abortion practices in pre and early European New Zealand. *NZ Med J* 1977;86:567–570.

60. Potts M: History of contraception, in Zatuchni GI, Laferla JJ, Sciarra JJ (eds.): *Gynecology and Obstetrics*, vol. 6. Philadelphia, JB Lippincott, 1990, pp 1–22.

61. Bloch H: Abandonment, infanticide, and filicide: An overview of inhumanity to children. *Am J Dis Child* 1988;142:1058–1060.

62. Chapman M: Infanticide and fertility among Eskimos: A computer simulation. *Am J Phys Anthropol* 1980;53:317–327.

63. Wilson JG, Fraser FC (eds.): *Handbook of Teratology*. New York, Plenum Press, 1977.

64. Lester D: The relation of twin infanticide to status of women, societal aggression, and material well-being. *J Soc Psychol* 1985;126:57–59.

65. Heiger AA: Filicide: An update. *Conn Med* 1986;50:387–389.

66. Langer WL: Infanticide: A historical survey. *Hist Child Q* 1974;1:353–366.

67. Grumfeld GR: Infanticide in history. *Hastings Cent Rep* 1989;19:48.

68. Forbes TR: Deadly parents: Child homicide in eighteenth- and nineteenth-century England. *J Hist Med Allied Sci* 1986;41:175–199.

69. Behlmer GK: Deadly motherhood: Infanticide and medical opinion in mid-Victorian England. *J Hist Med Allied Sci* 1979;34:403–427.

70. Funayama M, Sagisaka K: Consecutive infanticides in Japan. *Am J Forensic Med Pathol* 1988;9:9–11.

71. Scott PD: Parents who kill their children. *Med Sci Law* 1973;13:120–128.

72. d'Orban PT: Women who kill their children. *Br J Psychiatry* 1978;134:560–571.

73. Stern ES: The Medea complex: The mother's homicidal wishes to her child. *J Ment Sci* 1948;94:321–331.

74. Lesnik-Oberstein M: Multitherapeutic approach to clinical treatment for a child at

risk for maternal filicide. *Child Abuse Negl* 1986;10:407–440.

75. Bourget D, Bradford JMW: Affective disorders and homicide: A case of familial filicide. Theoretical and clinical considerations. *Can J Psychiatry* 1987;32:222–225.

76. Luchins DJ, Sherwood PM, Gillin JC, et al: Filicide during psychotropic-induced somnambulism: A case report. *J Psychiatry* 1978;135:1404–1405.

77. Foster HM, Narasimhachari N: Phencyclidine in CSF and serum: A case of attempted filicide by a mother without a history of substance abuse. *J Clin Psychiatry* 1986;47:428–429.

78. Margison F: The pathology of the mother-child relationship, in Brockington IF, Kumar R (eds.): *Motherhood and Mental Illness.* London, Academic Press, 1982, pp 191–219.

79. Chapman AH: Obsessions of infanticide. *Arch Gen Psychol* 1959;1:28–31.

80. Greger J, Hoffmeyer O: The killing of her own child by a schizophrenic mother. *Psychiatr Clin* (Basel) 1969;2:14–24.

81. Bascom I: Women who refuse to believe: Persistent denial of pregnancy. *Am J Matern Child Nurs* 1977;2:174–177.

82. Soloff P, Jewell S, Roth L: Civil commitment and the rights of the unborn. *Am J Psychiatry* 1979;126:114–115.

PART IV

Psychological Issues

Chapter 13

Somatoform Disorders

Therese M. Madden-Fitzsimons, MB, and
Lucy A. Bayer-Zwirello, MD

> We are not ourselves
> When Nature, being oppress'd,
> commands the mind
> To suffer with the body.
> —*King Lear* II, iv, 105
> William Shakespeare (1564-1616)

The somatoform disorders are complex conditions that are approached from the perspective of *abnormal illness behavior*, a notion which bridges the social, cultural, and psychopathological factors that interact in establishing a diagnosis such as hypochondriasis or somatization disorder.[1,2]

As first introduced by Pilowsky in 1969,[3] the concept of abnormal illness behavior included "the persistence of a maladaptive mode of experiencing, perceiving, evaluating, and responding to one's own health status, despite the fact that a doctor has provided a lucid and accurate appraisal of the situation and management to be followed (if any), with opportunities for discussion, negotiation, and clarification, based on adequate assessment of all relevant biological, psychological, social, and cultural factors"[4] (p. 77).

This definition emphasizes abnormal health behaviors serving a sociological function, ie, insofar as such activities are illness "affirming" one gains admission to the "sick role."[5] But, if these behaviors are interpreted as illness "denying," a myriad of potential complications can arise, including problems with compliance as well as self-defeating behaviors. Thus, one's behavior (here read one's symptoms) and perceived or communication discomforts are interpreted or not interpreted as evidence of "illness." From the psychological perspective, the motivation underlying the behavior may be either conscious or unconscious; this distinction being the difference between *factitious* versus *somatization disorders*.

Pilowsky makes usable and useful distinctions between these various disorders.[1] In our analysis it is important to remember that abnormal illness behaviors can be viewed as a spectrum with varying degrees of conscious motivation underlying behaviors or varying degrees of illness or illness denial.

Among pregnant women these uncommon disorders occur with sufficient frequency to merit attention by the clinician. Although exact statistics are not available, it is the firm conviction of psychiatric clinicians that the majority of pregnant women referred for psychiatric consultation have anxiety and mood disorders, both psychotic and nonpsychotic. Abnormal illness behavior, or as it is more commonly known, somatoform disorders including hysteria, hypochondriasis, and others, constitute less than 15% of requested consults.

Nevertheless it is this latter group that is overrepresented in terms of physician concern, office visits, and complaints. This latter group also represents a potential threat both to themselves as well as to their babies through overzealous physician response in unnecessary obstetrical interventions.

To conclude, when presented with a clinical situation where the illness behavior involved is abnormal, atypical, or anomalous in some other fashion, this framework can serve as a tool in the organization of one's thoughts before attempting to establish a diagnosis. The following sections will deal with some of these unusual disorders in the attempt to better equip the clinician with management possibilities.

Hysteria

Weir Mitchell likened *hysteria* to "the nosological limbo of all female maladies," an eternal chameleon whose roots can be traced as far back as 1900 BC, and whose legacy remains extant today even in the rarefied terms of the DSM-IIIR.[6] Taking its origins from the Greek *hysteron*, or womb, hysteria has been postulated as the classic "female" disease, mutable and enigmatic, a vast unstable repertoire of emotional and physical symptoms.

The earliest references to hysteria include a Kahun Papyrus, from dynastic Egypt (1900 BC), wherein is described "a woman ill in seeing" due to a malpositioned uterus.[7] Veith's[7] scholarly book, *Hysteria: the History of a Disease*, goes on to quote from the *Timeus* of Plato, which states, "The womb is an animal which longs to generate children. When it remains barren too long after puberty it is distressed and solely disturbed and straying about in the body and cutting off the passages of the breath, it impedes respiration . . . provokes all manner of diseases beside" (p. 546).

The notion that hysteria and femininity are exclusively allied has held sway over centuries; and the hunt for the origin(s) and etiology of hysteria has continued undaunted. At various times hysteria has been attributed to the presence or absence of a uterus, lack of relief of sexual frustration, demonic possession, lust, and numerous sources of pelvic and cerebral "congestion."[7-10]

It was not until the 19th century that hysteria was accepted more as a disease of the brain rather than the uterus.[11] The foremost exponent of this new hypothesis was Pierre Briquet (1796–1881), who published his *Treatise on Hysteria* in 1859.[12] Briquet defined hysteria as "a neurosis of the brain in which the observed phenomena consist chiefly as a perturbation of vital activities which serve as the manifestation of affective feeling and passions" (p. 57). Briquet contributed to the field by presenting a clinical epidemiological study of 430 patients seen over a 10-year period. Merskey,[9] a contemporary psychiatric writer, states that Briquet credits Carolus Piso (1563–1633), consulting physician to Duke Charles III of Lorraine, with having been the first to dissociate hysteria from the uterus, and to view hysterical symptoms as due to an idiopathic disorder with its origin within the head. However, it is

Sydenham (1624–1689) who generally gets the credit for being the first to relate hysteria to emotional causes.[13]

Whatever the true apportioning of credit, what is clear is that these men and a few others laid the groundwork for studying hysteria as a psychological disorder, in a time when the prevailing view was that it constituted a uterine disease. They set the stage for Charcot's seminal work in the Salpetrière with patients experiencing hysterical and epileptic fits.

Jean Charcot (1825–1893), the physician in charge of the Salpetriere Hospital in Paris, moved from his initial investigations of organic neurological disorders to a study of hysteria.[11] At his famous "Leçons de Mardi," he would present the hysterical symptomatology of a group of chronic women patients to an assembled group of male professors. While he believed that hysterics suffered from a hereditary weakness of their nervous system, he also developed a theory that hysteria had psychological origins. It was with Charcot that Sigmund Freud studied between October 1885 and February 1886. One cannot overestimate the importance to Freudian psychoanalysis of the fact that Freud's early theories were based on the study of hysterical middle-class women in late 19th century Europe. It was Freud who stated that "Charcot's work restored dignity to the subject: gradually the sneering attitude which the hysteric could reckon meeting with when she told her story, was given up"[14] (p. 18). Freud's early work on hysteria, as expounded in his "Studies on Hysteria," includes the story of Bertha Pappenheim, better known as "Anna O."[15] Bertha Pappenheim was a 21-year-old Viennese woman whom Josef Breuer treated for hysteria from 1880 to 1882. She was noted to have "a powerful intellect," "sharp and critical common sense," but no outlet for her mental talents. It was after her father's death from tuberculosis in 1880 that her complex hysterical symptoms began—anorexia, paralyses, speech disorders—culminating in mutism. In Breuer's analysis of the case, Anna O was offended and silenced by the conditions of her role as a dutiful daughter in an Orthodox Jewish family. He conceptualised her hysteria as a creative escape from her everyday boredom. Breur's treatment consisted of spending many hours with her, listening to her stories; thus was the origin of the "talking cure." The analysis ended abruptly when Anna O developed a hysterical pregnancy in which she imagined giving birth to Breuer's child. At this juncture he retreated in panic, unsure of how to deal with this most provocative of situations.

It was from case studies like Anna O and Dora that Freud formulated his theory of hysteria as a consequence of difficulties in psychosexual development.[15] Put simply, Freud believed that women were predisposed to developing hysteria because of an absence of a penis, thus requiring them to shift (at the time of puberty) from the clitoris to vagina as primary erogenous zone. As Chodoff so succinctly points out, "This explanation has a kind of nice symmetry with that advanced in the classical Greek world. For the Greeks, women were prone to hysteria because they were burdened with a uterus, for Freud because they were deprived of a penis"[11] (p. 548). However, it took two millennia to get from one formulation to the other!

It should be seen by now that "hysteria," a word with ancient and hazy origins, has, like a chameleon, passed through variously colored garbs over time; and what may be most universally accepted about it is its mutable quality. Also undeniable is its tendency to be used as a pejorative term.

Clinical Presentation

Hysteria has remained of interest to the psychiatric world, though in the last decade or so some decrease in interest has occurred, to the extent that the DSM-IIIR has abolished the term "hysterical personality," possibly out of concern for its jaded and historically overladen character.[16] But efforts remain ongoing in the psychiatric and psychoanalytic literature to come to a common ground of understanding of this "unicorn." As Chodoff and Lyons point out,[22] "hysteria" is generally used in at least five ways: (1) a pattern of habitual behavior by individuals deemed to have a hysterical personality, (2) a particular type of psychosomatic symptomatology called conversion hysteria, (3) a psychoneurotic disorder characterized by phobias and/or certain anxiety manifestations (anxiety hysteria), (4) a particular psychopathological pattern, and (5) a term of opprobrium or insult.

Today's stricter usage for the term can be narrowed into three major categories: (1) a pathological personality type—formerly hysterical personality— now termed the *histrionic personality disorder*, (2) certain physical symptoms of nonorganic origin, or conversion disorder (*hysterical neurosis, conversion type*); and (3) "hysteria" or *somatization disorder,* also known as Briquet's syndrome. It is to be hoped that the use of hysteria as a pejorative term, selectively reserved for women who evoke feelings of irritation and discomfort in the care giver, is now in abeyance.

In the interests of clarity, the three categories will be considered separately, from the perspectives of clinical presentation, diagnosis, pathology, clinical course, and treatment. These disorders are not specific to pregnancy, but we hope to illustrate, by the following cases, how they complicate the management of the pregnant woman.

Histrionic Personality Disorder

Clinical Presentation

Case 1

Ms. P, a 39-year-old, single Caucasian businesswoman was referred by her gynecologist for psychiatric consultation because of her inability to cope with recurrent cervical dysplasia requiring a cone biopsy, and several colposcopes and laser treatments. Her gynecologist stated, "She's angry, and all over the place. I like her but I can't seem to get through to her that she's not at any imminent risk."

On presentation, Ms. P revealed herself to be a vibrant, attractive, loquacious woman, dressed in a fashionable though dramatic way, who presented her plight in an urgent, compelling, and entertaining manner. "It's the end of everything. I'm almost 40, now I have to handle never having a baby. I need to get on with things or it's over for me." Further questioning revealed that Ms. P. had a long-standing "life script," which included prominence in her career by age 35, marriage by age 40, and two children (at least) by age 45. However, she had lost her job 4 years previously "because of jealousy," was remaking her way in an allied industry, and had never had a relationship with a man that lasted longer than 6 months. "I see through them and (snap of the fingers) that's it, over." She experienced her gynecological problems as a significant attack on her self. "I can't believe it was going on and I didn't know. It's all my family doctor's fault." She vacillated between stating that she would not let her gynecologist "touch me again," to weeping copiously, stating "he should do a hysterectomy now, I'm never going to meet a man anyway."

The past psychiatric and medical history was noncontributory. Her family history included a mother whose description strongly suggested a severe character disorder, and a father whose emotional repertoire was constricted and who was described as generally unavailable. The patient was the eldest of three children, and the only daughter. Her early memories were scant and vague. From age 10 to 18 years, she was in a series of boarding schools, where she captivated the teachers with her antics but made no long-term peer relationships. She failed to graduate from high school, dropping out to take a modeling course, and she describes the subsequent 3 years in a colorful and vivid way, "I could have had anyone I wanted—they all wanted me, but I knew I should get on and go into business. . . . I was raped three times on one job. I said nothing until 3 months later. . . . Since then I hate all men." From the age of 22 on, she embarked on a career in marketing, remaining with the same firm for 12 years. Her job suited her well, as it involved much traveling and numerous short-lived encounters. She worked hard and was often anxious that her performance would not be appreciated. At times her anxiety was so disabling she would smoke cannabis to "self-medicate": to enable herself to function in a "carefree, confident" way. After 12 years she was fired, which she exhaustively explained as being due to feelings of jealousy and embitterness she had inadvertently engendered in a boss. After that, she "fell apart for 6 months, I never left the house, everything had failed" until she decided to "try again" and embarked on a new career in a different area of marketing. She says she was "holding it together" until the realization that her cervical dysplasia would likely be "bothersome again," and "it was like pulling a card out of a house of cards, and I've fallen down." Since then, she describes herself as "raw," "tired of dancing," and trying to struggle with some realizations that have come to her such as, "I'm never going to get it all," "sometimes I think I can't keep friends," "what if it never gets any better?"

Case 2

Mrs R is a 32-year-old gravida 3 para 2. She came to the attention of psychiatry at 30 weeks gestation, when her obstetrician complained of her incessant telephone calls and visits, and her dramatically expressed and intense belief that the pregnancy was ill-fated. She would burst into his office, literally throwing a temper tantrum if not attended to immediately. She made frequent dramatic entrances and exits, usually dressed in an eye- catching, if not flamboyant way. The more her obstetrician attempted to alleviate her anxiety, the more demanding and emotional she became, eventually transferring her demands to the psychiatrist.

The prior case vignettes illustrate some of the aspects of the *hysterical* or *histrionic personality disorder* (DSM- IIIR, 301.50).[16] The essential feature of this disorder is a pervasive pattern of excessive emotionality and attention seeking, beginning by early adulthood and present in a variety of contexts.[16]

When delineating something as ubiquitous yet ephemeral as personality, it is best to look at observable behavioral characteristics. From the psychiatric literature, a distillation of characteristics can be made to describe this disorder. This behavioral description emphasized histrionic and emotional display, overt seductiveness, lability and shallowness of affect, verbal exaggeration and imprecision, and a tendency to be dependently demanding in interpersonal relationships.[17]

Words frequently used by authors to describe these characteristics include the following[17]: egoism, vanity, self-centered, exhibitionism, dramatization, exaggeration, self-display, labile affect, irrational emotional outbursts, inconsistency of reactions, emotional shallowness, sexualization of all nonsexual relations, provocative, intense fear of sexuality, demanding, and dependent.

Chodoff makes the point that the disorder of hysterical personality could usefully be considered as a caricature of femininity, and represents—as the more recent feminist writers profess—a behavioral response to a specific cultural context.[11,12,17]

It is a condition found far more often in women than men (in a ratio of 20:1). In addition to the descriptions given above, such people also tend to be impressionable, easily influenced and swayed. They are apt to be overly trusting and to show an initial positive response to any strong authority figure (eg, physician) who, they think, can provide a magical solution to their problems. There are frequent complaints of poor health, such as weakness or headaches, and conversion disorder and somatization disorder are frequently seen complications. Their initial presentation is generally attractive, even seductive, flamboyant, and inappropriate. Their speech tends to be expressionistic but vague. They are often perceived as superficially charming and appealing but, in time, as lacking genuineness. Their interpersonal relations are usually stormy and ungratifying. They are more vulnerable to experience dissociative disorders than average and are more susceptible to hypnosis, scoring higher than average on hypnotizability scales.

Differential Diagnosis

The following criteria are required for the diagnosis of histrionic personality disorder.[16]

There exists a pervasive pattern of excessive emotionality and attention seeking, beginning by early adulthood and present in a variety of contexts, as indicated by at least *four* of the following:

1. Constantly seeks or demands reassurance, approval, or praise
2. Is inappropriately sexually seductive in appearance or behavior
3. Is overly concerned with physical attractiveness
4. Expresses emotion with inappropriate exaggeration, eg, embraces casual acquaintances with excessive ardor, uncontrollable sobbing on minor sentimental occasions, has temper tantrums
5. Is uncomfortable in situations in which he or she is not the center of attention
6. Displays rapidly shifting and shallow expression of emotions
7. Is self-centered, actions being directed toward obtaining immediate satisfaction; has no tolerance for the frustration of delayed gratification
8. Has a style of speech that is excessively impressionistic and lacking in detail

Making the diagnosis is often assisted by the observer's mood after such an encounter. The feeling is frequently that of something slipping through the fingers—an entertaining, vibrant, even likeable person whose "staying" quality (in an interpersonal context) is superficial and shallow.

The differential diagnosis of this condition includes somatization disorder (they may coexist, as in Case 3); borderline personality disorder; narcissistic personality disorder; and dependent personality disorder.[16]

Pathophysiology and Psychopathology

The nature and "pathology" of hysteria have long been pursued, over a circuitous and often elaborate course. Like all other disorders of character, the pathology or defect is arrived at only with a high degree of inference and, given the nature of humanity, cannot be subjected to rigorous experimentation. However, more recent theorists would conceptualize the deficit in the hysterical personality as arising from an oral or even earlier stage (rather than phallic, as Freud believed) of psychosexual maturation. Many psychoanalysts today would describe a particular pattern of family dynamics believed to be influential in producing hysterical personalities. It goes something like this: the little girl in the first 4 to 5 years of life is deprived, for whatever reasons, of the mothering she needs, and so turns to, or is seduced into, an unusually close relationship with her father. To maintain this closeness and keep his interest, she adopts mannerisms and behavior to which he seems to respond, and learns to use these inviting maneuvers to elicit nurturing from future "father figures." Unfortunately the story is never straightforward and while that explanation fits some patients, it does not help us in understanding many others. Like any disorder of character, or like the development of personality itself, one must account for an immense number of variables, ranging from genetic, congenital, constitutional, to an entire range of social, familial, and environmental factors. It may be useful, too, to conceptualize the inner core of the hysteric as subjectively shaky, even, in some cases, empty. This allows an empathic view of their overdramatic posturings and behaviors as attempts to win validation, to capture a moment of admiration, and to experience a sense of being nurtured and gratified, however transiently. During pregnancy, the increased attention that the pregnant woman receives in our society serves to reduce these demands, though for some the pregnancy itself constitutes an increase in their psychological conflicts.

Clinical Course

Like all character disturbances, this condition is lifelong and pervasive. There are no longitudinal studies available to plot its course over time. We can, however, hypothesize that the behavioral pattern becomes more poignant (to the observer) with aging. It is clear that many hysterics embark on careers of chronic unhappiness and fleeting relationships, which may well take on a more desperate quality as their looks "go," and the aging process limits their perceived attractiveness and/or sexual desirability.

Treatment

Treatment consists of long-term psychotherapy (or analysis) to address the core deficits and defensive suprastructures. When seen in the general hospital or by the nonpsychiatric consultant, a supportive approach is best, with an emphasis on appreciating, validating, and consolidating strengths, while allowing ventilation of fears. The seductive and entertaining style is such that these patients can frequently evoke in the treating physician an intense response, including initial feelings of omnipotence and power, particularly in the early stages of an erotic transference, which these patients seem overly prone to develop. As this progresses, the physician's response slowly becomes more one of irritation, aversion, or downright hatred (see Chapter 6). This clearly poses a significant threat to both the doctor-patient relationship and the patient's best interests. It should also be noted that for the majority of people, medical illness constitutes a stressor, even a threat, which serves to exacerbate character styles and heighten defenses. It is not unusual, therefore, that the histrionic personality appears even more maladaptive and dysfunctional in these circumstances, particularly in circumstances that are perceived as threats to their sexual attractiveness and/or desirability, such as pregnancy.

Drug therapy has no place in the management of this personality disorder, other than for discrete superadded conditions. It should be noted, too, that these patients seem unduly prone to report complications with medication and drugs can indeed provide them with an additional tool in their interactions with their environment—noncompliance and abuse being risks.

There is no specific behavioral regimen that is indicated in the management of these patients. However, there are measures that can be useful in their day-to-day care. In the context of the physician-patient relationship, limit setting, clear boundary setting, and reiteration of reasonable expectations (of care givers, treatments, patient behavior) can provide a structure within which the patient-doctor relationship can be better contained. Validation of fears and concerns, when reasonable, and clarification of those fears deemed unreasonable, will assist these patients during crises.

Conversion Disorder:
Hysterical Neurosis, Conversion Type
Clinical Presentation

Case 3

Ms. A is a 34-year-old divorced woman, of Mediterranean background, with a 3-year-old child, who was hospitalized at 33 weeks gestation in an otherwise uncomplicated pregnancy. Her presenting complaint was an inability to walk. She stated that 2 weeks prior to admission, she had tripped over a cord at work and subsequent to that was unable to walk. She had remained at home until admission. She complained of weakness, loss of power, and marked fatigue in her legs, stating, "It's like I'm a little girl"; and required her parents to take care of her.

On admission, examination revealed no physical findings other than a normal pregnant woman at 33 weeks gestation. Several X rays of her hips were taken but she refused further investigation for fear that her baby would be harmed. She appeared emotionally unaffected by her disability, repeatedly stating, "In time I'll be able to walk."

Further history revealed that this was an unplanned pregnancy in a divorced Roman Catholic woman. The father of the baby was initially very angry at learning of the pregnancy and had increasingly distanced himself from the patient. On the morning of her fall, she had telephoned him and they had had a disagreement (she had told him she wanted a cesarean section).

Her personal history further revealed her to be an only child with a large extended and overprotective family. She described herself as quite spoiled until she had married and had her first child, who then became "the little princess." Her marriage had ended prior to the birth of this daughter and she had consistently refused her ex-husband access to their child. After her divorce, though she maintained her own home with her daughter, she remained closely entwined with her parents. This continued until she informed them of the present pregnancy and her father became irate because of its illegitimate status. He became withdrawn and seclusive where she was concerned, and had only resumed his former care and concern since her fall.

Of striking note was her nonchalant and blasé attitude to her disability, and her adamant refusal to acknowledge or consider any ambivalence or conflict about her situation. She consistently refused psychiatric intervention. She went on to have a spontaneous vaginal delivery of a live male infant, and returned home continuing to complain of difficulty walking, though moving about with a walker.

This vignette illustrates an example of a conversion disorder in a woman who also appeared to exhibit histrionic traits.

Conversion hysteria, or *conversion disorder*, has held an important place in the psychiatric literature since its inception. From its dramatic descriptions from literature of the middle ages[9] to the current reduction in the frequency of its diagnosis, it appeared to reach its zenith with the observations of Charcot, Janet, and Freud during the 19th century.[9] Now, like then, the essential feature is an alteration or loss of physical functioning that suggests physical disorder, but that instead is apparently an expression of a psychological conflict or need.[22] The symptoms are *not* intentionally produced and, after appropriate investigation, cannot be explained by any known physical or pathophysiological mechanism. The "classic" and most obvious symptoms are those that suggest neurologic disease such as paralysis, aphonia, seizures, coordination disturbance, blindness, anesthesia, paresthesia, etc. Symptoms can also include vomiting and possibly pseudocyesis (see Chapter 15).

The symptom(s) usually develop(s) in a setting of extreme psychological stress, and it appears suddenly. There is no consistent premorbid personality, though histrionic traits are common. *La belle indifference*, an attitude toward the symptom that suggests a relative lack of concern not in keeping with the severity of the impairment, is sometimes present but is not diagnostic.

It can occur at any age. Predisposing factors include preexisting or previous physical disorders that may provide a template for the symptom, exposure to other persons with the symptom(s), and extreme stress.

Differential Diagnosis

Diagnostic criteria for conversion disorder include[16]:

a. A loss of, or alteration in, physical functioning suggesting a physical disorder.
b. Psychological factors judged to be etiologically related to the symptom because of a temporal relationship between a psychosocial stressor that is apparently related to a psychological conflict or need, and initiation or exacerbation of the symptom.
c. The person is not conscious of intentionally producing the symptom.
d. The symptom is not a culturally sanctioned response pattern and cannot,

after appropriate investigation, be explained by a known physical disorder.

e. The symptom is not limited to pain or to a disturbance in sexual functioning.

The differential diagnosis includes a physical disorder, somatization disorder, hypochondriasis, factitious disorder, or malingering.[16]

Pathophysiology and Psychopathology

Current theory would attempt to explain conversion disorder in the following ways: an arrest of normal psychosexual development takes place at the stage where the young child has not yet learned to transfer his or her sexually tinged and guiltily held attachment to the parent of the opposite sex onto other attachment figures (or objects). Because this feeling retains its forbidden quality, it is subjected to repression, a defensive psychological mechanism that keeps it out of conscious awareness. In adulthood, a conflict over sexually related issues triggers the hysterical symptom, which not only protects the patient from conscious awareness of the conflict, but often permits a symbolic expression of the sexual desire or its derivative. This way of understanding the conversion disorder is reinforced by the difficulty patients have in relinquishing these symptoms. It is believed that this is due to, first, "primary gain," the gain involved by keeping an unbearable conflict or need out of awareness; and second, "secondary gain," the gain produced by the sick role such as avoidance of responsibility, deflection of anger and blame, evocation of nurturance, and support from an environment that ordinarily may not meet their dependency needs.

More recently, theoretical attention has focused on the conversion symptom as a form of interpersonal communication, communicating to the significant other that something is experienced as missing and needed.

From either standpoint, we can only approach this disorder with limited understanding, which will need to be modified with time and with better knowledge of the patient.

Clinical Course

Though the persistent and stubborn nature of the conversion symptom is known, its natural history is not clear. We do know that recurrent conversion symptoms suggest a relatively poorer prognosis for recovery. Slater's[18-20] work, a rare systematic study of prognosis, indicates that 50% of patients lost their symptom(s) within a year, 30% still had symptoms at the end of 5 years, and 20% retained them for 15 years or longer.

Treatment

Treatment depends not on the nature of the symptom(s) but on the personality structure of the patient. Positive results have been described using psychoanalysis, psychotherapy, supportive therapy, and hypnosis (see Chapter 22). Involvement of the patient's family and, possibly, environmental manipulation is also very important, and can effect change in the individual. A facilitative, nonconfrontative approach is usually best to help patients gently verbalize their concern and, in a sense, attempt to modify the need for the symptom and reduce the benefit from its persistence. Recovery needs to serve both the primary and secondary purposes more effectively than the symptomatic position. An attitude to be avoided is the punitive one, whereby support and care is withdrawn, as this may have the effect of not only perpetuating the symptom but further elaborating it.

Treatment and outcome are variable, and prognosis is basically dependent on the patient's personality structure and coping and relational styles, rather than on the severity (or otherwise) of the symptom. Like most other conditions, chronicity predicts poorer outcome. Drug therapy has no place, and there is no consensus on acceptable behavioral treatment.

Somatization Disorder: Briquet's Hysteria
Clinical Presentation

Case 4

Mrs. C is a 33-year-old nurse-practitioner who presented at 29 weeks gestation with the conviction that she must not receive her required Rh immune globulin because of an alleged risk of HIV transmission. She had recently read an allegation of an occurrence of HIV transmission following Rhogam administration and from that time had an intense dread of it. She was only dissuaded from this with great difficulty, and would only be reassured if she knew the Rh immune globulin she would receive came from a different batch than the one she believed was infected with HIV.

Her history was significant for multiple and long-standing physical complaints involving every organ system. She had sought numerous medical opinions, but no physical disorder had been found. Eventually she attributed the majority of these complaints to the "chronic yeast syndrome." Her complaints ran a chronic course, fluctuating in severity, and at times she experienced anxiety and depressed mood because of them. Her lifestyle was clearly affected due to her constant medical investigations and self-orchestrated attempts to "find an answer."

Personal history revealed she was the youngest in a sibline of two. Her parents had died when she was young. She had married a mild-mannered, self-effacing man who willingly took on all of her household chores and domestic functions. She was unable to work outside the home for several years due to the number and severity of her physical symptoms.

The dénouement was a normal vaginal delivery at term, with almost immediate resurgence of her physical symptoms and an extreme and inordinate fear for her child's health. Her husband did the majority of the child-rearing tasks. She refused to acknowledge any need for psychiatric intervention.

Differential Diagnosis

This brief vignette serves to illustrate some of the cardinal features of somatization disorder, namely the recurrent and multiple somatic complaints of several years' duration, for which medical attention is sought, but no physical disorder ever found. This disorder is marked by a 20:1 female to male ratio, and the majority of cases begin before the age of 20 years. The DSM-IIIR, in fact, does not recognize the onset of this condition after the age of 30.[16] Complaints are multiple and often presented in a dramatic, vague, or exaggerated way, generally as part of a complicated medical history where varied diagnoses have been entertained. The history is frequently noteworthy for the plethora of physicians involved, sometimes simultaneously, and for its multisystem nature. Complaints invariably involve conversion or neurologic-type symptoms, gastrointestinal disturbance, female reproductive difficulties (a typical presentation being menstrual problems), psychosexual problems, and cardiopulmonary symptoms.

Anxiety and depressed mood are frequent. Occupational, interpersonal, and marital difficulties are common. Antisocial problems can occur. Personality disorders, particularly histrionic, can coexist.

The lifetime prevalence is 0.2% to 2% among women, and is observed in 10% to 20% of female first-degree biological relatives of females with somatization disorder. Their male relatives show an increased risk of antisocial personality disorder and substance abuse.[21] Both genetic and environmental factors appear to be operative in this condition but little is known of the mechanisms involved.[17]

It is necessary to rule out any physical disorders that present with multiple, vague, or confusing complaints, such as hyperparathyroidism, acute intermittent porphyria, multiple sclerosis, and systemic lupus erythematosis, among others. Further possible diagnoses include conversion disorder, factitious disorder with physical symptoms, hypochondriasis, panic disorder, and (rarely) schizophrenia with somatic delusions.

Pathophysiology and Psychopathology

The etiology of the condition is unclear from a psychological perspective. However, it can be said that dissociative processes and psychological conflict contribute to the disorder. Strong interpersonal dependency needs are in evidence and, frequently, patient behavior is experienced as manipulative, with temper tantrums, ever-increasing insistence on having demands met, and even suicidal attempts aimed at influencing others. It is hypothesized that this is learned behavior, through childhood mimicry of adults or through reinforcement of illness behavior during development. Child abuse may result in somatization disorder in adulthood, particularly when the child never experiences validation of emotional states such as anger, fear, or sadness.[22]

Clinical Course

Although there are no systematic studies available on treatment or outcome, experience suggests the course is chronic and refractory, taxing the patient, her family, and the physicians involved.

Treatment

No specific treatment is available. However, treatment aimed at concurrent conditions such as depression can be instituted using the usual medications and psychological support. Serious attention to complaints is appreciated as are thorough physical examinations, which tend to reassure the patient. A reasonable goal would be the reduction of unnecessary and potentially hazardous investigations and treatments.

The initial step is to identify a primary treating physician and to consolidate that relationship as much as possible, preventing multiple involvements. The caveat in dealing with these patients always is, of course, to remain open to the possibility of "new" organic pathology which can be prematurely dismissed in a history of chronic unremitting complaints of pain and disability. Under the best of circumstances this is a difficult group of patients to work with and one in which the prognosis for cure is at best guarded (see Chapter 6).

The assistance of Dr. Mary V. Seeman, Professor of Psychiatry, University of Toronto, in the preparation of this chapter is gratefully acknowledged.

References

1. Pilowsky I: The concept of abnormal illness behavior. *Psychosomatics* 1990;31:207–213.
2. Mechanic D, Volkart EH: Stress, illness behavior, and the sick role. *Am Sociol Rev* 1961;26:51–58.
3. Pilowsky I: Abnormal illness behaviour. *Br J Med Psychol* 1969;42:347–351.
4. Pilowsky I: Abnormal illness behaviour. *Psychother Psychosom* 1986;46:76–84.
5. Pilowsky I: A general classification of abnormal illness behaviours. *Br J Med Psychol* 1978;51:131–137.
6. Mitchell SW: The uses of a diagnosis, in Sicherman B (ed.): *Doctors, Patients, and Neurasthenia. J Hist Med* 1977;32:41.
7. Veith I: *Hysteria: The History of a Disease.* Chicago, University of Chicago Press, 1965.
8. Mayou R: The social setting of hysteria. *Br J Psychiatry* 1975;127:466–469.
9. Merskey H: Hysteria: The history of an idea. *Can J Psychiatry* 1983;28:428–433.
10. Taylor DC: Hysteria, belief, and magic. *Br J Psychiatry* 1989;155:391–398.
11. Chodoff P: Hysteria and women. *Am J Psychiatry* 1982;139:545–551.
12. Chodoff P: The diagnosis of hysteria: An overview. *Am J Psychiatry* 1974;131:1073–1078.
13. Mai FM, Merskey H: Briquet's concept of hysteria: An historical perspective. *Can J Psychiatry* 1981;26:57–63.
14. Freud S, Charcot J: *Freud:Collected Papers*, in Jones E (ed.) London, Hogarth Press, 1948, vol. 1, p. 18.
15. Freud S, Breuer J: *Studies on Hysteria*, vol. 3. New York, Penguin Books, 1978, pp 73–102.
16. American Psychiatric Association: *Diagnostic and Statistical Manual of Mental Disorders* (ed. 3). Washington DC, American Psychiatric Association, 1987.
17. Nemian JC: Somatoform disorders, in Kaplan HI, Sadock E (eds.): *Comprehensive Textbook of Psychiatry* (ed. 4). pp 924–942.
18. Slater E: Diagnosis of 'hysteria'. *Br Med J* 1965;1:1395–1399.
19. Slater E: What is hysteria? in Roy A (ed.): *Hysteria.* Chicester, John Wiley.
20. Slater E, Glithero E: A follow-up of patients diagnosed as suffering from 'hysteria'. *J Psychosom Res* 1965;9:9–19.
21. Guze SB, Cloninger CR, Martin RL, et al: A follow-up and family study of Briquet's syndrome. *Br J Psychiatry* 1986;149:17–23.
22. Chodoff P, Lyons H: Hysteria, the hysterical personality, and 'hysterical' conversion. *Am J Psychiatry* 1958;114:734–740.

Suggested Reading

1. Taylor DC: Hysteria, play-acting and courage. *Br J Psychiatry* 1986;149:37–41.
2. Liskow BI, Clayton P, Woodruff R, et al: Briquet's syndrome, hysterical personality and the MMPI. *Am J Psychiatry* 1977;134:1137–1139.
3. Mersky H: The importance of hysteria. *Br J Psychiatry* 1986;149,23–28.
4. Fenton GW: Epilepsy and hysteria. *Br J Psychiatry* 1986;149:28–37.
5. Dongier M: Briquet and Briquet's syndrome viewed from France. *Can J Psychiatry* 1983;28:422–427.
6. Mai F: Pierre Briquet: 19th century savant with 20th century ideas. *Can J Psychiatry* 1983;28:418–421.
7. Mayou R: Sick role, illness behaviour and coping. *Br J Psychiatry* 1984;144:320–322.
8. Mai F, Mersky H: Briquet's 'Treatise on hysteria'. *Arch Gen Psychiatry* 1980;37:1401–1405.
9. Guze SB: Studies in hysteria. *Can J Psychiatry* 1983;28:434–437.
10. Guze SB: The validity and significance of the clinical diagnosis of hysteria (Briquet's syndrome). *Am J Psychiatry* 1975;132:138–142.
11. Sydenham T: *Dr. Sydenham's Complete Method of Curing Almost all Diseases, and Description of their Symptoms: To Which Are Now Added Five Discourses of the Same Author Concerning the Pleurisy, Gait, Hysterical Passion, Dropsy, and Rheumatism* (ed. 3). London, Newman and Rich Parker, 1697, pp 149–174.
12. Showalter E: *The Female Malady: Women, Madness, and English Culture, 1830–1980.* New York, Pantheon Books, 1985.
13. Miller A: *Thou Shalt Not Be Aware: Society's Betrayal of the Child.* New York, New American Library, 1984.

Chapter 14

Munchausen Syndrome

Lucy A. Bayer-Zwirello, MD

Strange things I have in head that will to hand,
Which must be acted ere they may be scann'd.
—*Macbeth,* III, iv, 139
William Shakespeare (1564–1616)

The study of factitious disorders opens an obscure chapter in psychiatric pathology. Factitious disorders have frustrated more physicians, nurses, and health care workers than any other health problem, yet little is known about these conditions. *Webster's Dictionary* defines the term factitious as: [L *factitius* pp. *facere* to make] 1: produced by man rather than by natural forces and 2: produced by special effort: sham. By extension, factitious disorders are characterized by either physical or psychological symptoms that are voluntarily produced by the individual. Although voluntary, the symptoms are nevertheless relatively uncontrollable. Patients presenting with these disorders are compulsively driven. They find it difficult to refrain from certain behaviors, as illustrated in the DSM-IIIR description: "Thus, in factitious disorders, behavior under voluntary control is used to pursue goals that are involuntarily adopted."[1]

Clinical Presentation and Differential Diagnosis

Before diagnosing a factitious disorder other possible causes of the apparent disorder or dysfunction must be excluded and a distinction made between *factitious disorders* and *true malingering.* In malingering not only are the symptoms voluntary but the intent is wholly conscious and the "patient" is not compulsively driven. Further, the person is goal-directed, determined to avoid a particular situation or to achieve some financial gain (ie, avoidance of active duty in the army, avoidance of jury duty, or desire for discharge from the hospital).

Factitious disorders can be subdivided into (a) *factitious disorders with psychological symptoms,* (b) *factitious disorders with physical symptoms* or the *Munchausen syndrome,* and (c) *atypical chronic factitious syndrome.*[1] Unfortunately, the three disorders are similar, although the presenting symptom may differ somewhat. All three disorders will be discussed under the Munchausen syndrome, an appellation that has gained considerable notoriety.[2,3]

Munchausen Syndrome

Although this condition is thought to be rare, Munchausen syndrome may simply be underreported due to identification failure. Several colorful synonyms can be found in the medical literature associated with this syndrome: hospital addiction syndrome,[4] hospital hoboes,[5] peregrinating hospital patients,[6] and chronic factitious disorders.[7] Subclasses have been described, such as an abdominal type, "laparotomophilia migrans"; a hemorrhagic type, "hemorrhagica histrionica"; a psychiatric type, "neurologica diabolica"; a fever type, "hyperpyrexia figmentatica"; and a dermatitis type, "dermatitis autogenica."[7-10] The French have a specific term for the syndrome of chronic self-inflicted anemia: "Lasthenie de Ferjol."[11] A proxy type of Munchausen syndrome has also been described as "Meadow syndrome."[9,12]

Mimicking the original Baron Munchausen, the cases reported from 1951 to the late 1960s involved male patients nearly exclusively. However, the early 1970s saw the publication of fewer reports, but proportionally more included both nonpregnant and pregnant women. Another evolutionary change seems to have been the limited American contribution to the newer articles, with the more recent cases reported from the Commonwealth countries such as Australia, Canada, Great Britain, and New Zealand. It is possible that easier access to medical care in these countries increases either the prevalence of the syndrome or perhaps its recognition.

Asher first described the Munchausen syndrome in 1951.[13] The following features are generally included in the clinical description: (a) appearance at the hospital with dramatic organic or psychiatric symptoms backed by a dramatic (but plausible) history but unsubstantiated by scientific testing; (b) evidence of surreptitious interference with diagnostic procedures, or self-inflicted wounds; (c) willingness to undergo physical examination and even invasive procedures such as major surgery; (d) concealment of prior admissions to other hospitals, sometimes in other cities, states, or provinces, sometimes using aliases; (e) evasiveness and truculence when confronted, even abusiveness when faced with hospital discharge; and (f) apparent absence of motive.

By 1973, 60 cases were reported in the world literature and since then a few more have been added, including more female patients. It is generally held that this entity is underreported as a result of the difficulty of making the diagnosis. Female patients may present in the emergency room with acute episodes of vaginal bleeding, urinary tract infection, severe abdominal pain, or any number of symptoms including those characteristic of such rare syndromes as caisson disease or acute intermittent porphyria.[4,9,14,15] Psychiatric illnesses may also be mimicked, with some patients being admitted to institutions with various psychiatric diagnoses or psychotic episodes.[7,10,13,16]

In most cases, a pattern emerges of an individual with more or less extensive knowledge of medical terminology and symptomatology thanks to an educational or social background in medicine, nursing, or associated health care. The patient often has fantastic tales to tell (*pseudologica fantastica*), and may have a history of vagrancy and peripatetic traveling from city to city, sometimes posing as a war veteran or hero. Although these patients often demand medication they are not necessarily drug dependent.[14] When confronted with the fact of their past admissions, they usually leave abruptly, often following an angry exchange. In general, they are difficult to handle, aggressive, and often disliked by nursing staff and other patients alike. They are frequently loners with few friends or family relationships. Most importantly, there seems to be no obvious reason for their behavior. If they are denied admission to hospital or otherwise confronted, they will leave and admit themselves to another hospital sometimes within hours, often with a different complaint. What motivates these patients is not well understood because so few have been studied in-depth. Less than half of the case reports include an in-depth psychiatric report.[7,9,14,17]

We will review several cases of female patients with presumed Munchausen syndrome derived from the world literature, adding several new patients from our own experience. It is anticipated that review of actual patient data will better outline the bizarre nature of this disorder and emphasize the difficulties faced by clinicians in handling these patients.

Gynecological and obstetrical symptoms are commonly reported in Munchausen syndrome, although they are not necessarily the only symptoms reported by these patients. Women with Munchausen syndrome have been seen with a variety of complaints including many mock obstetrical and gynecological disorders or apparent anginal pain, headache, loss of consciousness, fainting spells, arthralgia, fever, depression, and other, similar, nonspecific complaints.

Case 1

Miss D, a 21-year-old, single, Irish Catholic woman, presented herself to the emergency room of a large teaching hospital in Dublin, Ireland, with blood streaming down her legs. She related a history of passage of tissue, clots with severe abdominal cramping, and a last menstrual period of 6 weeks. She underwent an immediate dilation and curettage. No endometrial tissue was found in the uterus. A second physician recognized the patient and called a colleague at another institution who remembered the young woman. It appeared that this was her third admission in 5 weeks with a similar history and symptomatology. Due to these symptoms, she had undergone two other curettages. Finally, blood from her thighs was analyzed and found to be porcine in origin. Her β-HCG was negative.

Psychological profile: The patient was a mild-mannered, timid, passive young lady, studying art at a local university. Her boyfriend, who always accompanied her, was a second-year medical student. He was quite vociferous, truculent, and angry, always demanding the most senior clinician on duty. When confronted with the truth, the patient and her boyfriend both left and were lost to follow-up.

This couple may be better diagnosed as an early Munchausen by proxy (Meadow syndrome), or even a variant of a classic folie-à-deux. Nevertheless, this case illustrates some classic features of Munchausen's. The female Munchausen is often hospitalized with dramatic histories of hemorrhage either antepartum or postpartum, and sometimes gynecological hemorrhage or menorrhagia.[10,11,17] Several patients such as Rosalind (described by Sale and Kalucy[17]), Madame C (described by Boulanger and co-workers[11]), and the women with factitious trophoblastic disease (from Board and Hammond[18]) all presented with antenatal and/or postpartum vaginal bleeding. Our patient had gone to great lengths to procure animal blood. One reported patient stole blood from the blood bank in her hospital! Most of these patients had self-inflicted wounds, either vaginal or vulvar, to produce bleeding.[9] In unusual situations, they even stole needles and syringes with which to perform an au-tophlebotomy and then mimicked a hemorrhage using this aspirated blood. Virtually all these women were associated with the medical field either as nurses or daughters of doctors.

One patient was extensively analyzed by Gerstle and co-workers in 1957.[19] She went to extreme lengths in her symptoms, being admitted with antepartum hemorrhage and premature rupture of membranes and having had four cesar-ean sections for placenta previa and preterm labor. She self-inflicted her ob-stetrical complications with a variety of instruments including needles and hat pins, causing vaginal and/or cervical lacerations, and rupture of membranes. Her intent was to "have the baby as soon as possible because she was impa-tient to see its face" but not to cause abortion! Two of her children succumbed, one to prematurity (1418 gms) and one to anencephaly. Her first child survived (2125 gms). She was closely watched during her fourth pregnancy and fre-quently readmitted to the hospital whenever she reported the "urge" to ter-minate the pregnancy. She had several episodes of self-induced vaginal bleeding but none serious enough to jeopardize the last pregnancy. She was finally delivered by cesarean section at term of a healthy infant and she then accepted tubal ligation. This patient had been seen and evaluated by a psychi-atrist, which is relatively unusual for Munchausen patients, and her psycho-logical profile is known. She was the oldest child in a family of two, her younger brother had severe poliomyelitis, her father died of lung cancer when she was 7 years old, and her mother died in her presence when she was 18 of exsan-guination caused by a perimenopausal hemorrhage ("she died in one hour"). The patient was a high school graduate and she had trained for 2 years as a psychiatric occupational therapist.

This patient fits quite well the pattern of other Munchausen patients with a strong background in health care education and personal experience with ill health. She may not have traveled extensively, as did the original peripatetic patients described by Asher, but she nevertheless attended two or three dif-ferent hospitals for her various admissions.

Case 2

Mrs E is a 62-year-old retired nurse, married three times, with five adult children with whom she was estranged. She was referred to the psychiatry service after admission for recurrent chest pains. Her chief complaint was, "Doctors tell me nothing, I am in great pain, and I want to sign myself out!" Her past medical history as she described it was unrivaled in its complexity. She reported an episode of myocardial infarction, a 15-year history of coronary artery disease, five episodes of congestive heart failure, multiple deep vein thromboses and pulmonary embolisms, two laparotomies for diverticular disease, two fractured wrists, osteoarthritis, bad "nerves," and over 30 dilations and curettages for bleeding or miscarriages. She also reported several dozen spontaneous abortions. During her five known pregnancies she claimed that she was bedridden for the duration of each with fatigue and vaginal bleeding. She stated that she had delivered each child in a different state (records could not be found). She may once have been admitted to the Mayo Clinic with the diagnosis of Munchausen syndrome.

Psychological profile: The patient was born in Toronto, Canada, and lived there with her mother and two siblings. Her father lived in Detroit and visited only on the week-ends. She claims her mother died at the hands of a heart surgeon at the age of 42 and her father died also after some form of brain surgery, although this could not be confirmed. She also claimed that both her brother and sister died following heart surgery. Her own educational history was not any clearer, as she claimed to have graduated from the Mt. Sinai School of Nursing in "Kings, N.Y." She angrily demanded surgery and, when attempts were made to clarify her personal history, she became sullen and uninterested. She refused all psychological testing and constantly changed her story and symptoms. None of multiple discharge summaries from local hospitals described serious pathology related to her obstetrical and gynecological symptoms and curettages, nor was there any documented evidence of cardiopathy. The patient discharged herself before any further testing could be performed.

Although the patient presented with a nongynecological complaint, she related an extensive and complex history of pregnancy complications and miscarriages. She has five live children, but virtually all are alienated from her. Only her elder daughter would speak to us and she asked, "What was it now, another heart attack?" Many of her admissions had been in different hospitals both in the United States and in Canada. In this at least she was consistent with the syndrome, ie, seeking care in many different institutions.

In 1985, Goodlin[9] reported a series of cases of female patients that he diagnosed as Munchausens, a common disease entity in his estimation. Although in retrospect at least some of the cases related may be Munchausen variants, the diagnosis for several is at best unclear. Three of the 10 patients described had antenatal, recurrent self-inflicted vaginal bleeding. But he describes a variety of other presentations as well, such as recurrent preterm labor—factitious contractions on the monitor—with successful tocolysis in another hospital; severe hyperemesis and recurrent admissions for premature rupture of membranes—actually spontaneous bladder voiding—and factitious seizures.

Board and Hammond[18] also reported unusual cases. For example, they noted instances involving a history of reported recurrent urinary tract infections, presumably by self-contamination of urine samples, and recurrent vaginal bleeding postpartum with persistent presence of measurable β-HCG. The mimicking of actual disease was complex, even diabolical. The first patient was tampering with her blood samples, contaminating them with exogenous HCG. Because of this, only her outpatient blood work was positive for β-HCG. The patient was finally caught in a "sting" operation where known male blood was substituted for her own. This sample proved positive for exogenous β-HCG, while her own blood proved negative. She actually underwent unnecessary curettages for presumed persistent placental tissue and was to have more invasive procedures done when it was determined that she had a factitious disorder. Most interesting about this patient was her occupation. She was a second-year nursing student.

A second, similar case, also reported by Board and Hammond,[18] involved a woman who complained of persistent vaginal bleeding postabortion with a positive urine β-HCG which subsequently proved to be factitious. This patient was a medical student.

Both of these women, like our older patient, had previous hospital admissions at which they presented with a variety of gynecological and nongynecological symptoms and complaints, which resulted in several unnecessary surgeries for each.

Pathophysiology and Psychopathology

Many investigators have tried to find an explanation for the bizarre behavior found in these patients, but few have had the opportunity, as one of the main characteristics of Munchausen syndrome is their refusal to stay in care if confronted or denied treatment or invasive investigation.[13,20,21] These patients often seem to come from disturbed families, with one or both parents having been chronically ill. Past history may contain true illness accompanied by hospitalization and nurturing by a solicitous family doctor or nurse.[14] Many patients have a background in nursing, medicine, or medical technology, but rarely finish their schooling. Some patients have had parents or guardians who were doctors and it is possible that the symptoms represent an unconscious attempt to recreate the doctor-parent/child-patient relationship. Some authors report the IQ of their patients in the low-average to average range, but a few patients had a relatively high IQ.[14] It has been stated that these patients are often unattractive physically, that they are abusive, truculent, demanding, and generally disliked.[14] Several psychiatric- related disorders have been proposed to be associated with Munchausen syndrome such as schizophrenia, hysteria, and paranoid-delusional states but none has proven appropriate enough to gain acceptance.[7,10,22]

Thus, although the psychopathology behind factitious behavior has not been elucidated, a picture emerges of difficult childhoods, derouted personalities, and disfigured appearance. Perhaps these patients cannot elicit love and care from their entourage, so they search for it as best they can. They create an illness, sometimes going to great extremes, in order to find the support they need and otherwise cannot attain. Because menstruation and pregnancy is such a paramount and visible event in the life of a woman, it may well be an easy target of factitious illness.

Treatment

An interesting notion forwarded by Sale and Kalucy[17] is that the precipitating factor in the genesis of Munchausen syndrome is the denial on the part of the environment of the individual's "sick roles," which may lead to an escalation of behavior designed to reinstate it. If the patient's care is terminated too hastily, this in turn may encourage the patient to invent ever more serious situations. This hypothesis leads to an intervention strategy that permits a certain amount of acting out by the patient, provides care, and, therefore, arrests the behavior and prevents escalation. But other authors have shown that even with extensive support the chance of rehabilitation and arrest of the factitious behavior is slight.[4] All but three of the patients in the case reports seem to have been lost to follow-up, and only "Rosalind"[17] showed improvement. The two other patients described reverted back to hospital-seeking behavior within the year.

Conclusions

At present there is no known cure for Munchausen syndrome. As these patients cannot be prevented from continuing to arrive at institutions with symptoms, efforts have been made to protect against their admission by, for example, creating "black lists" as a warning for new or uninitiated emergency room staff[20]; but this has never been a widely accepted practice. Also, such patients may suffer from a true illness which must be considered at the time of any visit whenever acute symptoms are present.[10,14]

What is known concerning Munchausen patients is that confrontation usually leads to self-dismissal, referral to the psychiatry service results in denial, and investigations lead only to further hospital-seeking behavior.

References

1. American Psychiatric Association: *Diagnostic and Statistical Manual of Mental Disorders*, ed. 3, rev. Washington, DC, American Psychiatric Association, 1987, p 177.
2. Raspe RE: *Singular Travels, Campaigns and Adventures of Baron Munchausen*. New York, Dover Publications, 1960.
3. Ludwig J: MunchHausen versus Munchausen. *Mayo Clin Proc* 1983;58:767–769.
4. Barker JC: The syndrome of hospital addiction (Munchausen syndrome): A report on the investigation of seven cases. *J Ment Sci* 1962;108:167–182.
5. Clarke E, Melnick SC: The Munchausen syndrome and the problem of hospital hoboes. *Am J Med* 1958;25:6–10.
6. Chapman JS: Peregrinating problem patients—Munchausen's syndrome. *JAMA* 1957;165:925–927.
7. Spiro H: Chronic fictitious illness. *Arch Gen Psychiatry* 1968;18:569–580.
8. Ferrer-Iturralde J, Hernandez FJB, Sanchez JAM, et al: La fiebre ficticia como cause de fiebre de origen desconocido. *Med Clin* (Barcelona) 1982;78:221–225.
9. Goodlin RC: Pregnant women with Munchausen syndrome. *Am J Obstet Gynecol* 1985;153:207–210.
10. Sale I, Kalucy R: Munchausen's syndrome. *Med J Aust* 1978;2:523–525.
11. Boulanger JC, Delobel J, Delahousse J, et al: Le syndrome de Lasthenie de Ferjol. *Rev Fr Gynécol Obstet* 1985;80:279–283.
12. Meadow R: Munchausen by proxy: The hinterland of child abuse. *Lancet* 1977;2:343–345.
13. Asher R: Munchausen's syndrome. *Lancet* 1951;1:339–341.
14. Berney TP: A review of simulated illness. *S Afr Med J* 1973;47:1429–1434.
15. Engelhardt J: A new variant of Munchausen syndrome: Pregnancy complicated by urinary tract infection. *J Iowa Med Soc* 1979;40:318–322.
16. Gelenberg AJ: Munchausen's syndrome with a psychiatric presentation. *Dis Nerv Syst* 1977;38:378–380.
17. Sale I, Kalucy R: An observation on the genesis of Munchausen syndrome: A case report. *Aust NZ J Psychiatry* 1980;14:61–64.
18. Board JA, Hammond CB: Factitious trophoblast disease: Munchausen's mole. *South Med J* 1980;73:831–832.
19. Gerstel ML, Guttmacher AF, Brown F: A case of recurrent malingered placenta previa. *J Mt Sinai Hosp* 1957;24:641–646.
20. Bursten B: On Munchausen's syndrome. *Arch Gen Psychiatry* 1965;13:261–268.
21. Blackwell P: Munchausen at Guy's. *Guy's Hosp Rep* 1965;114:257–277.
22. Cheng L, Hummel L: The Munchausen syndrome as a psychiatric condition. *Br J Psychiatry* 1978;133:20–21.

Chapter 15

Pseudocyesis

John P. O'Grady, MD and Lewis M. Cohen, MD

Il n'y a pas de fausses grossesses,
Il n'y a que de faux diagnostiques.
—*Traveaux d'obstétrique
et de gynécologie,* 1882
C. Pajot

Pseudocyesis is a clinical syndrome in which a nonpsychotic woman firmly believes herself to be pregnant and develops objective signs and symptoms of pregnancy in the absence of true gestation. [1,2] Descriptions of this syndrome date back to antiquity, and more than 500 cases of pseudocyesis have been reported in the medical literature.[3] Numerous additional cases have doubtlessly gone unrecorded except in the clinical notes of practitioners. The number of published case reports has decreased in recent years, but it is uncertain if this represents a true decline in prevalence or simply an artifact of incomplete reporting.[1-6]

The term *pseudocyesis* is derived from the Greek root word *kyesis*, or pregnancy, and *pseudes*, meaning false. Several other less commonly used terms appear in the medical literature. These include: false pregnancy, hysterical pregnancy, spurious pregnancy, imaginary pregnancy, simulated pregnancy, and phantom pregnancy.[6-9] Pseudocyesis remains the best nonpejorative term for this condition.

There are several clinically important variants of pseudocyesis (Table 15.1).[1] "True" pseudocyesis (*pseudocyesis vera*) is by far the most common condition. It needs to be distinguished from *delusional pseudocyesis*, which may occur in psychotic individuals, and *factitious* or *simulated pseudocyesis*. In this latter and extremely rare circumstance, a woman professes to be pregnant, knowing that she is not.[10,11] Finally, *erroneous pseudocyesis* can result from organic disease in which signs or symptoms suggestive of pregnancy including amenorrhea, breast discharge, and abdominal enlargement precipitate a condition that the patient incorrectly interprets as pregnancy.[12-14] The latter condition is uncommon in modern practice.

In 300 BC Hippocrates described a number of clinical cases involving women "who imagine they are pregnant seeing that their menses are suppressed and their matrices swollen."[15] He believed the pathophysiology to consist of retention of menstrual fluid and gases, but did not suggest any specific therapy.

Table 15.1 Clinical Variants of Pseudopregnancy

Delusional pseudocyesis (psychotic patient)

Factitious pseudocyesis (deceptive patient)

Erroneous pseudocyesis (organic disease patient)

Pseudocyesis vera

A. Form fruste (amenorrhea/oligomenorrhea only)

B. Advanced form (amenorrhea/oligomenorrhea and major signs and symptoms)

William Harvey, the 18th century English scientist/physician, consulted on two cases of pseudocyesis[9] and stated that "no argument of mine could divest [the woman] of this belief." Harvey emphasized the psychological aspects of this condition, commenting on how a woman was "impregnated by the conception of a general immaterial idea and [thus] become[s] the artificer of generation."

In the 19th century, the writings of the noted English obstetrician Sir J. Simpson re-evoked interest in the disorder and its physiology.[16,17] Simpson's principal innovation in the evaluation of women for false pregnancy was the use of chloroform. Women with uncertain clinical presentations were anesthetized and then examined in the presence of family witnesses. Under anesthesia, marked decompression of abdominal distention usually occurred and palpation of a firm, normal-sized uterus became possible. This unusual and dramatic technique retained popularity well into the 20th century.[18–21]

In 1937, Bivin and Klinger collected 440 cases of pseudocyesis from the medical literature, largely from the period 1800–1900.[6] This collection of cases provides the basis used by virtually all later reports to discuss statistics concerning incidence, patient characteristics, and clinical presentation. Subsequent reviews, a number of case reports, and recently published neurophysiological data on selected patients and their response to therapy complete the material available for analysis and study. A modern, methodologically sound research study has yet to be performed that will provide us with the data to make meaningful statements concerning the prevalence or social patterning of pseudocyesis.

It appears that women who develop pseudocyesis display no consistent demographic or sociological characteristics. Further, pseudocyesis apparently has not ignored the famous or the privileged.[22–26] For example, Mary Tudor, queen of England, successor to Edward VI, half sister to Elizabeth I, and wife of Philip II of Spain, had two traumatic episodes of pseudocyesis that had national and international repercussions in the mid-16th century.[22–24] The literature on pseudocyesis includes women ranging from 5 to 79 years of age with a mean age of 33 years.[1,2,4,6,24,27–29] In Bivin and Klinger's series, three quarters of the cases fell in the childbearing age between 15 and 39 years.[6] All reviews note that pseudocyesis is uncommon among children and adolescents and most reviews take some note of the rare occurrence of this phenomenon among men.[1] These latter cases generally involve seriously disturbed individuals who have problems with sex identification, alcoholism, and psychosis.[30–33] However, if one assumes a global or anthropological perspective, the *couvade* syndrome, in which men mimic certain symptoms of pregnancy or labor, is a common occurrence.[3,34,35] In Western societies the term refers to the enactment of pregnancy behaviors (nausea, vomiting, depression, insomnia, etc) that parallel the female partner's symptoms during gestation.[35] In some social groups, the couvade syndrome is institutionalized by means of special ritual practices and restrictions performed by the father at the time of birth or soon thereafter.

Clinical Presentation

The similarity between pseudocyesis and actual gestation is often remarkable. As Table 15.2 indicates, the symptoms most commonly reported by these women are menstrual abnormalities and abdominal distention. The patient's history may also include reports of quickening, morning sickness, ptyalism, and even recurrent vomiting suggestive of hyperemesis gravidarum.[46] However, there always remain atypical features that are sufficient to alert an astute clinician to deviations from normal pregnancy.[9] Thus, while menstrual disturbances are universal, complete amenorrhea is not. Patients may complain of recurrent vaginal bleeding that suggests threatened abortion, abruptio placentae, or placenta previa. On close questioning, however, these episodes are atypical for the suspected pathology.

On careful palpation, the uterus is usually not enlarged beyond the size of a 6-week gestation, although Hegar's sign may be equivocal.[28] Variable abdominal distention occurs and can be convincing even to experienced examiners.[6,28] It is claimed that the umbilicus is virtually never protuberant in pseudocyesis, as it commonly is in true pregnancy.[2,47] The validity of this clin-

Table 15.2 Frequency of Presenting Signs and Symptoms in Pseudocyesis

	Selected Series* (%)	Bivin and Klinger[6] (%)
Belief in pregnancy	106/106 (100)	274/444 (62)
Abdominal enlargement	103/106 (97)	270/444 (61)
Menstrual disturbance	104/106 (98)	274/444 (62)
Quickening	79/106 (75)	270/444 (61)
History of infertility	63/106 (59)	—
Breast changes	63/106 (59)	—
Weight gain	47/106 (44)	—
Galactorrhea	59/106 (56)	173/444 (39)
Cervical softening	42/106 (40)	—
Uterine "enlargement"	27/106 (25)	—
Health personnel diagnosis of pregnancy	19/106 (18)	161/444 (36)
Fetal heart tones reportedly present	7/106 (7)	
False labor	1/106 (1)	133/444 (30)

*Fried et al,[28] Brenner,[36] Yen et al,[37] Daw,[38] Abram,[39] Kimball,[40] Lapido,[41] Starkman et al,[42] Zuber and Kelly,[5] Rosenberg et al,[43] O'Grady,[44] Schopbach et al.[45]

ical sign is uncertain. The abdomen is often moderately firm to palpation and tympanic to percussion with neither the uterus nor a fetal pole palpable. In markedly obese patients, where Leopold's maneuvers are more difficult, honest errors in palpation and resulting uncertainty in establishing the true diagnosis by physical examination alone are more likely. As already discussed, prior to the availability of reliable serological testing and ultrasound, anesthesia was employed to establish the correct diagnosis when abdominal examination proved difficult.[16,18-21] Modern methods of pregnancy diagnosis have superceded this potentially hazardous but dramatic technique.

The mechanism underlying the abdominal distention of pseudocyesis remains controversial. There are multiple causes related in the literature of varying validity or plausibility including: gaseous distention of the bowel[25,37,46,48,49] or uterus,[15,50] excessive omental fat,[13] retained feces/impaction,[48,50] urinary retention,[51-53] spasm of the diaphragm and/or abdominal muscles,[16,18,21,53] or combinations of these events.[10,18-20] While simple weight gain and lordosis of the spine will accentuate the lower abdomen, these are insufficient explanations for the marked distention that is often present in many women with pseudocyesis.

More modern investigations support the idea of a complex etiology for this observed distention. For example, a CAT scan was performed in a recent case and demonstrated a dilated colon, fat deposits in the abdominal wall, and a dilated/distended stomach extending all the way into the pelvis.[43]

Unrecognized pseudocyetic patients have been occasionally suspected of having obstetrical disorders and complications. Preeclampsia and eclampsia have been reported, but these instances are poorly documented and confounded by the inability to exclude preexisting conditions, such as epilepsy and chronic hypertension.[3,46,54] Exploratory laparotomy for presumed placenta separation has occurred on more than one occasion. Women have also been unsuccessfully explored for suspected ectopic or abdominal pregnancy. Serious errors were more common in the pre-ultrasound era, and erroneous laparotomy among patients with pseudocyesis is rare in recent times. However, hospital admission for another dramatic symptom, "pseudolabor," still occurs. Especially in multipara, pseudolabor is sometimes quite convincing to hospital staff. Such patients are occasionally admitted and even prepared for precipitous "delivery."

Reports of apparent fetal motion are common.[9,18] At times these motions are so violent as to be socially disruptive. Their presence can be confirmed by family, friends, and even physicians[55]; however, on close questioning and observation, the symptoms are usually atypical for their patterning, strength, or onset.[6] The motions presumably arise from the bowel and/or unconscious contractions of the woman's abdominal muscles. It is important to recognize that the presence of such motions during abdominal palpation, or their observation by other individuals, strongly reinforces the patient's conviction of the existence of true gestation.

Occasionally, maternal tachycardia can confuse the clinician into believing that the fetal heart has been heard, but it is impossible to excuse recurrent recordings of "fetal heart tones of 140 bpm in the left lower quadrant," even in busy clinical settings. Such reports can only represent wishful thinking, and inattention to detail on the part of the practitioner and/or assistants, and have the unfortunate effect of solidifying the patient's incorrect belief in her pregnancy.

Breast engorgement, galactorrhea, and tenderness are common in pseudocyesis.[5,56] The etiology of the breast discharge is not entirely clear. When prolactin levels are measured in these patients, they are variable. However, the secretion of prolactin is episodic and low levels may accompany established lactation. Galactorrhea and even true lactation can result from long-term breast stimulation, or more uncommonly from a constant irritative focus, such as a scar and/or inflammatory lesion in the breast or on the adjacent chest wall. Further, certain drugs, notably the phenothiazines, promote galactorrhea by their effect on dopamine and prolactin.[57] This can be confusing to patient and clinician alike if such drug therapy has been instituted.

The duration of pseudocyesis and the likelihood of recurrence is markedly variable. Some 43% of Bivin and Klinger's cases lasted 9 months.[6] Untreated cases may persist for 1 to 2 years and, under unusual circumstances, for even longer periods. One remarkable case attributed to Dupuytren reportedly lasted 18 years![18,28,58] Bivin and Klinger recorded 23 women with more than one episode of pseudocyesis, and one exceptional case of a woman who displayed pseudocyetic symptoms every 9 months from her marriage until her death.[6] The literature also reports a considerable number of cases of pseudocyesis followed or preceded by normal pregnancy, indicating that an episode of pseudopregnancy is by no means incompatible with normal reproductive function at some other time in life.[6,25,26,47,59,60]

Establishing the correct diagnosis by physical examination and medical history alone may tax the abilities of the best obstetrician, and the literature includes many instances of embarassing errors.[6,24,28] One or more physicians supported the diagnosis of pregnancy in 161 of Bivin and Klinger's 444 cases (36.3%).[6] Further, in the series of Fried and co-workers, nine patients of 27 (33.3%)[28] were thought to be pregnant by an examining physician and one woman was thought to be pregnant by no less than four separate physicians!

The failure to establish the correct diagnosis is due to incomplete examinations, or when no pelvic examination had been performed prior to the onset of the apparent labor. Poor patient compliance, obesity, inexperience, and/or wishful thinking by the examiner likely explain the remaining incorrect clinical diagnoses. Also, most of these erroneous diagnoses occurred in the pre-ultrasound era and before the development of highly accurate and reliable pregnancy testing.

Differential Diagnosis

While establishing the diagnosis of true pregnancy is considerably easier now than in the past, a number of medical conditions can still be confused with pseudocyesis (Table 15.3). It is also possible that individuals will present in settings where access to pregnancy testing or ultrasonography is not immediate, or does not immediately appear pertinent. In such circumstances, major diagnostic errors are possible, despite the availability of new technology.

In cases where early and often vague signs or symptoms of pregnancy occur, or if menses are irregular or scanty, pregnancy testing will establish the presence or absence of gestation. If spontaneous menses do not ensue, induc-

Table 15.3 Differential Diagnosis of Pseudocyesis

Complications of Pregnancy

1. Intrauterine fetal demise, missed or incomplete abortion
2. Ectopic, abdominal, or ovarian pregnancy
3. Rudimentary horn pregnancy or other Müllerian anomalies
4. Abruptio placentae
    a. Chronic/Breus' mole
    b. Acute placental separation
5. Placenta previa
6. Gestational trophoblastic disease or partial mole

Other Disorders

1. Hypothalamic galactorrhea/amenorrhea syndrome
2. Central nervous system tumors
3. Ovarian or uterine tumor
4. Morbid obesity
5. Ascites
6. Menopause or early ovarian failure
7. Drug side effects
8. Schizophrenia
9. Organic brain syndrome

tion by hormonal manipulation is common. Thus, under normal clinical circumstances, "erroneous" pregnancies are rapidly excluded and irregular menses promptly treated. As early diagnosis is established by home or office testing, it is unlikely in most cases that ignorance of true physiology influences or supports an erroneous belief in pregnancy. Thus, the incorrect assumption of pregnancy by otherwise normal women is uncommon except for relatively brief periods of time as the tools for correct diagnosis are accurate, relatively inexpensive, and commonly available. These innovations in clinical practice have meant that the dramatic cases reported with considerable frequency in prior years are now less common. In modern times, pseudocyesis has become a more subtle and complex disease, except in some subcultures where a more classic form of the disorder persists.

Ultrasonographic scanning provides an easy means of establishing the correct diagnosis and providing the patient with visible evidence that no fetus is present.[44,49] However, our experience and that of others has been that the use of either ultrasonography or, occasionally, radiography have their own unique pitfalls. One of our patients and two reported by Starkman[42] overheard discussions between the ultrasound technicians and/or visualized images on the screen, which they interpreted as indicating that a fetus was present. They then either mistook or ignored the official report. If ultrasonography is used as a means to exclude the diagnosis of pregnancy, an experienced person should be present during the procedure to point out the true anatomy and to answer any questions the patient has concerning unusual shadows or unclear images. It is critical that neither the clinician nor the technician provide any clues or suggestive statements during the course of the examination. The patient will assiduously listen for such verbal clues. Our common terminology in such cases is potentially problematic. The clinician and technician need to be vigilant with their remarks because an anxious woman hearing her uterus described as a "6- to 8-weeks size" may well interpret this as a confirmation of pregnancy.

Pathophysiology

Pseudocyesis is a psychoneuroendocrine disorder.[2,52,61] There is an extensive literature documenting the existence in animals of a similar condition termed *pseudopregnancy*. Pseudopregnancy occurs in dogs, mice, rats, rabbits, and other animals. Interestingly, the physical signs of pregnancy in such animals are usually noted in conjunction with complex maternal behaviors, such as grooming or nest building.[62] In these animal models, pseudopregnancy is commonly associated with a persistent corpus luteum[63] and can occur spontaneously or be induced by a variety of laboratory procedures. These include injections of chorionic gonadotropin, or cervical stimulation by sterile matings or small electrical shocks.[64,65] Pseudopregnancy in mice can even be induced by exposure to the pheromones contained in the urine of familiar stud males.[66]

In humans, it is theorized that psychic stress or an endogenous depression alters the function of hypothalamic biogenic amines and is the initiating event in pseudocyesis.[45,51,54,67-70] Thereafter, variable alterations in the regulation of gonadotropin- releasing hormone (Gn-RH), the hypothalamic releasing factor for luteinizing hormone (LH) and follicle-stimulating hormone (FSH), occur and menstrual disturbance results. However, the complex data available concerning the neurophysiology of pseudocyesis is both incomplete and often contradictory.[2] Much of the endocrine data in the human literature arises from case reports involving small numbers of women, and it is often left unclear how pronounced the signs and symptoms are in each case.

Despite these reservations, there have been several reports in recent years worthy of consideration. Endocrine findings have demonstrated variable elevations in prolactin, depressed levels of FSH, and the inconstant finding of a persisting corpus luteum.[3,4,10,28,37,67,71-74] For example, Ashe and coworkers[71] found normal basal serum levels of FSH, LH, growth hormone (GH), thyroid-stimulating hormone (TSH), estradiol, prolactin, and cortisol in patients with pseudocyesis. An exaggerated response of LH to Gn-RH was observed in five of nine patients tested. Drife[4] found a similar response of LH to the administration of Gn-RH and thyrotropin-releasing hormone (TRH).

Zarate and co-workers,[75] Yen and Rebar,[37] and other authors[4,28] have reported cases of pseudocyesis with galactorrhea and found elevated prolactin levels. However, in some instances, basal prolactin levels were normal. This finding might result from the sampling variation or alterations in receptor sensitivity. It is also at least theoretically possible that the galactorrhea of pseudocyesis is the result of a biologically active prolactin which is not specifically measured in standard assays.

Other authors have studied growth hormone secretion. Tulandi and co-workers[73,74] found an abnormal GH response to TRH during two episodes of pseudocyesis in the same patient. As growth hormone secretion is under the control of a dopamine neurotransmitter, they suggested that there may be a derangement in the hypothalamus caused by an abnormality in dopaminergic function.

Findings by other investigators have included abnormal dexamethasone suppression tests, low to normal levels of FSH, either low or elevated LH, elevated plasma testosterone and estradiol, and either normal or elevated serum progesterone.[4] Devane and co-workers,[72] for example, reported on five patients whose hormone profiles were most consistent with polycystic ovarian disease, except for an uncharacteristic elevation of progesterone levels.

Elevated serum progesterone has also been reported in other patients with pseudocyesis and might conceivably be due to a persisting corpus luteum. Moulton[76] and van Tongeren[77] reported three cases of pseudocyesis with apparent corpus lutea seen at surgery. However, when direct observation of the ovary has been undertaken in several additional cases, corpus lutea have not been observed.[27,75] In this regard the physiology of human pseudocyesis is probably different from the pseudopregnancy of other animals, especially those with reflex ovulation.

Other neuroactive substances have also been investigated. Endogenous opioid peptides are inhibitory for gonadotropin secretion.[72] Some women with hypothalamic amenorrhea respond to naloxone (Narcan) infusion with the release of LH. This suggests that hypothalamic opioid suppression may be involved in the amenorrhea of pseudocyesis. Opioid peptides also influence behavior and it has been postulated that production of endogenous opioid peptides may be an etiologic factor in pseudocyesis.[72] Unfortunately, recent data have not supported this attractive hypothesis. Devane and co-workers[72] administered naloxone to women with pseudocyesis but failed to induce release of either LH or prolactin. Thus a role for endogenous opioid peptides in the etiology of pseudocyesis remains speculative.

In summary, there is no single neurophysiological pattern that can be consistently demonstrated in patients with pseudocyesis.[42] Abnormalities in the hypothalamic-pituitary- ovarian axis are common, but nonspecific.[78] The bulk of data is consistent with an amenorrhea/oligomenorrhea syndrome of hypothalamic origin with variable prolactin secretion.

Pathophysiology and Psychopathology

Physical processes appear to be the trigger for pseudopregnancy in laboratory animals. A rough parallel occurs in humans, as in patients who arrive at the belief that they are pregnant after developing galactorrhea as a side effect of neuroleptic medications. In most instances, however, the basis for human pseudopregnancy is presumed to be psychological. Unfortunately, there are no characteristic psychopathologic processes in patients developing pseudocyesis. The majority of pseudocyetic women are *not* severely disturbed or psychotic, and this phenomenon usually occurs among women who would otherwise be considered psychologically normal.

Pseudocyesis is generally classified as a conversion disorder. This is a condition in which an aberration in physical function occurs that is not explicable by the usual mechanisms of pathophysiology. The essential feature of conversion disorder is that a psychologic conflict or need is expressed through somatic symptoms.[79,80] Conversion disorders are usually acute and ephemeral but may be recurrent or "permanent." Such reactions occur most often in individuals with immature, histrionic, or dependent personalities, but can also appear in the absence of any underlying psychopathology.[81] The symptoms may serve to reduce anxiety or other dysphoric affects, they may simultaneously symbolize or communicate an underlying conflict, and they are not intentionally produced.

The syndrome of pseudocyesis has often been attributed to a wish for and/or dread of pregnancy. Specific conflicts cited in cases of pseudocyetic women have included issues relating to unstable marital relationships,[3,27] desire for work compensation, more attention from family,[3] unfulfilled dependency needs,[3,44] proof of fertility,[36,41] establishing sexual identity,[40] and competition with parents.[28] Cohen[27] has emphasized the cultural pressures that impact on the incidence of pseudocyesis, such as the procreative imperative of the Bible, the need for large families in preindustrial societies, and the presence of customs such as the *lobola* or marriage dowry of South Africa.

What is unusual in considering pseudocyesis as a conversion disorder is the fact that the somatic "abnormality" is a parallel of normal reproductive physiology, and not a pathologic condition.[80] Also, symptoms such as galactorrhea and amenorrhea suggest involvement of the endocrine system, which is highly unusual for conversion disorders.

Although pseudocyesis is frequently cited as a conversion disorder, the syndrome has also been linked with other psychiatric disorders. Misinterpretation of bodily sensations is an essential aspect of pseudocyesis and it therefore resembles delusional disorders. Like other delusions it is not amenable to rational analysis. Because of the associated physical changes it commonly leads others to the same erroneous conviction, and family and friends join in a shared delusion (folie à deux). Pseudocyesis can also be viewed as being similar to a hypochondriacal state or an obsessional disorder, in which pregnancy is an *idée fixe*. According to this interpretation, the "pregnancy" is an idea or thought that constantly intrudes into the patient's conscious awareness and is beyond her control. In cases where the fear of pregnancy and sexuality are major components, pseudocyesis may appear to be related to anxiety disorders.

Some authors have suggested that pseudocyesis is a product of an affective disorder or major depression.[54,78] Emotional injuries or losses are not infrequent precipitants for pseudopregnancy and may include the death of a loved person, the end of childbearing ability, or other events that lower self-esteem.[54] It is appealing, but probably an oversimplification, to conceptualize pseudocyesis as being an affective disorder in which the pituitary-hypothalamic-ovarian axis is particularly involved.

Lastly, in a minority of cases, more profound associated psychopathology can be found.[82] The psychotic patient with pseudocyesis will evidence widespread loss of reality testing and associated unusual behavior. These patients are usually schizophrenic, but on occasion may have a major affective disorder with psychosis or an organic brain syndrome.

Treatment

The best recent review of pseudocyesis is by Miller and Maricle,[83] but their article is typical of the literature in devoting a total of seven sentences to treatment.[1,4,6,28,63,84] There are several logical reasons for the dearth of information regarding therapeutic management, the most pertinent being that with the exception of Bivin and Klinger's comprehensive monograph, the overwhelming majority of articles are literature reviews prompted by chance encounters with one or two patients. Most of these women are lost to follow-up and there are virtually no systematic studies. We are still in the early stages of our own investigation of pseudocyesis, and thus the following comments concerning clinical management are offered as guidelines (see Figure 15.1).

Working Alliance

It is worthwhile for the obstetrician to decide, before the first patient appears, the extent to which he or she is interested in treating this condition. In almost every sizable community there are obstetricians (most of whom will probably purchase this book!) who have developed reputations based on their curiosity and/or sensitivity to cases complicated by psychosocial factors. The general obstetrician should not hesitate in referring pseudocyetic patients to these colleagues if he or she does not wish to undertake their treatment. Treatment is ideally carried out with the collaboration of a psychiatrist, but direct and immediate referral for psychiatric services should be limited to those few pa-

Figure 15.1 Clinical management of suspected pseudocyesis

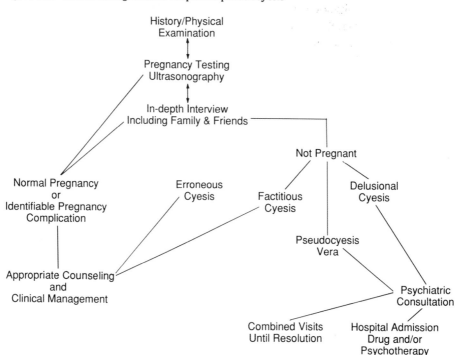

tients who have major affective disorders or are overtly psychotic.

Aside from their pseudocyetic syndrome, most of these women do not have major psychiatric disorders. The majority of these patients are probably either psychologically "normal" and subject to social pressures or, at worst, they have personality disorders. Rather than "crazy," the typical pseudocyetic patient seen in our medical center is more likely to be poor, uneducated, and an immigrant or child of immigrants. Her English may be rudimentary and communication is further disrupted because she is in acute distress. She is very likely surrounded by concerned and anxious relatives. Keeping this in mind, the obstetrician should make every effort to be aware of his or her own reactions, and focus on establishing a working alliance with these patients.

The physician needs to take every possible precaution to avoid an adversarial relationship—or the patient will simply leave. On some level, the pseudocyetic patient knows that she cannot trust her own bodily sensations or appearance, and it is an extraordinarily difficult task for a physician to foster a trusting relationship in this situation. If the woman can trust the physician she will return to his or her office or clinic, and definitive resolution of the syndrome is much more likely.

Another point worth considering is that while the clinician often feels the need to immediately clarify that the patient is not pregnant, this is likely to be greeted by both the patient and her family with incredulity or outright hostility. It is the patient's belief in her pregnancy that drives the social and physiologic changes and sustains the appearance of pregnancy. For the process to continue, the woman's belief in pregnancy is externally reinforced by the concurrence of others.

Reinforcement can be by friends, family, or physicians or other health workers who concur in the mistaken diagnosis. Patients who present with conversion disorders or hypochondriacal states cannot readily accept a psychological explanation. Such patients are simultaneously fearful and antagonistic, and they have a particular dread that they will be told by the physician that "it's all in your head." The author's clinical experience and the literature are consistent in concluding that confrontations are beneficial to neither physician nor patient.[28,44,78] The woman who is simply and directly told that she is not pregnant is usually unable and/or unwilling to believe the truth and often goes from doctor to doctor seeking confirmation of her supposed gestation.

A more rational strategy entails a clear statement that there are obvious *physiological* abnormalities present and, although they resemble pregnancy, they are unfortunately not signs of true pregnancy. The abnormalities merit a thorough evaluation in which the physician will also pay attention to the stresses in the patient's life, since stress can affect people's bodies. The physician explicitly states that he or she is aware that the woman and her family are undoubtably disappointed by this finding and may even have some trouble believing it to be true. The emphasis in this approach is on initially acknowledging the physical symptoms, and on avoiding the conflict that would follow a premature focus on psychosocial issues.

Immediate involvement of the family is ideal. Social pressures are major etiologic forces in the genesis of this syndrome. Therapy should take full advantage of the influence of friends and family and employ their assistance in encouraging the patient to attend follow-up appointments. They should be allowed and even encouraged to participate in the procedures that establish the correct diagnosis.

Establishing the Diagnosis

Patients with pseudocyesis may appear in the office seeking prenatal care or questioning some complication of gestation such as bleeding or postdatism. Usually, there is sufficient time for the obstetrician to foster at least an initial working alliance. Unfortunately, it is becoming more common for pseudocyetic patients to arrive at an emergency room in the middle of the night in the throes of apparent labor. The patients typically are strangers to the obstetrician, and are anxious, frightened, and in acute distress. Even in this tense setting, however, both the gross psychiatric and obstetrical diagnoses are usually ascertained with little difficulty. A brief examination coupled with some minimal background information should also establish whether the patient is severely depressed or psychotic.

For example, we recently saw in consultation a 52-year-old woman who presented to our emergency room with the belief that she was about to deliver a child. The patient had a history of multiple psychiatric hospitalizations and carried a diagnosis of chronic paranoid schizophrenia. She was promptly admitted to our psychiatric unit, where her delusion responded to treatment with neuroleptic medications. Neither the psychiatric nor the obstetric diagnoses were ever seriously questioned.

Identification of the Psychosocial Stresses

While information can also be gathered from friends and from family, it is essential that the patient be given the opportunity to tell her own story in privacy. This is often the most difficult part of the entire process, as the obstetrician is invariably constrained by time limitations. The art of listening to one's patients can only develop with time and practice.

Perhaps the biggest problem that obstetricians experience in trying to elicit these histories is their own propensity to actively intervene or to make recommendations. Such interventions usually derail the patient from recounting the story, and also prove mutually frustrating when they are ineffective. It is safer for the obstetrican to assume that patients have both common sense and a greater awareness of their own circumstances. The thrust of the interview is directed toward eliciting the underlying situation, and not in rectifying it.

The inclusion of psychiatric assistance has to be delicately managed, and in most cases the challenge remains for the obstetrician to discover the issues without the assistance of psychiatric consultation. Women with pseudocyesis rarely wish to see a psychiatrist, much less get psychological treatment. However, if a psychiatrist can be involved, he can facilitate communication and assist in explaining how the apparent pregnancy developed, pointing out the patient's strengths and what environmental stresses and internal conflicts contribute to the condition.

We conceptualize pseudocyesis as a product of both social forces and unconscious dynamic forces. The influence of friends and family is tremendously important in either reinforcing error or promoting symptom resolution. Most patients with a firm conviction of pregnancy will not follow through with psychiatric care unless pressed by others. Furthermore, these patients are often very provocative and a psychiatrist can be helpful in preventing their care takers from dismissing them as simple malingerers. It is often not a simple matter to accept the unconscious elements of this disorder and recognize that the symptoms are outside of the patient's control. This is partly because pseudocyetic patients also usually have clearly defined external pressures that they are trying to cope with.

One such patient, a Portuguese-American woman, had moved in with her married boyfriend, to the dismay of her family and community. Frantic efforts were made to separate the lovers until finally, her "pregnancy" became manifest. The pseudocyesis served to calm the social situation, but it also was a product of unconscious conflicts related to early childhood abuse, and led her physicians to provide analgesic and anxiolytic medications and eventually to perform an unnecessary surgical exploration. The above case is illustrative of women who have characterological problems and whose lives are chronically tumultuous.[83] It is unrealistic to expect that their lives will change appreciably with obstetrical or psychiatric intervention or that they will not develop other complaints and symptoms. This is especially true when there is a history of drug, medication, or alcohol abuse. Such cases are often frustrating and complex. As a general rule, individuals who have a long history of hysterical symptoms, impaired social relations, drug abuse, or other evidence of personality disorders, are unlikely to accept psychological exploration, and recurrences of the original problem are to be expected. On the other hand, patients who have had good psychosocial adjustments prior to their pseudocyesis, close relationships with others, and an obvious precipitating stressor, will be likely to have a successful treatment course.

Conclusions

The classic conversion disorders, such as pseudocyesis, are gratifying to treat because of their rapid amelioration to most psychotherapeutic interventions.[84] It was these disorders that led Freud and Breuer to the discovery of the "talking cure" in which hypnosis and analytic techniques were used to reveal underlying conflicts. We are not alone in the impression that many individuals who develop conversion disorders have an impairment of their ability to communicate the psychosocial situation and attendant feelings.[84] When the obstetrician or psychiatrist helps the patient to put her story into words, this is often followed by a rapid reversal of symptoms. While the conflict itself does not necessarily abate or disappear, openly talking about it serves to lessen some of its power. Sometimes this will be sufficient to suggest some other means of resolution for the underlying situation.

There are some physical measures that can play a role in helping patients and their families accept their nongravid condition. As an adjunct to psychotherapy, hormonal manipulations to induce menses, or, more rarely, uterine curettage, can help convince a patient that she is not pregnant. It needs to be emphasized that any such therapy should *accompany and not precede* psychological evaluation and treatment. Otherwise, vaginal bleeding may be interpreted as being an induced or spontaneous abortion or another pregnancy complication. This will likely prompt the patient to panic and/or seek help elsewhere. Most but not all patients with pseudocyesis will respond by having a withdrawal flow to administration of progestational agents (eg, medroxyprogesterone acetate 10 mg qd for 10 days). However, if menstrual function has been suppressed for a prolonged period progesterone alone can be ineffectual and administration of combined estrogen and progestin may be necessary to initiate menstrual bleeding. We recommend using conjugated equine estrogens 1.25 mg qd for 21 days with medroxyprogesterone acetate 10 mg qd for the last 7 days. These physical interventions should never supplant the emphasis on understanding the psychosocial factors that contribute to the development of the pseudocyesis.

There are few more dramatic clinical conditions than pseudocyesis. Rarely is the desire or the fear of an individual more concentrated, intense, and remarkable. Pseudocyesis is one of the most singular symptom complexes encountered by clinicians who practice obstetrics and it indelibly impresses upon us the importance of emotional control over human physiology.

References

1. Hardwick PG, Fitzpatrick C: Fear, folie, and phantom pregnancy: Pseudocyesis in a 15-year-old girl. *Br J Psychiatry* 1981;139:558–560.
2. Murray JL, Abraham GE: Pseudocyesis: A review. *Obstet Gynecol* 1978;51:627–631.
3. Small GW: Pseudocyesis: An overview. *Can J Psychiatry* 1986;31:452–457.
4. Drife JO: Phantom pregnancy. *Br Med J* 1985;291:687–688.
5. Zuber T, Kelly J: Pseudocyesis. *Am Fam Physician* 1984;30:131–134.
6. Bivin GD, Klinger M: *Pseudocyesis*. Bloomington, IN, Principia Press, 1937.
7. Gueniot P: Fausses grossesses et grossesse nerveuses. *La Méd* 1932;13:270–274.
8. Eustasche G: Des fausses grossesses ou grossesses par illusion. *Nouv Arch d'Obstet Gynécol* 1894;9:481–493.
9. Paddock R: Spurious pregnancy. *Am J Obstet Gynecol* 1928;16:845–854.
10. Madden TM: On spurious, feigned and concealed pregnancy. *Dub J Med Sci* 1872;53:255–264.
11. Lever JCA: Malingered pregnancy and delivery—hysteria. *Guy's Hosp Rep* 1848;6:239–240.
12. Chambers WR: Brain tumor simulating pregnancy. *Am J Obstet Gynecol* 1955;70:212–213.
13. Paulowski EJ, Pawlowski MMF: Unconscious and abortive aspects of pseudocyesis. *Wis Med J* 1958;57:437–440.
14. Steinberg A, Pastor N, Winheld EB, Segal HI, Shechter FR, Colton NH: Psychoendocrine relationships in pseudocyesis. *Psychosom Med* 1946;8:176–181.
15. Hippocrates, in Littre E (ed.): *Oeûvres complètes d'Hippocrate*, Volume IX. Paris, JB Baillière et Fils, 1861.
16. Simpson J: *Clinical Lectures on the Diseases of Women*, vol. 3. Edinburgh, Black, 1871.
17. Simpson J: Spurious pregnancy—its frequency and nature. *Month J Med Sci* 1850;11:90–91.
18. Daley MD: Pseudocyesis. *Postgrad Med J* 1946;22:395–399.
19. Haultain FWN: Spurious pregnancy. *Am J Med Sci* 1891;101:342–345.
20. Markoe JW: Pseudocyesis. *Int Clin* 1918;2:34–37.
21. Vinay C: Grossesse nerveuse et menopause. *Bull Lyon Méd* 1906;107:1124–1127.

22. Aldrich CK: A case of recurrent pseudocyesis. *Perspect Biol Med* 1972;16:11–21.

23. Barnes AC: Mary Tudor. *Obstet Gynecol* 1953;1:585–590.

24. Hunter QW: Pseudocyesis. *Med Age* 1905;23:326–333.

25. Cunningham JL: Phantom tumors, simulating pregnancy. *Tex Cour Rec Méd* 1890;8:64–67.

26. Caulet D: La fausse grossesse de la Reine de Serbie. *Semin Méd* 1901;21:173–176.

27. Cohen LM: A current perspective of pseudocyesis. *Am J Psychiatry* 1984;139:1140–1144.

28. Fried PH, Rakoff AE, Schopbach RR, Kaplan AJ: Pseudocyesis: A psychosomatic study in gynecology. *JAMA* 1951;145:1329–1335.

29. Selzer JG: Pseudocyesis in a six year-old girl. *J Am Acad Child Psychiatry* 1968;7:693–720.

30. Aronson GJ: Delusion of pregnancy in a male homosexual with an abdominal cancer. *Bull Meninger Clin* 1952;16:159–166.

31. Silva JA, Leong GB, Weinstock R: Misidentification syndrome and male pseudocyesis. *Psychosomatics* 1991;32:228–230.

32. Bitton G, Thibaut F, Lefevre-Lesage I: Delusions of pregnancy in a man. *Am J Psychiatr* 1991;148:811–812.

33. Evans DL, Seely TJ: Pseudocyesis in the male. *J Nerv Ment Dis* 1984;172:37–40.

34. Trethowan WH: The couvade syndrome, in Howells JL (ed.): *Modern Perspectives in Psycho-Obstetrics*. New York, Brunner- Mazel, 1972, pp 67–93.

35. Trethowan WH, Conlon M: The couvade syndrome. *Br J Psychiatry* 1965;111:57–66.

36. Brenner BN: Pseudocyesis in blacks. *S Afr Med J* 1976;50:1757–1759.

37. Yen SSC, Rebar RW, Quesenberry W: Pituitary function in pseudocyesis. *J Clin Endocrinol Metab* 1976;43:132–136.

38. Daw E: Pseudocyesis. *Br J Clin Pract* 1973;27:181–183.

39. Abram HS: Pseudocyesis followed by true pregnancy in the termination phase of an analysis. *Br J Med Psycho* 1969;42:255–262.

40. Kimball CP: A case of pseudocyesis caused by "roots." *Am J Obstet Gynecol* 1970;107:801–803.

41. Lapido OA: Pseudocyesis in infertile patients. *Int J Gynecol Obstet* 1979;16:427–429.

42. Starkman MN, Marshall JC, Ferla JL, Kelch RP: Pseudocyesis: Psychologic and neuroendocrine interrelationships. *Psychosom Med* 1985;47:46–57.

43. Rosenberg HK, Coleman BG, Kroop J, Granowetter L, Evans : Pseudocyesis in an adolescent patient. *Clin Pediatr* 1983;22:708–712.

44. O'Grady JP: Pseudocyesis. *Obstet Gynecol Surv* 1989;44:500–511.

45. Schopbach RR, Fried PH, Rokoff AE: Pseudocyesis: A psychosomatic disorder. *Psychosom Med* 1952;14:129–134.

46. Ryan WB: Spurious pregnancy. *Lancet* 1855;381,429–430,532–534.

47. Rutherford RN: Pseudocyesis. *N Engl J Med* 1941;224:639–644.

48. LaMotte GM: *A General Treatise of Midwifery*. London, Waugh, 1746.

49. Guzinski GM, Conrad SH: Pseudocyesis and sonography. *Am J Obstet Gynecol* 1980;138:230–232.

50. Mauriceau F: *Traité des Maladies des Femmes Grossesse, Quatrième Edition*. Paris, L D'Houry, 1694.

51. Greaves DC, Green PE, West LJ: Psychodynamic and psychophysiological aspects of pseudocyesis. *Psychosom Med* 1960;22:24–31.

52. Bouchacourt A: Sur la grossesse nerveuse ou imaginaire. *Lyon Méd* 1892;69:19–21.

53. Berkeley C: *Diseases of Women by Ten Teachers*. London, Edward Arnold, 1922, p 621.

54. Brown E, Barglow P: Pseudocyesis: A paradigm for psychophysiological interactions. *Arch Gen Psychiatry* 1971;24:221–229.

55. Chapman EN: Spurious pregnancy. *Am Med Times* 1864;9:50–51,62–63.

56. Briehl W, Kulka EW: Lactation in a virgin. *Psychoanal Q* 1935;4:484–512.

57. Cramer B: Delusion of pregnancy in a girl with drug-induced lactation. *Am J Psychiatry* 1971;127:960–963.

58. Mitchell SW: Pseudocyesis—spurious pregnancy. *Med News* 1895;66:393–395.

59. Jana AP: Case of pseudocyesis followed by true pregnancy. *Ind Med Gaz* 1934;69:445–446.

60. Clifford JL: Spurious pregnancy with report of case. *Old Dom J Med Surg* 1911;13:160–167.

61. Reifenstein EC: Psychogenic or "hypothalamic" amenorrhea. *Med Clin North Am* 1946;30:1103–1114.

62. Saito TR: Plasma progesterone levels and maternal nest building behavior during pseudopregnancy and early pregnancy in the IVCS mouse. *Ann Anim Psychol* 1986;36L10:1–5.

63. Barglow P, Brown E: Pseudocyesis: To be and not to be pregnant: A psychosomatic question. In Howells JC (ed.): *Modern Perspectives in Psycho-Obstetrics*. New York, Brunner Mazel, 1972, pp 53–67.

64. Caillol M, Martinet L, Lacroix M: Relative roles of oestradiol and of the uterus in the maintenance of the corpus luteum in the pseudopregnant brown hare (*Lepus europaeus*). *J Reprod Fert* 1989;87:603–612

65. Morehead MH, Gala RR: The restraint stress-induced decrease of the nocturnal prolactin surge and the physiology of pseudopregnancy and pregnancy in the rat. *Life Sci* 1989;45:201–215.

66. Thomas KJ, Dominic CJ: Induction of pseudopregnancy in pregnancy-blocked mice by re-exposure to stud males. *Physiol Behav* 1987;41:515–517.

67. Ayers JWT, Seiler JC: Neuroendocrine indicies of depression in pseudocyesis. *J Reprod Med* 1984;29:67–70.

68. Forsbach G, Guitron A, Munoz M, Bustos H: Pituitary function in human pseudocyesis. *J Endocrinol Invest* 1987;10:39–43.

69. Osotimehin BO, Ladipo OA, Adejuwon CA, Otolorin EO: Pituitary and placental hormone levels in pseudocyesis. *Int J Obstet Gynaecol* 1981;19:399–402.

70. Yoshida T, Hattori Y, Takashima Y, Noda K: Serum oxytocin concentrations in women under pseudopregnancy therapy. *J Exp Med* 1982;137:347–348.

71. Ashe RG, Padayachee T, Moodley J, et al: *Study of Presenting Features and Pituitary Function in Pseudocyesis*. XII World Congress on Fertility and Sterility, Singapore, October 26–31, 1986, p 670.

72. Devane GW, Zera MI, Buhi WC, Kalra PS: Opioid peptides in pseudocyesis. *Obstet Gynecol* 1985;65:183–188.

73. Tulandi T, McInnes RA, Metah A, Tolis G: Pseudocyesis: Pituitary function before and after resolution of symptoms. *Obstet Gynecol* 1982;59:119–121.

74. Tulandi T, McInnes RA, Lal S: Altered pituitary hormone secretion in patients with pseudocyesis. *Fertil Steril* 1983;40:637–641.

75. Zarate A, Canales ES, Soria J, et al: Gonadotropin and prolactin secretion in human pseudocyesis. *Ann d'Endocrinol* (Paris) 1974;35:445–450.

76. Moulton R: The psychosomatic implications of pseudocyesis. *Psychosom Med* 1942;4:376–389.

77. van Tongeren FC: Pseudo-gravidité par les Kystes luteiniques. *Gynécol Obstet* 1936;34:350–362.

78. Rubman S, Goreczny AJ, Brantley PJ, Pevey WJ: Pseudocyesis and depression: Etiological and treatment considerations. *J La State Med Soc* 1989:141:39–41.

79. Task Force on Nomenclature and Statistics: *Diagnostic and Statistical Manual of Mental Disorders*, ed. 3, rev. Washington, DC, American Psychiatric Association, 1987, pp 244–247.

80. Ziegler FJ, Imboden JB, Rodgers DA: Contemporary conversion reactions. III. Diagnostic considerations. *JAMA* 1963;186:307–311.

81. Lazare A: Conversion symptoms. *N Engl J Med* 1981;305:745–748.

82. Bressler B, Nyhus P, Magnussen F: Pregnancy fantasies in psychosomatic illness and symptom formation. *Psychosom Med* 1958;20:187–202.

83. Miller WH, Maricle R: Pseudocyesis: A model for cultural, psychological, and biological interplay. *J Psychosom Obstet Gynaecol* 1988;8:183–190.

84. Ford CV, Folks DG: Conversion disorders: An overview. *Psychosomatics* 1985;26: 371–383.

Chapter 16

Early Reproductive Loss

Halina Wiczyk, MD

> If the seed is ejected, . . . there will be corrective measures . . . if . . . bodily
> agitation, . . . remove it; . . . appease the soul, if the worries of life have troubled
> it; and if atony exists in . . . the uterus . . . strengthen these parts together with
> the whole body.
> —*Gynecology* I,47
> Soranus (AD78–117)

Spontaneous abortion is a common gynecologic event now recognized to have profound psychological impact. Recent research has broadened our understanding of the etiology of such pregnancy failures and has helped to identify new therapies. In this chapter the problems of both sporadic and recurrent pregnancy loss are reviewed with emphasis on both the psychological effects of such losses on the patient and the appropriate response of the clinician.

Clinical Presentation

Spontaneous or *sporadic abortion* occurs in one of six clinically recognized pregnancies.[1] Most of these early losses are due to chromosomal abnormalities and recurrence is uncommon.[2] Such pregnancy failures are to be distinguished from the syndrome of *recurrent* spontaneous abortion. In this latter condition, abnormal chromosome analyses are uncommon.[3,4] Coulam[5] estimates that the cause for such recurrent spontaneous abortion losses are immunologic (40%), hormonal (29%), anatomic (10%), and chromosomal (6%).

A major problem in interpretation of such data is that not all pregnancy losses are clinically evident. There is evidence that silent, unrecognized abortion of an unbalanced zygote is a frequent phenomenon both in humans and in other species.[6] Further, as many as 85% of all abortions occur prior to the clinical awareness of pregnancy.[1,7–9] Edmonds and co-workers[7] observed an embryonic premenstrual mortality rate of fully 34%. In their study, embryos lost after fertilization but before nidation could not be detected since testing was begun 7 days after ovulation. Thus, the true incidence of early pregnancy loss is probably even higher than estimated.

Differential Diagnosis

Recurrent spontaneous abortions are classified as either *primary* or *secondary*. *Primary aborters* are women who have experienced three or more consecutive spontaneous abortions and have no pregnancies continuing beyond the 20th week of gestation. To fulfill the definition, these pregnancies must have occurred with the same partner. Such abortions account for approximately 6% of pregnancy failures.[10] *Secondary aborters* are women who have experienced a live birth or stillbirth and subsequently have three or more spontaneous abortions, again, all with the same partner. Such abortions account for approximately 1.5% of all pregnancy losses. When both the primary and secondary abortion patients are fully investigated, half are found to have an underlying immunologic abnormality.[5]

Among the features distinguishing spontaneous from recurrent losses are the associated chromosomal abnormalities.[11] Trisomies and monosomy for the X chromosome are found in the sporadic type of miscarriages, while Robertsonian translocations are seen more often in recurrent losses. It is important to remember that the risk for repeated abortion is not increased if a chromosomal error is found in abortus material. In fact, the likelihood for subsequent abortion is actually greater in patients who experience a chromosomally normal pregnancy loss.[12]

History alone is insufficient to establish a correct diagnosis when the possibility of *recurrent* spontaneous abortion is suspected. A complete investigation is required including chromosome analysis of both partners, hysteroscopy or hysterosalpingography to evaluate the anatomy of the uterus, determination of the adequacy of the luteal phase through endometrial biopsy and/or serum progesterone determinations, and specialized immunologic testing.[3–5,13] Unfortunately, despite careful study in many patients no specific diagnosis will be possible, emphasizing the limitations of current knowledge.

Pathophysiology

Distinct anatomic abnormalities are common in aborted pregnancies. In a detailed morphologic study of the products of conception in 472 failed pregnancies, 60% of the embryos were abnormal with severe disorganization of growth.[7] Fully 32.5% had focal anomalies of the central nervous system, heart, or musculoskeletal or digestive systems. Many early abortions involve abnormal karyotypes but, increasingly, other distinct etiologies are being identified, including immunologic, Müllerian, metabolic, and infectious causes.

Immunologic mechanisms are important in many recurrent abortions but not in sporadic abortions. A primary aborter will often have normal pregnancies if another partner is substituted, indicating a mate-specific problem.[14] In contrast, secondary aborters will continue to miscarry in pregnancies conceived with other men. In normal pregnancy, the gestation stimulates the mother's immune system to generate an immunologic response that prevents maternal rejection of the fetus and placenta largely by production of blocking antibody.[15,16] It is hypothesized that the primary aborter is unable to recognize and mount this expected immunologic response to the conceptus produced with a specific mate, leading to pregnancy failure.

Primary aborters apparently fail to adequately recognize and mount the protective immunologic responses to trophoblast antigens.[20] Mixed lymphocyte culture (MLC) reactions are used to evaluate the absence of blocking factors in such cases.[21] In mixed lymphocyte cultures, maternal lymphocytes are used as responder cells with irradiated paternal lymphocytes as stimulator cells. When such studies are performed, lymphocytes from couples with primary abortion sometimes have depressed stimulation indexes as compared to fertile couples.[18,21]

Normal blocking antibody production is to be differentiated from the lymphocytotoxic antibodies occasionally found in secondary aborters.[10,17] McIntyre and Faulk[18] suggest that secondary aborters may lose their pregnancies by mounting antibodies in excessively high titers to such fetopaternal antigens, an aberration of the expected response. In this specific instance, leukocyte immunotherapy is contraindicated as with this type of therapy the situation may be made worse.[18,19]

Thus, normally pregnancy-blocking antibodies develop, preventing maternal lymphocyte responses to paternal antigens expressed on trophoblast cells.[22,23] Primary aborters who express either a lack of immunologic response or an abnormal response are candidates for seminal plasma sensitization or leukocyte immunotherapy as a method of evoking blocking antibody production.[23,24]

There are other rare immunologic causes for recurrent losses: at least some couples with unexplained recurrent abortions share various HLA antigens and are therefore histocompatible at several discrete loci.[25,26] Such HLA or histocompatibility antigens are present on almost all human tissues except trophoblast.[11] Other investigators have not found this association, but claim that family size is smaller among such histocompatible couples and that the interval between their children is longer.[27–29] Primary aborters who share HLA antigens with the father of their pregnancies occasionally benefit from leukocyte immunotherapy, again thought to stimulate maternal blocking antibody production.[11]

Various other autoantibodies are now recognized to be increased in abnormal or failed pregnancies.[30] The lupus anticoagulant (LAC) is a phospholipid antibody originally found in patients with systemic lupus erythematosus but now also identified in spontaneous aborters who do not have clinical lupus.[31–33] Patients with circulating LAC antibodies who abort usually do so after the 20th week of gestation. A characteristic finding in such cases is massive fibrin deposition and infarction in the placenta. Other phospholipid autoantibodies found in habitual aborters are the anticardiolipin (ACL) and antiphosphoserine (APS) antibodies.[34] It is not known if these antiphospholipid antibodies are produced as a response to pregnancy or if they predate gestation. Treatment for these miscarriage/antibody syndromes is either low dose aspirin (80 mg/day) and prednisone (30–70 mg/day) or full anticoagulation with heparin.[35]

Anatomic defects account for approximately 15% of repeated pregnancy losses. Cervical insufficiency (incompetence) is associated with painless dilatation and second-trimester losses. Among such patients treated with cerclage or bed rest and pessary, the successful pregnancy rate is usually greater than 70%. Other anatomic defects including submucous fibroids, multiple polyps, and uterine synechiae are also implicated in reproductive losses.[36]

Müllerian duct anomalies are associated in specific instances with both pregnancy wastage and preterm delivery. Uterine septae can be treated with transabdominal metroplasty or hysteroscopic excision with success rates of 80% to 90%.[37,38] A bicornuate uterus can also be surgically reunited by metroplasty. However, in a study comparing fetal salvage rates both before and after metroplasty, the live birthrate was essentially equal, emphasizing the importance of case selection for surgery.[5]

Endocrinologic abnormalities related to ovulation are frequently causes for early abortion. If a luteal phase defect is diagnosed, treatment with either clomiphene citrate or progesterone results in successful pregnancies in over 90%.[11] However, the actual existence of luteal phase defects has been debated and the incidence in a given review is dependent upon the criterion used for diagnosis. The likelihood of making the diagnosis decreases when basal body temperature charts and endometrial biopsy data are combined with menstrual dating versus when accurate documentation of ovulation using serial ultrasonic examinations is used as a basis for selection.[39]

Chronic metabolic abnormalities are also an occasional etiology for abortion. Uncommonly, maternal thyroid disease or malnutrition can be causes of pregnancy loss. However, the number of these cases is generally overestimated and they account for only a minute percentage of spontaneous pregnancy losses.

It is not known to what extent exposure to environmental pollutants, drugs, and/or ionizing radiation contribute to pregnancy losses. The correlations between such exposures and pregnancy losses are usually complex and are highly controversial.

Finally, various pathogenic bacteria and parasites are rarely implicated in miscarriage. Such agents include but are not limited to toxoplasmosis, rubella, cytomegalovirus, parvovirus, herpesvirus, *Listeria monocytogenes*, and various mycoplasma species. It is presumed that such infections either kill the conceptus or, alternatively, damage it leading to disordered growth, eventual abortion, or immediate loss.[36]

Treatment

Medical therapy for recurrent abortion depends upon cause. The most important step is a complete evaluation (Table 16.1). A couple undergoing study for recurrent abortions should have a pedigree analysis as well as chromosomal

Table 16.1 Work-Up of Recurrent Pregnancy Loss

1. Complete history and physical examination
2. Chromosomal studies of both partners and a full pedigree analysis
3. Hysteroscopy/hysterosalpingogram
4. Luteal phase evaluation with endometrial biopsy/serum progesterone/ultrasound
5. Immunologic testing: autoimmune and alloimmune testing
6. Screening for systemic disease as clinically indicated (eg, diabetes mellitus testing, thyroid series)
7. Appropriate cultures

Table 16.2 Immunologic Testing

1. HLA testing for histocompatibility antigens
2. Lymphocytoxic antibody titers
3. Mixed lymphocyte cultures for evaluation of blocking factors
4. Partial thromboplastin time, protime determinations
5. Screening for autoantibodies (lupus anticoagulant, anticardiolipin, antiphosphoserine antibody titers, antinuclear antibody titers)

studies of their peripheral blood. As there is no available treatment for either a parental chromosomal translocation or multifactorial genetic disorders, if such defects are found to be responsible for the observed abortions, artificial insemination by donor semen or adoption is the best therapy. The likelihood for a spontaneous full-term, living child for couples with such abnormalities is only 20% to 30%.[40,41]

In evaluating a woman for recurrent pregnancy losses, an immunologic screen consisting of tests for antinuclear antibodies, the lupus anticoagulant, the anticardiolipin antibody, and the antiphosphoserine antibody should be performed (Table 16.2). Included in this testing should be cytotoxic antibodies as well as evaluation of blocking factors. Also, a panel of basic laboratory tests is appropriate (eg, hemoglobin, hematocrit, urea nitrogen, creatinine, and thyroid panel) along with a complete physical/pelvic examination as well as a review of any medical records for prior therapies and/or surgery.

Different treatment modalities for recurrent pregnancy losses are summarized in Table 16.3.[42,43]

Ectopic pregnancy must also be viewed as early pregnancy loss. In the past, salpingectomy via laparotomy was the treatment of choice. However, with progressively earlier diagnosis and a rapidly increasing incidence of the disorder, conservative management is considered best. Both subsequent normal pregnancy rates and repeat ectopic rates are similar in those patients who are treated conservatively by salpingostomy or salpingectomy.[44] In two studies evaluating patients with a sole remaining tube who were treated conservatively, intrauterine pregnancy rates of 53% and 47.6% were reported, with repeat ectopic rates of 20% and 42.8%.[45,46] Recently, laparoscopic techniques for the treatment of ectopic pregnancy have been developed. Using this new technique, both intrauterine pregnancy and repeat ectopic rates are similar to those observed among patients undergoing a standard laparotomy.[47] The

Table 16.3 Treatment for Recurrent Pregnancy Loss

Abnormality	Possible therapy
Chromosomal	Artificial insemination (AID)
Luteal phase defect	Clomiphene citrate/progesterone
Structural defects	Metroplasty, hysteroscopic resection, cervical cerclage
Immunologic	ASA/prednisone, heparin, WBC immunotherapy, or seminal plasma therapy

obvious advantage of the laparoscopic method is reduced patient morbidity with subsequent early hospital discharge. However, if this technique is performed, it is essential that patients be monitored with weekly β-HCG titers until the levels are negative, to exclude persistent trophoblastic tissue.[48] Patients whose titers plateau or rise can be treated with the antimetabolite methotrexate as an alternative to a repeat surgical procedure.[49]

Psychological Aspects

In general, clinicians do not give the same status to early pregnancy losses as to losses occurring later in gestation. It is commonly believed that the grief and mourning that occur for an early abortion is not as profound as that associated with a third-trimester stillborn. However, women who have a spontaneous miscarriage experience the same feelings and go through the same stages of mourning as those with later losses. This process becomes even more pronounced if a pattern of repeated abortions occurs.

Men and women have different responses to early pregnancy loss, occasionally leading to conflict. Further, such losses are commonly associated with a prolonged period of emotional adjustment. While the grief period for an involuntary pregnancy loss is extremely variable, it is usually 6 months to 1 year and the type of loss does not affect this period of mourning.[50] Thus, couples often consider health care professionals insensitive to their needs when early trimester losses occur, as the clinician assumes that psychological resolution occurs as rapidly as physical recovery.[51] The needs and expectations of women and their physicians commonly differ. For example, if the woman requires a dilatation and curettage, the goal for the clinician is to have her discharged from the hospital as quickly as possible. Unfortunately, such rapid intervention often leaves no time for discussion or reflection. Not surprisingly, couples are commonly dissatisfied with the reasons and explanations given to them for the cause of their miscarriage and the clinician is mystified by their apparent hostility. Anger may be a part of the loss reaction and displacement of this anger can be a mechanism whereby the doctor becomes the object of such anger and hostility. In some women, a prolonged or morbid grief reaction can ensue as they are unable to progress through the stages of grief, reach acceptance of the loss, and continue with their lives.

During the first trimester, a woman is most vulnerable psychologically. It is the narcissistic stage of pregnancy, when she perceives the fetus to be part of herself.[52,53] It is not unusual for women who wanted to be pregnant and who desired to have a child to experience second thoughts or misgivings, once they are pregnant, about what they have gotten themselves into. These feelings of ambivalence are felt to be quite normal. But, when the pregnancy is unsuccessful, the woman may feel that her ambivalence contributed in some way to her unfortunate outcome.[54]

Spontaneous abortion often occurs rapidly and unexpectantly. Thus, the woman usually has no psychological preparation for the loss of her pregnancy. She may not understand the abortive process.[55] Cramps and bleeding can precede the miscarriage by hours, days, or weeks. During this time, she may be fearful of what can happen as well as helpless as to any intervention. There may be little or no time for anticipatory grieving.[56] The woman may blame herself. Did she do something wrong? Did she not seek medical attention soon enough? Did she take some medication prior to her knowledge of pregnancy that may have caused the miscarriage? She may feel inadequate or a failure as a woman.[56]

There is little physical evidence of pregnancy in the first trimester. Thus, when a loss occurs, it is usually unrecognized by others and therefore it becomes more difficult for normal grieving to take place. Parents are often unable to admit fantasies, thoughts, and feelings to each other, family, and friends, and they feel isolated.[53] The significance of the loss may be unrecognized by helpful friends, relatives, and professionals. Comments such as, "You can try again," "You didn't get to know it," "It would have been deformed anyway," are not helpful, and encourage denial and intellectualization.[55,57] Also, the normal ambivalence about the pregnancy and a sense of privacy may have prevented the woman from telling others.[53]

Couples have few concrete details about the pregnancy. They did not see, hold, know the sex, or experience the child in a physical form.[58] Attachment to the pregnancy begins at different times in the pregnancy for different women.[54] After one successful pregnancy, the attachment will occur earlier in a subsequent gestation. The inexperienced mother's attachment forms later in the pregnancy, usually after quickening is felt. After a loss, the woman will hold back on forming an emotional attachment with a subsequent pregnancy. She will not allow herself to think about the child inside and will protect herself from the pain of loss should the pregnancy fail.[54] Such women will be exceptionally concerned throughout the pregnancy, especially in the first few weeks. They will call their physicians with any or all symptoms that might be signaling the onset of another miscarriage. They usually cannot begin to relax until they have passed the period of gestation when the previous loss occurred.

Women who undergo therapeutic (ie, induced) abortions are initially relieved, but later may experience anxiety, ambivalence, and depression, although such reactions are commonly transitory.[53] A woman with a history of therapeutic abortions who has problems with subsequent pregnancies may view this as punishment for a decision to abort. The unresolved grief of a previous abortion (whether spontaneous or therapeutic) may contribute to postpartum mental problems after the birth of a subsequently healthy baby.[53,59] No relationship exists between the number of previous losses and the intensity of grief.[60]

Six key signs of mourning have been identified by Kennell et al.[61] They are *sadness, loss of appetite, inability to sleep, increased irritability, preoccupation with the lost infant,* and *inability to return to normal activities.* With the possible exception of the preoccupation variable, these characteristics mimic those of depression. Costello and others have discussed the expression of grief and the process of mourning, which is similar to normal grief responses following the death of any loved one.[50,53,62,63] Initially, there is a brief self- protective period of shock and disbelief. Parents have an inability to concentrate and their decision making is impaired. They can cry uncontrollably, stare into space, and become either manic or stoic. Then, yearning and searching begin with a struggle between the conscious and unconscious to accept the loss. Anxiety, anger, guilt, confusion, and sadness can all occur. Disorganization is the third phase and is characterized by disorientation and feelings of weakness, guilt, and depression. However, it occurs several months after the loss when everyone else thinks they should be over this process.

Grieving does take time. A prolonged or morbid grief reaction can occur if the couple is unable to progress through the stages of grief, reach acceptance of their loss, and continue with their lives[51] (see Chapter 17).

Pathological grief can be defined as the intensification of a normal grief reaction to a level at which the person becomes overwhelmed and resorts to maladaptive behavior or remains interminably in a state of grief without progression of the mourning process toward resolution.[64]

Men and women have different responses. The man is expected to be in control, make decisions, protect and support the woman emotionally, recover quickly, and return to work to earn a living.[53] Although the man does grieve, it is usually at a different pace and in a different manner. The sense of guilt and question of responsibility is resolved sooner by the man.[51] He may also be afraid to discuss the loss and a change may occur within the relationship.[56] Grieving parents are often using so much of their own energy for grieving that they cannot reach out to one another and marital problems may result.[53] Leppert and Pahlka[65] found the husband's reaction and depth of emotion related to the length of pregnancy. Men were more distraught if the loss occurred in the second trimester. Children and grandparents are affected by the loss and their emotional needs should be recognized. Also, it is not unusual for the woman to be resentful of other pregnant women, especially her friends.

Flandermeyer[66] interviewed women experiencing early pregnancy loss and identified stressors and coping behaviors. The stressors included (1) the perceptions of the conceptus as a potential child, (2) the intangible nature of the loss, (3) feelings of inadequacy in the reproductive role, and (4) the stress of telling acquaintances who know of the pregnancy that it was miscarried. The five coping behaviors were (1) communication or discussing the miscarriage with significant others, (2) emotional catharsis, (3) searching for causality of the loss, (4) putting the experience in perspective, and (5) justifying their reproductive worth by past reproductive achievements, either conception or previous pregnancies.

Parents who have experienced previous perinatal loss or losses are especially vulnerable to grieving. Their grief may be complicated by unresolved grief from a previous loss or losses, and by mourning over the increasing likelihood that they will never be able to have a healthy baby.[51] Guilt is the stage of grief that is the strongest. It also takes the longest time to resolve.[57,61]

Physicians and other care givers need to be able to recognize the indicators of an unresolved grief reaction.[57] Signs and symptoms suggesting unresolved grief include (1) vivid memory of events surrounding the period of loss; (2) frequent back-flashing to events of the day or specific scenes of the loss, even furniture and position of people in the room; (3) anniversary effects recurring on the date of miscarriage or the original due date; (4) persistence of affect such as sadness or anger when talking about the loss, even if it occurred many years ago; and (5) flooding of emotion at time of a subsequent crisis. When the response to a current crisis is excessive, it is frequently an indication of unresolved grief.

The incidence of pathological grief after spontaneous abortion is not known but several predisposing factors have been identified.[67] Agitated depression is more likely to occur in patients with an obsessive personality dis-order and in those with a previous history of depressive reactions. Patholog-ical mourning is more likely to occur in mothers who have previously lost children and those who had high expectations for the most recent (but now lost) pregnancy. Women who are in ambivalent relationships with their hus-bands and parents, particularly their mothers, are at higher risk, as are pa-tients who have recently lost a parent, especially if that relationship was marked by hostility. It has also been shown that patients who have recently changed their socioeconomic status or are facing severe financial burdens are also at high risk.[68,69] Strong ambivalent feelings about the pregnancy and being raised in a culture or religion that has a strong social prohibition against "inadequate" mothering are also risk factors.

If the loss of an early pregnancy is acknowledged by the woman and others, the normal process of mourning can and usually does take place.[57] Care givers, friends, and loved ones "give permission" for the grieving person to experi-ence and express a sense of loss. Many women do not realize that the feelings they are experiencing are normal. There is an extreme sense of relief in being able to talk about their loss with others, especially those who have had similar experiences. This can be accomplished in individual therapy or support groups, either professionally run or run by a lay group.

The woman should be encouraged to talk about her feelings with her doc-tor, family, and, most of all, her partner. Any sense of blame, self-devaluation, helplessness, anger, or hostility should be specifically acknowledged and dis-cussed. If anger is directed toward the physician, a sense of equanimity and willingness to accept and discuss it as part of the grief process are important.[67] The physician should also be alert to pathological grief and mourning that may be taking place and provide appropriate psychological or psychiatric referral.

Clyman and co-workers[70] showed that patients who received ongoing fol-low-up by their physicians were more likely to be satisfied with the nature and type of information provided and care they received than women who were not followed. Individual professional attention and psychotherapy diminish the incidence and severity of subsequent grief reaction as well as psychiatric and psychosomatic disorders that result from acute bereavement.[71]

Rituals of bereavement and burial are of benefit to the couple in accepting their loss. Unfortunately, they are commonly absent when early abortion is concerned. If a curettage is performed, the specimen is sent to pathology. Thus the couple has no "tangible evidence" of their pregnancy if miscarriage or fetal loss occurs. Friends and relatives should be encouraged to send cards or flow-ers to acknowledge the couple's experience. A religious ceremony can be re-quested and performed, but most religious groups do not have specific services for early pregnancy losses when no body is available for burial.

If the pregnancy was found to be genetically abnormal, the couple needs to be counseled regarding their risks in a future pregnancy.[11] They may benefit from formal consultation with a genetics expert who can allay their fears as well as provide them with valuable information.

These problems are compounded when losses occur repeatedly. Couples who experience habitual abortions (three or more) need to have a formal eval-uation. Many physicians prefer to institute a work-up following two spontane-ous miscarriages. The risk of pregnancy loss after a second spontaneous abortion rises considerably and can only be improved if a diagnosis is made and treatment instituted.[40]

The infertility experience is a stressful life crisis whether or not the involved couples eventually achieve pregnancy.[72,73] It places tremendous stress on the parents in their individual as well as their joint life.[74] Anxiety, depression, frustration, guilt, and isolation are common among infertile couples.[75] Forty-nine percent of women and 15% of men state that infertility is the most upsetting experience of their lives.[76]

Once treatment is initiated, each cycle becomes a roller coaster of highs and lows. Patients grasp at signs suggesting pregnancy. For those couples undergoing ovulation induction with human menopausal gonadotropins (hMG) with or without inseminations, it becomes especially difficult to start a menstrual period. The emotional as well as financial investment in each cycle is tremendous. Many of these couples eventually find themselves undergoing assisted reproductive technologies.

It should be kept in mind that the couple that is infertile, becomes pregnant, and then suffers an early pregnancy loss grieves profoundly.[77] Initially, the news of finally achieving a pregnancy is shared with everyone and there is a state of disbelief. But when the pregnancy fails, intense support is needed. It has been recommended to have mental health professionals within the infertility clinic setting.[78] This avoids outside referral and represents a potentially less stigmitizing option for infertile patients, particularly when such services are considered a normal part of general infertility treatment.

Most recently, Corsan and Kemmann[79] evaluated women who aborted after an hMG-induced pregnancy. In this group, he observed a high risk for repeat spontaneous abortion in a subsequent hMG pregnancy (48%). Conversely, those women with a successful first hMG pregnancy were at much lower risk for a loss in their second attempted pregnancy.

The grief reaction after an unsuccessful in vitro fertilization (IVF) cycle can be severe.[80–82] Greenfeld and co-workers[81] have described this type of grief experience as being analogous to the emotional reactions of women who have suffered spontaneous abortion.

Women who become pregnant through assisted reproductive technologies are monitored frequently with various blood studies as well as serial ultrasonic scans. The woman who fails to see a fetal heartbeat on ultrasound defers her attachment to the pregnancy and becomes very concerned.[81] Campbell has shown the benefit of ultrasound feedback on women's attitudes toward the pregnancy.[83] It is speculated that unresolved anxiety may confer an increased risk for complications.[84] This might occur either through a direct effect on maternal and, by implication, intrauterine physiology or through indirect promotion of health-damaging behaviors, such as substance abuse, poor compliance, or impaired nutrition.[85]

Conclusions

Unexplained infertility is an especially difficult diagnosis for couples to accept. They look for an answer as to why they are not getting pregnant. Each month at the menses with or without treatment, the woman grieves over her inability to conceive. It becomes difficult for her to be around pregnant women or women with young children. Marital relationships become strained. Intercourse becomes planned according to a schedule demanded by the plan of treatment. Intercourse can also be eliminated and substituted for by inseminations. Not surprisingly, adverse emotional reactions by the partners are common. On the other hand, the relationship can become strengthened as the couple progresses together through evaluations and treatments. The role for the clinician is to support the family, provide advice, and assist in the necessary procedures, maintaining a stance of determined optimism throughout the vicissitudes of treatment, regardless of the eventual outcome.

References

1. Miller JF, Williamson E, Glue J, et al: Fetal loss after implantation: A prospective study. *Lancet* 1980;2:554–556.
2. Hassold T, Chen N, Funkhouser J, Jooss T, Manuel B, Matsuura J, et al: A cytogenetic study of 1000 spontaneous abortions. *Ann Hum Genet* 1980;44:151–178.
3. Harger JH, Archer DF, Marchese SG, Muracca-Clemmens M, Garver KL: Etiology of recurrent pregnancy losses and outcome of subsequent pregnancies. *Obstet Gynecol* 1983;62:574–581.
4. Stray-Pedersen B, Stray-Pedersen S: Etiologic factors and subsequent reproductive performance in 195 couples with a prior history of habitual abortion. *Am J Obstet Gynecol* 1984;148:140–146.
5. Coulam CB: Unexplained recurrent pregnancy loss: Epilogue. *Clin Obstet Gynecol* 1986;29:999–1004.
6. McDonough PG: Repeated first-trimester pregnancy loss: Evaluation and management. *Am J Obstet Gynecol* 1985;153:1–20.
7. Edmonds DK, Lindsay KS, Miller JF, Williamson E, Wood PJ: Early embryonic mortality in women. *Fertil Steril* 1982;38:447–453.
8. Whittaker PG, Taylor A, Lind T: Unsuspected pregnancy loss in healthy women. *Lancet* 1983;1:1126–1127.
9. Poland BJ, Miller JR, Harris M, Livingston J: Spontaneous abortion. A study of 1961 women and their conceptuses. *Acta Obstet Gynecol Scand* [Suppl] 1981;102:1–32.
10. McIntyre JA, McConnachie PR, Taylor CS, Faulk WP: Clinical immunologic and genetic definitions of primary and secondary recurrent spontaneous abortion. *Fertil Steril* 1984;42:849–855.
11. Dudley DJ, Branch DW: New approaches to recurrent pregnancy loss. *Clin Obstet Gynecol* 1989;32:520–532.
12. Faulk WP, Coulam CB, McIntyre JA: Recurrent pregnancy loss, in Seibel M (ed.): *Infertility: A Comprehensive Text*. Norwalk, CT, Appleton and Lange, 1990, pp 273–284.
13. Tho PT, Byrd JR, McDonough PG: Etiologies and subsequent reproductive performance of 100 couples with recurrent abortion. *Fertil Steril* 1979;32:389–395.
14. Beer AE: New horizons in the diagnosis, evaluation and therapy of recurrent spontaneous abortion. *Clin Obstet Gynecol* 1986;13:115–124.
15. Scott JR, Rote NS, Branch DW: Immunologic aspects of recurrent abortion and fetal death. *Obstet Gynecol* 1987;70:645–656.
16. Rocklin RE, Kitzmiller JL, Garvoy MR: Maternal-fetal relation. II. Further characterization of immunologic blocking factor that develops during pregnancy. *Clin Immunol Immunopathol* 1982;22:305–315.
17. Mowbray JF, Underwood JL: Immunology of abortion. *Clin Exp Immunol* 1985;60:1–7.

18. McIntyre JA, Faulk WP: Recurrent spontaneous abortion in human pregnancy: Results of immunogenetical, cellular and humoral studies. *Am J Reprod Immunol Microbiol* 1983;4:165–170.

19. Mowbray JF: Genetic and immunological factors in human recurrent abortion. *Am J Reprod Immunol Microbiol* 1987;15:138–140.

20. Faulk WP, McIntyre JA: Trophoblast survival. *Transplantation* 1981;32:1–5.

21. McIntyre JA, Faulk WP: A cell-mediated immune defect in recurrent spontaneous abortion. *Trophoblast Res* 1983;1:315–321.

22. Rocklin RE, Kitzmiller JL, Carpenter CB, Garovoy MR, David JR: Maternal-fetal relation: Absence of an immunologic blocking factor from the serum of women with chronic abortions. *N Engl J Med* 1976;295:1209–1213.

23. Sargent IL, Redman CWG: Maternal cell-mediated immunity to the fetus in human pregnancy. *J Reprod Immunol* 1985;7:95–104.

24. Kajino T, Torry DS, McIntyre JA, Faulk WP: Trophoblast antigens in human seminal plasma. *Am J Reprod Immunol Microbiol* 1988;17:91–95.

25. Roman E: Fetal loss rates and their relation to pregnancy order. *J Epidemiol Commun Health* 1984;38:29–35.

26. McIntyre JA, Faulk WP, Nichols-Johnson VR, Taylor CF: Immunological testing and immunotherapy in recurrent spontaneous abortion. *Obstet Gynecol* 1986;67:169–175.

27. Jeannet M, Bischof P, Bourrit B, Vuagnat P: Sharing of HLA antigens in fertile, subfertile and infertile couples. *Transplant Proc* 1985;17:903–904.

28. Lauritsen JG, Jorgensen K, Kissmeyer-Nielsen F: Significance of HLA and blood-group incompatibility in spontaneous abortion. *Clin Genet* 1976;9:575–582.

29. MacQueen JM, Sanfilippo FP: The effect of parental HLA compatibility on the expression of paternal haplotypes in offspring. *Hum Immunol* 1984;11:155–161.

30. Faulk WP, vanLoghem E, Stickler GB: Maternal antibody to fetal light chain (Inv) antigens. *Am J Med* 1974;56:393–397.

31. Hughes GRV: Autoantibodies in lupus and its variants: Experience in 1000 patients. *Br Med J* 1984;289:339–342.

32. Harris EN, Chan JK, Asherson RA, Aber VR, Gharavi AE, Hughes GRV: Thrombosis, recurrent fetal loss and thrombocytopenia. *Arch Intern Med* 1986;146:2153–2156.

33. Branch DW, Scott JR, Kochenour NR, Hershgold E: Obstetric complications associated with the lupus anticoagulant. *N Engl J Med* 1985;313:1322–1326.

34. Unander M, Morberg R, Hahn L, Arfors L: Anticardiolipin antibodies and complement in ninety-nine women with habitual abortion. *Am J Obstet Gynecol* 1987;156:114–119.

35. Lubbe WF, Butler WS, Palmer SJ, Liggins GC: Fetal survival after prednisone suppression of maternal lupus-anticoagulant. *Lancet* 1983;1:1361–1363.

36. DeCherney AH: Habitual abortion, in Kase NG, Weingold AB, Gershenson DM (eds.): *Principals and Practice of Clinical Gynecology*, ed. 2. New York, Churchill Livingstone, 1990, pp 471–476.

37. DeCherney AH, Russell JB, Graebe RA, Polan ML: Resectoscopic management of Müllerian fusion defects. *Fertil Steril* 1986;45:726–728.

38. Perino A, Mencaglia L, Hamou J, Cittadini E: Hysteroscopy for metroplasty of uterine septa: Report of 24 cases. *Fertil Steril* 1987;48:321–323.

39. Lloyd R, Coulam CB: Role of endometrial biopsy in diagnosing luteal phase defect. *Fertil Steril* 1988;50:S57–S58.

40. Poland BJ, Miller JR, Jones DC, Trimble BK: Reproductive counseling in patients who have had a spontaneous abortion. *Am J Obstet Gynecol* 1977;127:685–691.

41. Dewald GW, Michels VV: Recurrent miscarriages. Cytogenetic causes and genetic counseling of affected families. *Clin Obstet Gynecol* 1986;29:865–885.

42. Coulam CB, McIntyre JA, Faulk WP: Reproductive performance in women with repeated pregnancy losses and multiple partners. *Am J Reprod Immunol Microbiol* 1986;12:10–12.

43. Taylor CG, Faulk WP, McIntyre JA: Prevention of recurrent spontaneous abortions by leukocyte transfusions. *J R Soc Med* 1985;78:623–627.

44. DeCherney AH, Kase N: The conservative surgical management of unruptured ectopic pregnancy. *Obstet Gynecol* 1979;54:451–455.

45. DeCherney AH, Maheaux R, Naftolin F: Salpingostomy for ectopic pregnancy in the sole patent oviduct: Reproductive outcome. *Fertil Steril* 1982;37:619–622.

46. Oelsner G, Rabinowitch O, Morad J, Masiach S, Serr DM: Reproductive outcome after microsurgical treatment of tubal pregnancy in women with a single fallopian tube. *J Reprod Med* 1986;31:483–486.

47. Pouly JL, Mahnes H, Mage G, Canis M, Bruhat MA: Conservative laparoscopic treatment of 321 ectopic pregnancies. *Fertil Steril* 1986;46:1093–1097.

48. Tanaka T, Hayashi H, Kutsuzawa T, Fujimoto S, Ichinoe K: Treatment of interstitial ectopic pregnancy with methotrexate: Report of a successful case. *Fertil Steril* 1982;37:851–852.

49. Ory SJ, Villaneuva AL, Sand PK, Tamura R: Conservative treatment of ectopic pregnancy with methotrexate. *Am J Obstet Gynecol* 1986;154:L1299–L1306.

50. Peppers LG, Knapp RJ: Maternal reactions to involuntary fetal/infant death. *Psychiatry* 1980;43:155–159.

51. Reed KS: Involuntary pregnancy loss research and the implications for nursing. *Issues Ment Health Nurs* 1984;6:209–217.

52. Stack JM: Spontaneous abortion and grieving. *Am Fam Practice* 1980;21:99–102.

53. Costello A, Gardner SL, Merenstein GB: Perinatal grief and loss. *J Perinatol* 1988;8:361–370.

54. Friedman R, Gradstein B: *Surviving Pregnancy Loss*. Boston, Little, Brown, 1982.

55. Wall-Haas CL: Women's perceptions of first trimester spontaneous abortion. *J Obstet Gynecol Neonatal Nurs* 1985;14:50–53.

56. Stirtzinger R, Robinson GE: The psychological effects of spontaneous abortion. *CMA J* 1989;140:799–801, 805.

57. Stack JM: The psychodynamics of spontaneous abortion. *Am J Orthopsychiatry* 1984;54:162–167.

58. Theut SK, Pedersen FA, Zaslow MJ, et al: Perinatal loss and parental bereavement. *Am J Psychiatry* 1989;146:635–639.

59. Kaij L, Malnquist A, Nilsson A: Psychiatric aspects of spontaneous abortion. II. The importance of bereavement attachment and neurosis in early life. *J Psychosom Res* 1969;13:53–59.

60. Toedter LJ, Lasker JN, Alhadeff JM: The perinatal grief scale. *Am J Orthopsychiatry* 1988;58:435–439.

61. Kennell JH, Slyter H, Klaus MH: The mourning response of parents to the death of a newborn infant. *N Engl J Med* 1970;283:344–349.

62. Kubler-Ross E: *On Death and Dying*. New York, Macmillan, 1969.

63. Bowlby J, Parkes CM: Separation and loss within the family, in Anthony EJ, Kouperik D (eds.): *The Child in His Family*. New York, Wiley, 1970, pp 219–230.

64. Horowity MJ, Wiler N, Marmar C, et al: Pathological grief and the activation of latent self-images. *Am J Psychiatry* 1980;137:1152–1157.

65. Leppert PC, Pahlka BS: Grieving characteristics after spontaneous abortion: A management approach. *Obstet Gynecol* 1984;64:119–122.

66. Flandermeyer AA: Women's coping with a spontaneous abortion occurring in early pregnancy. *Chart* 1987;84:7.

67. Hall RCW, Beresford TP, Quinones JE: Grief following spontaneous abortion. *Psy-*

chiatr Clin North Am 1987;10:405–420.

68. David CJ: Grief, mourning, and pathological mourning. *Primary Care* 1975;2:81–92.

69. Lovell A: Some questions of identity: Late miscarriage, stillbirth and perinatal loss. *Soc Sci Med* 1983;17:755–761.

70. Clyman RF, Green C, Mikkelsen C, et al: Do patients utilize physician follow up after the death of their newborn? *Pediatrics* 1979;64:665–667.

71. Parkes CM: Bereavement counseling: Does it work? *Br Med J* 1980;281:3–6.

72. Seibel MM, Taymor ML: Emotional aspects of infertility. *Fertil Steril* 1982;37:137–145.

73. Bibring G, Dwyer T, Huntington D, Vakenstein A: A study of the psychological processes in pregnancy and of the earliest mother-child relationship. II. Methodological considerations. *Psychoanal Study Child* 1961;16:25–31.

74. Rosenfeld DL, Mitchell E: Testing the emotional aspects of infertility. Counseling services in an infertility clinic. *Am J Obstet Gynecol* 1979;135:177–180.

75. Bresnick E, Taymor ML: The role of counseling in infertility. *Fertil Steril* 1979;32:154–158.

76. Freeman EW, Boxer AS, Rickels K Tureck R, Mastroianni L: Psychological evaluation and support in a program of in vitro fertilization and embryo transfer. *Fertil Steril* 1985;43:48–53.

77. Bowers NA: Early pregnancy loss in the infertile couple. *J Obstet Gynecol Neonatal Nurs* 1985;14:55s–57s.

78. Berg BJ, Wilson JF: Psychiatric morbidity in the infertile population: A reconceptualization. *Fertil Steril* 1990;53:654–661.

79. Corsan GH, Kemmann E: Risk of a second consecutive first-trimester spontaneous abortion in women who conceive with menotropins. *Fertil Steril* 1990;53:817–821.

80. Mazure CM, Greenfeld DA: Psychological studies of in vitro fertilization/embryo transfer participants. *J Vitro Fert Embryo Transfer* 1989;6:242–255.

81. Greenfeld DA, Diamond MP, DeCherney AH: Grief reactions following a failed cycle of IVF. *J Psychosom Obstet Gynecol* 1988;8:169–174.

82. Reading AE, Chang LC, Kerin JF: Attitudes and anxiety levels in women conceiving through in vitro fertilization and gamete intrafallopian transfer. *Fertil Steril* 1989;52:95–99.

83. Campbell S, Reading AR, Cox DN, et al: Ultrasound scanning in pregnancy: The short-term psychological effects of early real-time scans. *J Psychosom Obstet Gynecol* 1982;1:57–61.

84. Istvan J: Stress, anxiety, and birth outcomes: A critical review of the evidence. *Psychol Bull* 1986;100:331–348.

85. Reading AE, Campbell S, Cox DN, et al: Health beliefs and health care behavior in pregnancy. *Psychol Med* 1982;12:379–383.

Suggested Reading for Patients

1. Berezin N: *After a Loss in Pregnancy.* New York, Simon & Schuster, 1982.

2. Brody J: The new and often reassuring information about miscarriage. *Redbook* 1983;160:52, 54, 57.

3. Borg BJ, Lasker J: *When Pregnancy Fails.* Boston, Beacon Press, 1981.

4. Falacci O: *Letter to a Child Never Born.* New York, Simon & Schuster, 1976.

5. Friedman R: *Surviving Pregnancy Loss.* Waltham, MA, Little, Brown, 1982.

6. Hales D, Creasy RK: *New Hope for Problem Pregnancies.* New York, Harper & Row, 1982.

7. Hillard PA: Ectopic pregnancy. *Parents* 1983;58:116.

8. McDonald-Grandin M: *Will I Ever be a Mother?* Portland, OR, Celeste Books, 1983.
9. Pizer H, O'Brien-Palinski C: *Coping with a Miscarriage.* New York, New American Library, 1981.
10. Rando TA: *Parental Loss of a Child.* Champaign, IL, Research Press Company, 1986.
11. Schweibert P, Kirk P: *Still to be Born.* Portland, OR, Perinatal Loss Press, 1986.

Chapter 17

Perinatal Grief and Mourning

Paul Kirk, MD and Patricia Schwiebert, RN

And now remains
That we find out the cause of this effect
or rather the cause of this defect,
For this effect defective comes by cause.
    —*Hamlet* II,ii,100
    William Shakespeare (1564–1616)

The modern era in obstetrics can be characterized in many different ways. It is an era of reliance on technology, of quick resort to cesarean section, of a glimpse into the future of genetic manipulation, of litigation, of remarkable progress in neonatal care, of visible family involvement in the process of delivery, and of a steady, albeit uneven and still reducible, drop in perinatal death rates. Social planners and public health officials continue, appropriately, to draw attention to the relationship between social issues such as housing, nutrition, education, access to health care, substance abuse and pregnancy outcome, while obstetricians and perinatologists study and describe the more technical aspects of obstetrical care which are designed to continue the improvement in outcome. Both disciplines use perinatal or infant mortality rates as indices of progress.

These indices tend to hide other important characteristics of the modern era. These include the relatively new awareness that each perinatal death represents an individual personal tragedy for the mother and family with a potential for significant difficulties with personal relationships or the development of psychopathologies. There is as well a growing realization of the responsibility of the obstetrical and hospital team to acknowledge the importance of perinatal losses and to react appropriately and constructively to these events.

This chapter describes the general characteristics of the experience of perinatal loss, relates these characteristics to other similar experiences such as abortion and adoption, and suggests various strategies for dealing with particular circumstances.

Perinatal Loss

Important Viewpoints

At the outset, it is important to emphasize that the subject of perinatal loss does not lend itself well to formal scientific study.[1-3] The available literature is limited and, not surprisingly, is anecdotal, descriptive, and experiential. Nevertheless, the observations recorded by professionals and stated by bereaved family members are consistent and may be summarized as follows:

1. The attitude prevalent among health professionals a generation ago—that a perinatal loss was a relatively minor event and was best quickly forgotten by all concerned—was not only an ignorant attitude, but was always hurtful and often harmful to the bereaved parents.

2. Health professionals do not automatically recognize the dynamics of the loss reaction. Indeed, they are likely to shy away from the discomfort of death. Therefore, they need to be educated about the process and helped and encouraged to become involved, often to the extent of understanding and dealing with their own feelings and experiences of loss.[4-6]

3. Whenever a strong bond is broken, a loss reaction occurs. Although these loss reactions may take on many different forms, the recognition and appreciation of the reaction is an essential first step in the grief work that has to be done in order to lead to the resolution of the loss and a "letting-go" of the attachment. In time, this will permit strengthening of existing bonds and the development of new and secure attachments in the future.[7-9]

4. The importance of the maternal-child bond has long been recognized. The security of this bond is fundamental to successful childhood development. However, it was not until the 1970s that it was appreciated that this attachment preceded delivery and the arrival of a viable, tangible (and audible) infant. Bond development begins relatively early in the pregnancy, commencing at least from the time that quickening occurs.[9] It is likely that this process commences even earlier in pregnancy now that the remarkable images produced by modern ultrasound equipment reveal features of the fetus as soon as it develops its human form.[10] The recognition of this early maternal-fetal attachment is especially important in the management of perinatal loss. The bond exists. When a death occurs, the bond is broken and a bereavement response, normal or abnormal, is inevitable.

5. The nature of bereavement and the characteristics of grief reactions are experiences common to the human condition. They have been recognized and described not only over the centuries in cultural and religious behaviors and ceremony and in literature, but also they have recently been described and documented as a type of clinical syndrome.[11]

6. Although the general characteristics of a loss reaction are well described and apply to perinatal loss as well as the other losses, there are some peculiar features. Most important, and a particular problem with stillbirths, is the disordering of the natural and, therefore, expected pattern of conception, birth, and death. The appearance of death before birth is an unusually confusing situation and one that is difficult to assimilate.[12]

7. The emotional reaction to a loss requires weeks, months, perhaps years to resolve and will always be a part of the individual's experience and psyche. But the health professionals' involvement is brief. While this appearance occurs at a critical time, it provides little more than an opportunity—an opportunity on the one hand for facilitating the early grief reaction and, on the other, for obstructing and obscuring a healthy response.

8. Most health professionals are involved with the parents and family at a very early stage of the process, for instance, at the time of the diagnosis of intrauterine death or during the mother's hospital stay during the initial care of an acutely sick neonate. Inevitably, the parents are distracted either by anxiety for an extremely sick infant or by the shock, numbness, emptiness, and, sometimes, denial that occurs immediately after the death. Often these parents have had little personal experience of loss and may make decisions within the disastrous context of ignorance and numbness. This situation frequently leads to regret for wasted opportunities unless the health professionals step in with the right balance of support, education, and persuasion.[8,13]

9. It is at the time of a perinatal loss that unthinking health professionals may lose sight of their principal responsibility—that of patient advocate. All too often, the obstetrician and nurse may themselves be confused by their own feelings. Their own sense of loss or disappointment; a suggestion of guilt leading to denial or defensiveness; or an embarrassment, unease, or discomfort with the obvious emotional pain and hurt that the family are experiencing clouds their judgment or causes them to recoil from the anger that some or all of the family express.[1,13,14] When both the family and the health providers are confused, the inevitable happens: the "system" takes over and decisions are made by those least connected to the family, from the pathologist who wants to complete the autopsy "as quickly as possible," to the clerk in the admission office who "wants to get the paperwork out of the way." When this happens, opportunities for preparing for constructive grief work are lost and decisions are made that are later regretted.

The challenge for the health professional is clear. The clinician must recognize the need, identify a role to play, understand the dynamics, and direct the workings of the health system on behalf of the bereaved mother and her family.

Important Behaviors

An important decision has to be made at the time of the mother's discharge from the hospital: what form of follow-up should be provided, what its content should be, and who should provide the care. Various models have been suggested, from individual follow-up by the physician directly involved in the obstetric care, to a separation of the physical component (physician) from the emotional component (provided by the expert counselor such as a medical social worker or psychologist), to referral to lay mutual support organizations such as The Compassionate Friends. Particular difficulties arise when the delivery and death have occurred in a tertiary center, often distant from the patient's home. The staff have to temper their enthusiasm for providing direct follow-up with the inconvenience to the mother and her family and the possible misunderstandings that can occur if the referring physician feels excluded or even threatened if there are accusations, real or imagined, of error in the poor outcome.

The behaviors that apply in the management of the immediate period after death of an infant apply equally to later follow-up. This behavior can be listed as follows:

1. An emphasis on the infant as an individual who has the concern, attention, and respect that this designation implies.
2. An appreciation of, and an ability to respond to, the particular phase and characteristics of the grief response that the patient and her family have reached. In this the clinician should recognize that individual family members are unlikely to be demonstrating the same response or to be at the same stage of response.
3. A willingness of the professional to become involved or to stay involved as long as is necessary. It is unlikely that a single, traditional postpartum visit is sufficient. This willingness requires an examination of the professional's own feelings and attitudes; an appreciation of the cost to the professional, particularly his or her time; professional pride and image; and a readiness to refer, not abandon, the mother or other members of the family when they demonstrate signs of pathological grief or have a need for more expert or prolonged counseling than the professional can offer.

It is our view that the initial follow-up should be provided by the professionals who were present at the time of the death. For stillbirths this may mean obstetricians and obstetric nurses, and for neonatal deaths, neonatologists and neonatal nurses. The potential for confusion clearly exists when the real cause of a neonatal death is obstetric rather than neonatal, and when the death occurs in the nursery after the mother has been discharged from the obstetric ward.

Clinical Presentation

Perinatal Grief

Grief is defined as a cognitive, physiological, and behavioral response elicited by a significant loss.[8] The process of grief involves the readjusting of one's life to accommodate that loss. It is now accepted that a pregnancy loss is indeed significant to parents, and it is expected that a predictable grieving process will occur. Each person reacts to this death in his or her own style. The parents' ages, their experience with previous losses, concurrent life stresses, personal insights, the particular meaning of this loss to the individuals involved, as well as the support system available to them, are among factors that will be major impacts on how the parents will integrate this unexpected tragedy.

The behaviors that accompany grief are part of what Lindemann terms "grief work."[11] This grief work enables the bereaved to achieve emancipation from bondage with the dead infant and to readjust to the environment in which the dead infant is missing, and allows the formation of new relationships. Kubler-Ross first identified *stages* of grief, leaving an impression that the bereaved moved along a predetermined path.[15] Harm has been done to parents in the past when it has been suggested that their grief should follow a set schedule and direction. It is now recognized that grief is not a linear process and that regression is likely at times. Grief is best reinterpreted as including four tasks of mourning, as described by Worden.[16] This formulation is more helpful and less confining than a rigid model in attempting to understand the process that parents undergo in order to resolve a perinatal loss.

The Four Tasks of Mourning

Task I: Accepting Reality

At the immediate time of diagnosis of the death, parents may display shock and disbelief. This may last anywhere from hours to weeks. A large percentage of mothers know the baby is dead even before the physician's diagnosis. On one level of consciousness she is aware her baby is dead; on another level she appears unable to grasp the meaning of carrying a dead infant. The intense bonding between mother and child does not permit the easy acceptance of fetal death.[14] The physical and mental stress of the labor process, possibly compounded by heavy sedation, can enhance the sense of unreality. Women have admitted that even weeks after coming home from the hospital, when they heard the phone ring, they imagined that someone from the hospital staff was calling to say a mistake had been made and that their baby was not dead after all.[7]

Task 2: Experiencing the Pain of Grief

The sensations of grief are both physical and emotional. Physical sensations accompanying grief are often overlooked, but they play a significant role in the grief process. Examples of physical pain include tenseness, aching arms, tightness in the throat, dry throat, oversensitivity to noise, headaches, altered sleep patterns, fatigue, diminished appetite, a sense of depersonalization, digestive upsets, and the emergence of worsening medical problems such as ulcers, rashes, high blood pressure, allergies, etc. In many cases, alarming physical sensations and reactions will prod the bereaved parent to seek medical advice.

The emotional pain of grief is displayed by crying, anger, feelings of powerlessness and fear, emptiness and loneliness, guilt and self-reproach, yearning, depression, and marital discord.[16-18]

Task 3: Adjusting to an Environment in Which the Deceased is Missing

This task involves a sense of practical issues. These include notifying relatives and friends about the loss, deciding what to do with the baby's belongings or nursery, deciding how often to visit the cemetery, adjusting to "planned holidays" without the new baby, learning how to deal with music and locations that remind the parent of the baby, and relinquishing hopes and dreams connected with the dead infant.

Task 4: Withdrawing Emotional Energy and Reinvesting in Another Relationship

This task takes place over a long period of time and is characterized by both successes and setbacks. Signs that reinvestment is taking place include a lessening of the frequency, intensity, and duration of pain; the realization that the good days outbalance the bad ones; the ability to enjoy old activities or take on new ones without overload; the ability to see options and possibilities for the future without the child; the capacity for encountering grief and pain in another person without re-emergence of one's own pain; and the ability to reinvest in new and old relationships. Finally, as grief "softens," there is an ability to remember the joy of the time with the child, even if only intrauterine, as opposed to a focus restricted to the death.[19]

The process of incorporating the reality of a perinatal loss into one's psyche is not easy. It demands that both the death of the infant and the failure to achieve parenthood be accepted by the parents.[20] To compound the problem, bereaved parents are doing their grief work amidst an audience that often fails to recognize the loss as real or significant. For some, this task will be especially burdensome. Some of the psychosocial issues of pregnancy that may make this task difficult are: motivation for pregnancy and parenthood, ambivalence, and the relationship with the fetus during pregnancy.[20,21]

Problems for the Bereaved

1. The parent is grieving a nonevent.[22] Since no one else knows the child it is difficult for others to offer the sustained support and understanding the parents need during their bereavement.
2. Most mourning is retrospective—recalling and giving up a past relationship which can no longer continue. Perinatal bereavement is prospective mourning—giving up the wishes, hopes, and fantasies about a future relationship that can never unfold as planned.[6]
3. The process is chronologically out of order. Parents expect to die before their children. Death before birth is a reversal of the natural order of life.
4. Perinatal death may be seen as a statement to the woman that her body has failed her. Since a woman is conditioned to think of her body as a vehicle equipped to foster new life, she may experience a sense of shame, perceiving that her body is inadequate.[3,23]
5. The parents may feel that they have let the baby down. The parents have been led to accept that it is their responsibility to provide for, protect, and nurture their child. If the baby dies, the mother commonly assumes liability for having "failed" the child.
6. Perinatal death is still widely regarded more as a medical misfortune than as a human tragedy. In general, the impact of perinatal death has been diminished rather than acknowledged. Replacement is often suggested as a way to lessen this loss.
7. Perinatal death involves a narcissistic loss for the mother. Losing a child at an early stage of development can feel like losing a part of one's body. This sense of loss is more difficult to mourn than when the lost object is clearly identified as a separate person.[6]
8. Perinatal death is usually sudden and unexpected. Psychological preparation is important. Not surprisingly, bereaved parents of unanticipated versus anticipated child losses experience more severe grief reactions.

Treatment

Basic Principles

For 15 years we have been openly exploring and learning the best ways to help families cope with the tragedy of perinatal loss and putting these concepts into practice. Most of what we have learned has come through listening to parents and challenging ourselves to question what we do.

Following are some guidelines for practitioners, with our rationale for each. These are only guidelines. Each case needs to be approached with the specific experiences of the parents in mind.

Support

We cannot prevent parents from experiencing pain, but we can support them through it.[24] In the past, we have been guilty of not confronting the reality that death of a child has occurred. Perinatal death was seen as a medical misfortune rather than a personal tragedy. Until recently, unnecessary cesarean sections or heavy sedation were common practice in dealing with stillbirths. This encouraged the notion that we were dealing, not with the death of human being, but with a routine medical procedure. Parents were not given opportunities to see or hold their baby. It did not occur to most of us to suggest that a memorial service might be conducted for the stillborn child. Parents who had just suffered a loss were encouraged to jump quickly into another pregnancy. Nearly everything we did supported the idea that these parents had not lost anything of real or permanent value to them, that severe emotional distress was unwarranted, and that their lives would be disrupted only briefly. While we meant no harm by such practices, we failed to perceive that our not dealing with the reality of perinatal death did not make the parents' pain go away. Parents followed our lead, assuming we knew best, but they remained confused by their own conflicting feelings and by the need, they felt, to do the opposite of what we suggested. We are now learning how we can help the family to confront the reality of their loss; for example, by holding the baby, by formally acknowledging the baby through naming and memorializing, and by talking openly about their pain.[12] No longer do we cooperate in the conspiracy of silence in the face of death.

We now know how important it is to let the family know that we have not abandoned them, that we appreciate the difficulty of what they are going through, and that we know that it will take time for them to recover from their grief.[25]

Education

Educate parents about what to expect. The practitioner needs to have a sense of the full range of options open to the grieving parent, or at least a knowledge of who in the community has helpful information. If we acknowledge to parents that we understand grief to be a major component of their experience, they will be more likely to deal with their grief up front rather than letting it catch them off guard later on.

Control

Give parents as much control as possible. As practitioners, we have sometimes attempted to make decisions for parents and to persuade them to act in prescribed ways based upon our experience. By doing this we are likely to recreate the past by, again, enforcing our preconceived rules. It is better to explain our rationale, slow down the decision-making process, and let parents catch up. We need to give them a chance to change their mind, and to allow them to make the final decision even if, from our point of view, the decision is wrong. Most parents deal more easily with having made the wrong decision than with having been forced to do something they did not feel right about at the time. Finally, parents should be given the opportunity to make these important decisions in their own time frame, not ours.[5,21]

Individualization

Parents should be treated as individuals, recognizing that there are many different ways to experience grief. Men and women grieve differently. People from different cultures, ethnic groups, or religious affiliations practice dissimilar styles of grieving or turn to unique rituals to help them through their sorrow. Moreover, individuals commonly defy stereotypes. We are caring for parents in the midst of a highly emotional event and we should create a safe environment in which parents are able to be vulnerable and express their emotions in ways appropriate to them. Our success is a better indicator of quality of care than when we try to squelch intense or unusual forms of emotional expression.[25]

Parents may not be able to embrace the opportunity to confront the reality of the death of their baby even if it is offered to them. There are barriers impeding parents from taking advantage of their opportunities at the immediate time of death.

Common Problems

Inexperience

The life experience of many people has not included seeing a dead person, much less a dead baby. Where once both birth and death occurred at home, these beginnings and endings now usually take place in the sheltered and unfamiliar environment of the hospital. As a result, parents may be afraid of what they imagine death looks like. In addition, technological advances have decreased the incidence of perinatal loss to the point where most families suppose it to be virtually nonexistent.

The "window of opportunity" for parents to get the emotional and logistical support they need is limited. The staff's discomfort in confronting grief combined with a family in shock limits the effective use of this period of opportunity. The parents can be harmed by rushing through this process.

The Uncomfortable Practitioner

The comfort level of the clinician often affects how the parents respond to this initial experience of grief. The physician is in an influential position. Parents tend to trust professionals and look to them for direction. Because they are stunned by the immediate experience of their loss they will most likely follow the clinicians' lead and do whatever is suggested. If the practitioner appears uncomfortable in the presence of the death of their child, the parents are also likely to feel ill at ease.

Ignorance

Most parents have been preparing for the birth of their child, not the child's death, and so they will probably be ignorant of what they can do to make this time special. They will not automatically know that they are allowed to hold the baby, name the baby, and unwrap the baby. Nor will they know their legal rights concerning taking the baby home or transporting the baby to the funeral home. You may feel uncomfortable discussing such matters, or that such discussion is unnecessary. What we have learned, however, is that these matters are of utmost importance to the family. It is not our personal feeling or experience that counts here, but theirs. We need to trust parents to do what their intuition tells them they need to do, given a full range of options. This will happen if we help to create an atmosphere of acceptance and openness. By allowing and encouraging parents to make decisions in matters affecting them we offer to them a sense of control at a time when they otherwise feel desperately out of control.[5]

The Desire for Normality

A strong survival skill is the "art of appearing unaffected by whatever is happening around us." Parents may attempt to look unaffected for a number of reasons. They want to take care of you. They do not want you to feel guilty and they may feel embarrassed for exposing you to what they experience as their failure. They may be afraid that you will abandon them or lose respect for them if you see them behaving in ways that reflect the depth of their feelings. As their grief is confusing to them, they may think of it as abnormal and thus feel the need to hide it. They want you to think they can handle this tragedy. This is especially true if they believe this will be the deciding factor as to whether you will encourage another pregnancy soon.

Complications of Induction/Intervention

It is unusual for a fetal death to occur during the course of labor. The majority of deaths are neonatal, most often associated with extreme immaturity. Occasionally a death will occur soon after birth, at a time when the family is all but forgotten in the midst of heroic efforts at resuscitation. In both circumstances, the mother has labored with the *expectation* of the birth of the live baby. This is, of course, not the case where there has been an intrauterine demise, and where the mother, therefore, labors with a sense of dread rather than excitement. In in utero demise, the principal responsibility for the practitioner is precise diagnosis and immediate communication with the family. This is no time for pretense, avoidance, obfuscation, or procrastination. With modern equipment a correct diagnosis can be made swiftly. It often seems that the mother has already made her diagnosis, or at least has a strong intuition that something is seriously wrong. Although the diagnosis should be established without delay,[26] there is usually no urgency in delivery.

Parents have been planning and preparing for a birth, not a death. The shock of the news of their baby's death added to their lack of knowledge of grief can complicate the outcome unless the practitioner becomes a grief advocate for these parents. Although some parents are in a hurry "to get it over with," most benefit from some solitude in preparation for the separation from this person they have never had a chance to know. Kellner and co-workers[5] report that when given the opportunity 53% of the patients chose to wait before proceeding to delivery. Too often in the past, practitioners have behaved intrusively, agitating for some form of action, when in fact the family's main needs are for quiet, privacy, and the support provided by staff who are willing to remain available but aside. Our booklet, *When Hello Means Goodbye*,[24] includes suggestions about how parents can use the brief time they will have with their baby. Our experience has shown that just handing them the book may not be enough; prior to labor it is helpful to encourage them to read the pages which discuss seeing the baby and gathering mementos.

Once the family is emotionally prepared, induction is planned. Relatively rarely, a medical emergency exists requiring immediate induction. Induction is often not easy, particularly when associated with immaturity, an unprepared cervix/uterus, and primiparity. The mother must be granted the same degree of attention that every laboring mother has a right to expect. Birth plans should be reviewed and respected and adequate levels of pain control guaranteed. In the past, inappropriately aggressive steps have been taken to "save the mother the distress" of labor and delivery. Elective cesarean sections have been performed, deep (amnesic) sedation provided, or even general anesthetic administered for delivery. Like many other well-meaning interventions, these steps are misguided. Such interventions should be avoided because they tend to treat the mother as if she were a patient preparing for removal of an abdominal tumor; they fail to respect the infant as an individual, and they obliterate the consciousness so that experiences that would otherwise become valuable memories are lost.

An intrapartum fetal demise is a rare event. More frequent is the circumstance in which the baby is severely depressed at birth, requiring urgent attention, or is delivered with serious, unanticipated anomalies. Neither circumstance is easy to deal with, and both carry the risk of leaving the mother feeling abandoned. There can be no hard and fast rule about the right location for the resuscitation. Whether or not the baby is within sight of the mother, it is essential that someone knowledgeable is assigned to the mother to keep her informed, explaining the interventions and involving her as the resuscitation is carried out. To exclude her at a time when others are frantically working on her infant is to invite speculation and resentment, particularly if the eventual outcome is bad.

Labor and Delivery

Practical Steps in General Management

Labor and delivery can be a time of special strain for both patient and practitioner. Reasonable plans for parturition include the following measures:

1. Have a support person with the mother during labor and delivery.
2. Offer verbal assurance, as the mother enters labor, that those caring for her in labor are fully aware of her situation and will try to maintain open communication in a tension-filled predicament. Be available to talk with the woman and allow her to express her feelings during labor so that she may begin to accomplish her mourning tasks. A comfortable atmosphere that promotes expression of feelings is critical.
3. Provide pain relief, but assure that the mother is alert enough to experience the reality of the birth and death, and to participate in necessary decision making.
4. Do not assume that the father is automatically aware of what is happening. Keep him informed and provide emotional support to him also.
5. Let the mother know what she can expect. Pushing may be particularly difficult, and an unbearable task for her under the circumstances. Unconsciously she may think that as long as the baby remains unborn she does not have to face the reality of the baby's death.
6. Involve her in making decisions about how she wants her care to be received. For example, does she want to hold the baby immediately after birth, or wait till she is in postpartum care? Does she want the father to hold the baby until the third stage of labor is completed and she is then free to devote her full attention to the baby?

Showing the Baby to the Parents

There are no situations where it is unwise to give the parents the option of seeing and spending time with their dead baby. In the past, practitioners have often assumed the contrary. But, in our experience not seeing the infant is more disruptive to the parents than seeing it. The act of viewing and touching helps parents confront the reality of this untimely death and relieves parents' anxiety about the appearance of the baby. When it was less common for the parents to view their dead infant, fantasies rather than facts sometimes took over in the minds of the parents. Parents who did not see and touch their baby have reported such illusions as phantom crying, belief that the baby was not dead but adopted out, or the notion that what they delivered was a disfigured "monster" rather than a real child.[12]

Whether the baby is normal or abnormal in appearance, it is important to prepare parents ahead of time for what they can expect to see. Descriptions should include the baby's weight, length, color, general appearance, any malformations, and how the baby will feel (cold, stiff, floppy, heavy, etc) The term "macerated," is confusing and frightening to parents and should be avoided.

Parents focus more on the normal features of the baby than the anomalies, a refreshing reminder of how parents in general accept their live children even with their imperfections.

Whether the parents choose to see the baby or not, pictures should be taken of the baby and offered to them. If the parents choose not to accept these photographs, the pictures should be kept with the child's medical records for possible later retrieval.

Other helpful hints for showing the baby to the parents include the following:

1. Make the baby look as presentable as possible. Bathe, diaper, and dress the baby as a routine newborn. Wrap the baby in a warm blanket when taking him to his parents.
2. Placing a bonnet on an anencephalic baby helps soften the facial features.
3. Do not point out the anomaly that caused the baby's death, as if to justify or minimize the loss. Comment on positive characteristics of the baby's appearance (eg, long fingers, lots of hair).
4. Hold the baby close to you as you would a live baby and refer to the baby by name. If the baby has not been named refer to the baby as "your son" or "your daughter."
5. Allow the parents to spend as much time as they need with their baby. Offer them the opportunity to show the baby to siblings, grandparents, and close friends.
6. Ask the family if they want to be alone with the baby without other relatives or staff present.

Postpartum Management

In the past, mothers of stillborns or critically ill babies were often routinely placed on a ward away from the usual postpartum ward. This was done in an effort to protect the grieving mother from the harsh reminder that her baby died while other babies lived. That practice was consistent with our general approach to perinatal death—that of denial. By our actions we pretended—and encouraged the mothers also to pretend—that they had lost nothing of real value. We now believe we can give the most helpful and compassionate care to these parents in the postpartum care area, if certain conditions are met. The very placement of the woman in this setting is a way of affirming and valuing her role as a mother, even though her maternity was short-lived. Also, in the postpartum care area we have a much better chance of maintaining a therapeutic environment for the grieving parent, through the development of helpful protocols, than we would have in other areas of the hospital over which we have less control.

It would indeed be cruel and uncaring to assign a mother to a postpartum ward where, for example, she would be exposed to the crying of healthy babies, without making every effort to acknowledge and support her in her grief. It would be equally heartless to place her in another area of the hospital if the staff there are insensitive to her situation and treat her like they would any other patient has who has only had a "piece of tissue" removed. The most important factor in either case is that the staff be trained in grief management and that they be primed to give attention to her specialized grief needs.[24]

The staff will probably have a limited time available for preparing parents for the grief that still lies ahead. These patients tend to leave within the first day of a perinatal death unless there are medical complications.

Practical Steps in General Management

There are a number of suggestions that we have found helpful in our clinical experience dealing with these cases.[2,12,21]

1. Mark the patient's room and chart so that every person who comes in contact with the family is mindful that this is a mother whose baby has died.
2. Provide a cot so that the patient's support person can stay with her through the night.
3. Provide a private room, if possible.
4. Let the family know why you are caring for her in the postpartum area. They may otherwise assume that you are uncaring and indifferent to the mother's emotional needs.
5. If the mother insists on a room away from the postpartum area, be sure a float nurse from postpartum is assigned to provide the necessary grief support.
6. Do not assume that the best solution is to discharge the mother as soon as possible. The longer the mother is in the hospital the more support she can receive from knowledgeable people.
7. Speak with grandparents and acknowledge their loss of their grandchild. Gain their support in offering a listening ear to the parents.
8. Sit down when talking with parents. Plan to spend time listening and answering questions. Be prepared to repeat information if necessary.
9. Ask questions about the parents' past experiences with death, and about how they plan to say good-bye to this baby.
10. Schedule a follow-up appointment within a month (or sooner if necessary).
11. Provide parents with take-home literature about the grief process.
12. Give telephone numbers of local support groups to the parents or ask them if they would like you to make a referral to a group.
13. Prepare parents for the fact that they will grieve in their own unique way. Tell them that there is no right or wrong way to grieve.
14. Discourage parents from attempting another pregnancy right away. They need the time and energy to deal with the loss, before they can enter fully into the new pregnancy.
15. Gather mementos of the baby for the parents (lock of hair, wrist band, footprints, pictures, blanket, monitor strip, etc).
16. Be alert for overprotective interference of fathers and grandparents.

Special Problems

Fathers

"How's your wife doing?" is an all too familiar question heard by bereaved fathers. For some the question brings resentment and a reminder of the lack of support they have felt in the grieving process. Others accept it as just part of their role.[27] Quite often the father has been seen more as a part of the support team for the mother rather than as a parent who is also grieving.

Men are as likely as their wives to be emotionally distraught at the immediate time of death. However, bereaved fathers may try to fill a role expectation which requires that they appear strong and "in control" so as not to let their own grief add to that of their partner.[28] Women cry; men become angry. Women seek relationships and support. Men seek to provide support and turn to action.[27] These behaviors are consistent with what we generally see in our bereaved families.

Though the father probably will not experience the loss as deeply as the mother in the period following the initial event,[1,18,29] he will grieve in his own way and needs to be acknowledged for his loss.

Occasionally, a father will obstruct the grief work of his wife by trying to prevent her from seeing and touching their dead baby. If he is honestly trying to protect her he needs to be respected for his good intention, even as he is encouraged to see that this course of action will not prove to be helpful in the long run. If his wife goes along with him and submits to his wishes, he may have a price to pay down the road for having denied her the opportunity to see her child. She may be very resentful as she realizes that he was able to view the baby and she was not. The mother needs to be supported to make her own decision about viewing or holding the child.

The Children

If there are siblings in the family, they will not escape the impact of the death of the infant upon the whole family. This is true in spite of the usual attempts, in our society, to protect children from the harsh realities of death.[8,31] The younger the child the greater will be the temptation to avoid painful and difficult references to the loss. What harm can there be, we wonder, in concealing the death, if the young child had been told little or nothing about the birth anyway and was therefore not eagerly expecting a new brother or sister? Emanuel Lewis and others have documented cases where young children later developed psychosomatic disorders that could be traced back to the loss of a sibling they had never been told about.[32-34]

Parents may ask for the practitioner's guidance in how to tell the child about their dead sibling and whether or not the child should see the baby. Some parents will be comforted by the practitioner's being present, and even participating in the discussion with the child.

Speaking to children is difficult for many practitioners. Our suggestions and clinical observations include:

1. The child should always be told that there is a sibling and that the sibling has died. How much the child is told about the death, and the level of the child's participation in the immediate experience, will depend on the child's age, their communication skills, and the parents' level of coping.
2. A child will be more disturbed by disruptions in his life (people around him talking in hushed tones or crying, being suddenly cared for by strangers, not having the attention of a parent who is too consumed by grief to be able to attend to the normal care-giving role) than by the death of the baby itself.[12] Most children find it much easier to deal with the sadness of the adults in their life than with the emotional withdrawal of those they normally look to to meet their own comfort needs. The child needs to be offered reassurance that he has not been forgotten during this confusing and difficult time.

3. Many parents do not speak to their children about death because they do not understand death themselves. These parents need to be reassured that it is okay to tell the child that they also have unanswered questions. Reading books together helps both parent and child to deal with the subject at the child's level of understanding.

4. The choice of words in describing death is critical. It is better not to use euphemisms for death. If a child is told that her brother is "asleep" she could confuse sleep with death and later develop a sleep disorder related to her fears about death. If a sibling's death is explained by saying, "God wanted her because she was such a good little girl" the surviving child may later act "bad" so he will not risk being taken by God.[35,36]

5. In most cases, the surviving sibling will benefit from having a chance to see and hold the dead baby. It is good to prepare the child ahead of time by describing what the baby will look and feel like. If the child demonstrates a lack of interest in seeing or holding the dead baby, he or she should not be forced to do so. If the child does not view the baby, showing the child the pictures of the baby at a later date and seeing mementos of the baby's short life will provide tangible evidence of the sibling that was and will always be a part of the child's life.[35]

   Surviving children may want to cling to their parents for fear that they too, or their parents, may die. Other problems such as enuresis, nightmares, acting-out behaviors, punishment seeking, or problems in school may be indicators that the sibling has some distorted concepts of death.[8,25] The parents need to be encouraged to allow the child to discuss their grief reactions, to convey the message that it is all right to cry, to wonder and question, and to express feelings, including feelings of anger or relief.

6. The siblings need to be in the care of an adult who can provide the emotional support and understanding required of the child at that time. The adult should realize that the child will not grieve in the same way as an adult and that the child may ask questions that may make others uncomfortable, or even sound disrespectful.

Cultural Differences

Expressions of grief vary from person to person but are almost always influenced by a person's ethnic and cultural background. Cultural and ethnic diversity is a reality we must deal with in this society. No socioeconomic, racial, religious, or cultural group is spared the tragedy of perinatal loss. Thus, it is essential for practitioners to acquaint themselves with the variety of customs and traditions that may govern patient expectations. Practitioners who do not take these variations into account risk having their personal approach to care misunderstood.[37]

Cultural differences may be bridged, but only as we are willing to explore our own attitudes about grief, what death means to us, how the death of an infant affects us, and how we expect a person to grieve. For example, you may want to consider how your own family of origin customarily behaves when a family member dies and who you would most likely turn to for help if you were grieving. In order to care for parents of other cultures it helps to separate your own values and expectations about death from the values and expectations you may find in parents of other cultures.

It is as potentially harmful to stereotype or to use a "cookbook approach" for all members of a particular cultural group as it would be to assume, for instance, that all men, no matter what their cultural background, will not cry. While it is helpful to become familiar with different cultural norms, it is also appropriate to be open to variations. Remember, too, that parents coming out of such cultures may already have adapted to American ways. The important thing is to ask questions and listen carefully for what each patient will reveal about their own unique style and set of needs.

Some questions that may help to reveal the cultural dynamics of grief within a particular family are as follows: What do you think may have caused your infant's death? Since your infant died, what has been happening to you and your family? What do you think might help you in your grief?[37]

Keep in mind that medical diagnoses that we consider normal and acceptable may not be similarly viewed in other cultures. Some cultures seek a spiritual rationale for the death of their loved one. For example, it is a common Native American belief that, while the fontanels remain open, an infant may choose to die if its spirit is not happy in this life. Thus the physiological explanations to which we have become accustomed may not have the same meaning to these families. Another factor to consider when caring for Native Americans is that they may appear to be very stoic, and apparently unaffected by the loss. This attitude may be misunderstood if the practitioner is not aware that some Native Americans believe that talking about the death distracts from its spirituality and risks bad luck.[38] Italians, by contrast, may be extremely demonstrative and cry loud, hard, and long. In such cases a well-meaning, but uncomfortable practitioner may resort unnecessarily to prescribing drugs as a means of controlling what is actually a normal and appropriate expression of grief.

Southeast Asians consider the family as the basis of society. The oldest male in the family generally is the one who makes decisions about health care.[38] When working with Southeast Asians it is important to acknowledge the key role of the eldest and to include the whole family in the care plan. Also, Southeast Asians may scold the dead child for causing grief to the family.

For some of us, accepting the grief patterns of another culture may be difficult and challenging. This will be especially true when the bereaved parents request procedures that are unfamiliar to us. As a rule such requests should be honored as long as they do not cause physical or emotional harm to anyone.

The practitioner does not need esoteric skills in order to provide culturally sensitive care to grieving parents. The most important thing we can bring to their situation is a willingness to accept their unique qualities and their customs of respect for their dead and a readiness to listen and support them through their grieving process.

Autopsies

The state of perinatal autopsy is today where adult autopsy was two generations age. Although most neonatal deaths can be explained by neonatal events, and although most fatal congenital anomalies are recognized and understood, most stillbirths remain unexplained. The responsibility of the practitioner is threefold: first, to seek permission for the autopsy after an explanation as to why the information should be of value; second, to notify the pathology department that permission for an autopsy was obtained; and third, and most important, to educate the pathologists as to the clinical circumstances. The clinician should act as an advocate for a thorough examination, and seek to identify an explanation for the death that will be of value in later counseling. If the practitioner does not fill this role, nobody else will, and the current dismal 50% rate of negative findings at necropsy will continue.[39]

Clinicians should recall that unpleasant situations have occurred when pathology departments have not been apprised of new protocols for managing perinatal death. Because viewing the baby was not common practice until recently, pathologists have not always taken care to perform necropsies with the possibility of another viewing by the family.

Follow-Up Appointment

A follow-up visit after a perinatal death is usually characterized by considerable anxiety for both patient and conciliate. But there are some things that the practitioner can do to help reduce this anxiety and turn an otherwise difficult ordeal into a supportive encounter.

Part of the patient's dread may have to do with the office environment itself. If this office was the place where the mother heard the confirmation of her baby's death, the return visit may be clouded by that memory. If the office staff does not verbally acknowledge her loss, the mother may assume that either they have not heard the news or that they are insensitive. The fear that she will have to sit in a crowded waiting room with pregnant women or with women holding their healthy infants, and that she will have to respond to innocent questions and comments, may be overwhelming.

The following simple procedures will help create a less threatening and more supportive environment, both at the initial postpartum appointment and in subsequent visits:

1. Arrange for the mother's appointment to be at the end of the day when you will not feel rushed and she will not be waiting with others. If she must come when other patients are around, ask your staff to seat her in an examining room or office away from others even if she must wait longer. Be sure you explain why you are doing this.
2. Flag the chart so everyone on your staff will be aware of the death and so that insensitive remarks can be avoided. Note the name given to the baby and encourage the staff to refer to the baby by name.
3. Make sure your office staff are familiar with the grieving process and that they understand how important it is to acknowledge the mother in her grief.
4. Send the parents a sympathy card signed by the office staff. Mark the first anniversary of the baby's death on your calendar as a reminder to send another card a year later.
5. Telephone the mother, or have someone from your office call her, while she is still in the hospital, or within the first week at home to see how she is doing and to offer condolences.[14,26]

6. On follow-up visits continue to offer her opportunities to share her grief experience with you.
7. Have perinatal bereavement pamphlets or books available in your office. This will help bereaved parents realize that they are not the only ones who are going through this experience and that you are sensitive to this aspect of their care.
8. Know the resources available in your community, such as support groups and counselors who are knowledgeable about perinatal bereavement.
9. Be prepared ahead of time to provide the mother with names and telephone numbers of other patients who have experienced a perinatal death and who are willing to talk with her.
10. Remember that these women will probably have limited emotional reserves and a low threshold of tolerance for others' mistakes or oversights, no matter how insignificant.

It is not only the patient who comes to the visit with feelings of anxiety. Even those most experienced in medical practice seldom escape the discomfort of that first visit with a bereaved parent.

Your fear of the unknown (ie, how the patient will behave toward you), your own discomfort in the face of deep grief, your inability to explain adequately what happened and to give reasonable assurances that it will not happen again, and your own feelings of guilt in having not been able to provide the parents with a healthy baby may all interfere with your ability to support this parent in her grief. Simply be aware of these tendencies and try not to be overcome by them.

Walking into the patient's room may be the hardest part of the encounter. Once there, if you can resist the inclination to avoid the difficult issues of death and grief and if you can remain open to the experience in which you are about to engage, the outcome will probably be positive.

If you have not spoken to the mother since the death occurred she may be feeling a certain anxiety about how you will respond to her during the visit. She may be afraid that you will blame her for the death, that you will be uncomfortable in the presence of the intense grief she is feeling, or that you will find fault with the ways she is expressing her grief.[25] No matter how irrational or unnecessary her fears and concerns may seem to you, you need to be aware and respectful of them.

By the time she keeps her first postpartum appointment the bereaved mother may already have undergone much emotional abuse from family and friends who have been trying to "help" her get over this tragic event as quickly as possible.[18] She may be desperate for someone to acknowledge the significance of her loss and to validate how hard it must be to endure it.

Offering this acknowledgment and validation is a good way to begin the interview. Encourage the mother to talk about her sense of loss. Let her needs form the agenda for the encounter and avoid the temptation to try to maintain control of the conversation. Above all, do not try to "fix" her pain by suggesting solutions such as subsequent pregnancy or adoption.[22]

Allow time for the grief process to run its own course and do not attempt to rush it. Accept the fact that the process will take longer than both you and she will want it to.

Having done what you can to create an atmosphere of acceptance and trust you will be in a better position to help the patient deal with the medical issues surrounding the death of her child.

From this point on, the follow-up appointment can be viewed from two different perspectives: that of the physician or designee, or that of the mother. The mother is likely to want answers or explanations as to the possible causes of the death.[13,14] She may want confirmation or denial of a particular explanation. She is unlikely to be aware of the inadequacies of many autopsies and may be disappointed and frustrated by the lack of certainty that the autopsy provides. Parents often think "knowing" why the baby died will remove some of the pain of grief. Such relief is minimal at best, and an effort to prepare parents for this disappointment is appropriate.

In addition to the "clinical-pathological aspect" of the visit, the patient and her family may need reassurance that the sometimes dramatic mood and behavior changes that she is exhibiting are normal behaviors and are not indications that she is going mad.

From the physician's point of view, the purposes of the follow-up appointment include an attempt to inform the patient and her family as to cause of death and an appreciation of the mother and her support system's ability to cope with the difficulties of the grief reaction, an opportunity to support her in that process, and, rarely, an opportunity to diagnosis a truly distorted and pathological response. Even allowing for the frustrations of incomplete understanding in individual situations, these visits are often rewarding and constructive as long as they are built on openness. We have to make it quite clear to the mother that all the information that we have will be made available to her. It is equally important to distinguish between information that can be classed as *certain* and information that should be classed as *speculative*. It is reasonable to allow some speculation as to cause and consequence, but it is absolutely essential that when the discussion is speculative, it is identified as such. It is particularly easy to become unreasonably speculative when the autopsy report is lacking. Although it is tempting to offer the mother and her family more information than one has immediately available, this is not a constructive response. Not only does it undermine the confidence of the professional relationship, when information presented as certain later turns out to be uncertain; it also potentially compromises management in a subsequent pregnancy. Fantasies will have to be unraveled. We have been particularly impressed that although families are often disappointed in their early response to the autopsy, they do in fact appreciate a simple "we don't know" more than an elaborate obfuscation.

The most difficult area is the question of guilt.[25] Although there is an element of guilt in any grief reaction, it is not unusual for a mother to become obsessed with some behavior in the pregnancy which she imagines to be the cause of her catastrophe. It is not helpful to discount this association as being ridiculous. However, a slow and deliberate dismantling of the association, with appropriate data to support such a dismantling, is necessary. Perhaps more difficult is the situation where it *is* known that a particular behavior in the pregnancy contributed to the poor outcome. On occasion, the mother will be open and verbal about the association. It is necessary, and important, for us to confirm the association, and help her work through the painful guilt to an experience of forgiveness rather than to suggest that such an association did not exist or that it was not important.

When the patient denies an association, it is often tempting to enter into collusion with her, in an attempt to protect her from further pain. Collusion may seem charitable, but it is not constructive. A relationship must be established between patient and practitioner for the provisions of the facts, the breaking down of the denial, and the start of the work towards eventual resolution of the guilt. Convenient fables do not contribute to this process.

Some physicians are concerned that open review such as we are recommending may increase the risk of malpractice litigation. We have two responses to this concern. The first is that there is no evidence that honest exchange of information increases the risk; in fact, it probably *reduces* the risk. A better understanding of the circumstances—even in the face of bad outcome—along with a demonstration of concern by the provider will help the bereaved appreciate the impossibility of truly assigning blame. Our second response is that on those rare occasions when errors have been made, a suit is probably inevitable. To turn our backs on the inevitable probably invites further reaction from the bereaved and angry family.

What to Do and Not Do

As we cast about for ways to support the bereaved, our natural inclination is to search for words that we think will make the bereaved "feel better." Out of our deep desire to "say something" that will diminish their pain and "fix" their grief, we may turn to platitudes which, though well meaning, are in fact paternalistic and hurtful. Though parents may not openly express their resentment of our shallow offerings, their sense that we do not really understand their pain will tend to make them skeptical about receiving much support and help from us in the future.

The truth is that the only thing that could diminish the sorrow of these parents would be to have their child back alive. There is nothing we can say that will take away the pain of an irreversible loss. On the other hand, our silent presence with the bereaved will bring them more comfort than our careless and ill-conceived words could ever do.

Words to Avoid

The following platitudes are not helpful and should be avoided when speaking to bereaved parents[26,36]:

"You're young. You can always have other children."
"It's just as well the child died, considering his condition had he lived."
"It's better this way."
"It was God's will" or "God has his reasons."
"You'll be a better person for having gone through this."
"You're lucky to have other children."
"It could have been worse."
"At least you didn't lose both of the twins."
"Don't cry."

"I know just how you feel."
"You're standing up well."
"Keep a stiff upper lip."
"Life is for the living."
"At least you didn't get to know him."

If you recognize that you did say something that might have been interpreted as uncaring or insensitive to the family, discuss it openly with them. Acknowledging your regret will most likely be received by the bereaved parents as a positive expression of caring.

Words to Use

The following statements or questions will be perceived by bereaved parents as caring and helpful:

"You must feel terrible."
"It's okay to cry."
"I don't know what to say, but I'll be glad to listen."
"How can I help?"
"Tell me about how you are feeling."

The practitioner can help greatly by encouraging parents to talk freely and openly without fear of censure or criticism. Most parents will not automatically share intimately unless you give them permission and encouragement to do so.

Danger Signs of Pathological Grief

Parents will experience grief in their own way. They need to understand that the degree of intensity of their grief may be quite normal and appropriate for them. But there are danger signs that will tell us when certain bereaved parents need more help to resolve their grief. Such warning signs include:[16,17]

1. Persistent thoughts of self-destruction.
2. Persistent mourning or long-term depression.
3. Failure to attend to the five basic survival needs: daily nutritional intake, appropriate amount of sleep, adequate fluid intake, regular range of motion exercise, and the maintenance of a nurturing social network.
4. Abuse of controlling substances such as alcohol or drugs.
5. Recurrence of mental illness.
6. Refusing to be consoled.
7. Inability to speak of the dead infant without experiencing fresh grief.
8. The triggering of an intense grief reaction by some minor event.
9. Radical changes in lifestyle.

Support Groups

Good support groups should be able to encourage the parents to face the reality of their loss, provide a safe environment for parents to express their feelings honestly, recommend ways for coping with their feelings and with relationships to others, and challenge them to look at life beyond their loss.[40] Talking with others who have shared a similar experience ranks high on the list of what helped most in parents' recovery.[26,40–43] For example, the tension that develops within a marriage due to the incongruence of husband-wife grief seems to diminish when couples observe this as a common problem within families.[44] Thus support groups can provide an arena for the recovery process.

Parents admit that their decision to attend their first meeting is often an act of desperation, a willingness to try anything that might relieve some of the tension that had built up inside them. Physicians are sometimes concerned that the group experience introduces a bereaved couple to the wider range of possible causes of perinatal loss, which they could face in a subsequent pregnancy, thus exacerbating their fears. Most parents deal matter of factly with this reality, however, and believe that the value of the support they receive outweighs the possible uneasiness that accompanies a greater awareness of other potential risks.

There are a number of nationwide, infant loss support groups available to parents, all of which can be valuable referral sources (see Appendix 17.1). Giving to the bereaved family telephone numbers to contact, or making the referral yourself, with their permission, validates that what they are experiencing is normal and adds credence to the suggestion that it helps to talk with others—even strangers—who have had a similar experience.

Special Circumstances

Miscarriage

Women experiencing multiple early pregnancy losses used to be considered "illegitimate mourners." The ending of an early pregnancy was considered a blessing in that it would protect parents from the sorrow of their later delivering an imperfect child. This fact did not necessarily provide comfort to them at the time of the miscarriage, however. Because the cause of miscarriage is still a mystery in many cases, myths fill the void of knowledge and tend to heap further blame, usually on the mother.[45] Miscarriage continues to be clouded by feelings of shame, disappointment, and envy (see Chapter 16).

Family planning, which contributes to a sense of control in one's life; advanced technology, which permits earlier recognition of a pregnancy; and improved visualization, which promotes bonding, all intensify the potential for grief that we now see surrounding early pregnancy loss.

Because of doubts cast on the mother's reproductive capacity and her femininity, there is a tendency to search for a justification for punishment within herself or her partner, and a generalized anger seems to permeate her life.[23]

The grief these parents are feeling is legitimate, though different from that of parents who have experienced a full-term loss. These parents grieve a failure, a fear of the future without children, and the loss of a sense of purpose in their lives. And because there is fear of not receiving adequate recognition for their pain, much of their grief remains private.

It remains difficult for parents to believe that a hard-earned pregnancy that is at risk of miscarriage cannot be saved. After years of waiting for a successful outcome their experience of loss can be devastating, and the woman's reaction, especially, may seem extreme to the practitioner.

The lives of these parents are consumed with becoming and staying pregnant. It becomes difficult for them to be around old friends who have borne healthy children. Family gatherings become, for them, reflections of everyone else's success.

By now sexual intercourse may have become a means to an end rather than a loving expression of the couple's life together. Unfortunately, this occurs at the very time when they need this expression more than ever.

This group of parents demands the best from the medical practitioner, and they demand it with a vengeance. It is essential that you and your office personnel be compassionate and tolerant of what at times seem to be unreasonable demands. Clear explanations and directions may need to be repeated. It is helpful to remember that these persons probably have a limited emotional reserve, and to take this into account when dealing with them. Support groups that acknowledge grief instead of focusing on the latest developments in reproductive technology will help discharge some of the intense emotions these couples carry.

Therapeutic Abortion

The decision to terminate a pregnancy, although accepted by most of society as a solution to an unwanted pregnancy, presents conflicts for the woman. The decision to terminate is usually an intellectual process, but the aftermath is an emotional one. Epidemiological studies do not suggest that widespread psychopathology follows abortion, but such a sweeping statement tends to obscure the struggles that many women experience.[17,46] The pattern of grief after abortion will be similar to that of a woman experiencing a miscarriage, except that suppression and inhibition of grief are more likely. Stigma, shame, and secrecy still surround this decision. Society sends subtle messages, such as that the woman should be pleased and relieved after the abortion rather than sad. The woman may feel she does not have the right to feel sad because abortion was her choice. Conflicts may not surface until many years later when she becomes aware of other losses in her life (see Chapter 19).

To echo the recurrent theme of this chapter, we believe the optimum method of management with abortion is one of openness and directness, rather than denial and subterfuge. Women who tend to have difficulty resolving grief after an abortion and who may need special attention include those who have had a previous mental illness, those who felt coerced into making the decision, those who underwent a second-trimester abortion, and those who terminated pregnancy due to medical reasons.

Adoption

In recent years we have come to appreciate more fully the extent of perinatal bereavement experienced by the woman who relinquishes a child for adoption. Our earlier assumption, that the birth mother would soon get on with her life after this minor interruption, has been challenged by birth mothers who are refusing to remain anonymous and who are beginning to speak openly about their experience of grief.[7,47,48]

For too long we have looked at adoption primarily as a solution to a societal problem, without recognizing that it also has created internal psychological problems which we have not yet adequately addressed.[47] We are not against adoption, but we oppose any institution that creates or encourages pathology. Surely a system such as adoption, if built on lack of trust and secrecy, has that potential.

There are two major, undeniable factors that distinguish a birth parent's experience from that of the parent of a dead baby. First, the birth mother can change her mind and decide to keep her baby and, second, the child is not dead. It is because of this first factor that mothers in the past have been denied opportunities to get to know and then say good-bye to their offspring.

It is essential, in counseling with the birth mother, to help her examine her personal reasons for considering relinquishment. It is not enough merely to inform her of her "rights."

We recommend the following ways for supporting the birth mother in her grief:

1. The birth mother should be treated the same as other bereaved parents, and given every opportunity, at her request, to be with and relate to her baby (naming, bathing, dressing, rooming- in, breast-feeding, etc).
2. Mementos should be gathered for the birth mother.
3. The birth mother should not be rushed to sign adoption papers, nor made to feel guilty if she changes her mind.
4. The birth mother's needs should be the ones considered at the birth, not the adoptive family's. Birth mothers tend to want to please others rather than be their own advocates.
5. If the birth mother appears to be wavering in her decision to relinquish the child, the person who has been counseling her should be notified. This person is the most qualified to help her sort through her initial reasons for relinquishment and to help determine if these reasons are still valid.
6. The physician's primary responsibility is to the birth mother. Obviously, the adoptive family will experience grief if the adoption fails. Their grief will continue most likely until a successful adoption is achieved. But the grief of the birth mother will be lifelong and, therefore, it merits particular consideration by the practitioner in the period immediately following the birth of the child.

It is understandable why infertile parents will grieve for the loss of their ability to bring forth life, and for the loss of the biological child they can never have. Ultimately, however, acceptance and resolution are necessary, especially if the couple chooses adoption as a means of building a family. The trouble starts when adoption is used to avoid resolving the sense of loss infertility brings. The adoptive parents' sense of loss often resurrects itself in the form of deep fears that somehow the child's birth parents will come back and take the child away, leaving them childless again. This dynamic of unresolved grief, fear, insecurity, and denial is intimately related to many of the emotional and behavioral problems the adopted child may face in the course of growth and development. Parental anxiety is easily communicated. As practitioners, we need to help families recognize the possibility of unresolved grief surrounding infertility and the potential problems it carries into the future.[47]

Open adoption presents new challenges and unmarked territory. It is our hope that this new form of adoption will prove to be healthier and prevent less pathology than the previous method of adoption, which was couched in secrecy and fear. Families entering into adoption need to understand that it is a lifelong process and they must be willing to invest the time it will take to make it a positive experience for everyone.

We have earlier emphasized the importance of patient advocacy and the importance of protecting the grieving mother from the insensitivities of the medical system. The birth mother who is about to relinquish her baby is particularly vulnerable when her attending physician is a party to or has perhaps helped to arrange the adoption. Too often the physician becomes a stronger advocate for the adopting family in helping them acquire the baby as quickly as possible, thus ostensibly limiting the risk of the birth mother changing her mind. Favoritism in advocating for the family with whom the professional relationship is specious, at the expense of the interests of the birth mother with whom a professional relationship already exists, is a phenomenon of the "business" of adoption that reflects poorly on our professional ethics and must be avoided.

Multiple Gestation Losses

Wilson and co-workers[49] found that losing one of a set of twins (multiple) involves as much grief as losing a single newborn. In some ways such a loss is even more difficult because there is usually less grief support available and the recognition of being a special family vanishes. Most people tend to think (and say) "Be thankful, at least one survived," assuming therefore that the parent can just forget about the one who died. These parents feel guilty for grieving, feeling they do not have a right to feel sad. At the same time they find it difficult to celebrate the life of the surviving baby. Here, as in hasty subsequent pregnancies, the processes of attachment-detachment do not always occur simultaneously. Parents will find it difficult to mourn completely the baby who died and at the same time feel attached to the survivor.[21]

After a death of one of a pair of twins, parents describe a sense of falling from grace into a deep sense of shame. Lewis and Bryan[34] report a mother of twins saying "I've come to terms with S's death; I shall never come to terms with not being a mother of twins."

Suggestions for handling the problems of loss of one of a twin pair include the following :

1. While the surviving twin is in the hospital keep the bassinet marked as you would if both twins had survived (Twin A).
2. Take a photograph of the babies together and alone.
3. Be careful not to make statements that negate the baby's loss.
4. Encourage the parents to talk about the dead baby.

Subsequent Pregnancy

The purpose of an adequate grief response is to allow resolution, to separate bonds, and to make room for new relationships. Ideally the loss will be well on the way to resolution and acceptance before another pregnancy is attempted, but sometimes the next pregnancy occurs quickly and sometimes the grief response is prolonged. In either event, the grief work is likely to be postponed during pregnancy only to be resumed after the delivery, often with surprising results.[22,33]

The key behavior in managing a subsequent pregnancy is *acknowledgment*.[19] It is necessary to acknowledge anxiety that is inevitable, to acknowledge the anniversaries that are inevitable, to acknowledge the anniversaries that relate to the previous loss, to acknowledge the particular sensitivities that accompany the memories of the previous pregnancy, and to acknowledge the special need for reassurance that characterized these pregnancies.

The previous pregnancy must be treated seriously. No mother is going to be reassured by the trite dismissal that "lightning never strikes twice." A clear surveillance strategy should be developed early in the new pregnancy. This plan must pay attention to the previous cause, recognize times of special stress and anxiety, yet not assume that the anxiety is automatically going to be relieved once the landmark is passed, ie, when maturity is reached in a mother with a history of preterm birth. Most often these subsequent pregnancies result in a happy outcome, and a sense of relief attached to the delivery. The mother may have true ambivalence in her feelings toward the new infant and her memories of the one that died. This ambivalence may result in surprising and, sometimes, disturbing behaviors and may be seriously misinterpreted if not understood.[3,50,51]

Conclusions

There is little evidence that the management, as outlined herein, does anything to reduce psychopathology caused directly or indirectly by perinatal loss. However, on theoretical grounds and with the analogy to other loss situations, it would seem that effective grief work is bound to reduce other problems and that active supportive intervention helps make the work effective. Support for this type of intervention comes from our clinical experience of interviews with hundreds of families seen in personal follow-up or in association with The Compassionate Friends.

Without exception, these families have expressed appreciation of the encouragement, permission, and opportunity to grieve in the hospital setting. They affirm that they need direction, that without it they simply would not know what to do, would flounder, and would have made some bad choices. They do not resent the emotional pain, and they empathize with the provider who is obviously hurting too, although they have no time for posturing, unreasonable solicitude, or patronizing. They value freely given time, particularly when they recognize that time is short, but over and over again, and seemingly without exception, they say, "Thank you for letting me spend time with our baby." Early doubts that we had about this important part of our management have long since gone.

The right preparation is essential; skilled nursing is a must. Every recollection has been welcomed; even parents with severely macerated or grossly anomalous babies have welcomed the opportunity to see the baby and have reassured us. It has been our experience in this area, as in no other in our medical and nursing careers, that we have learned most from our patients. This was illustrated by the mother of the baby with cyclopia who, when asked how she felt about the time she had spent with him after his stillbirth, said simply, "Fine. After all, he was my baby."

References

1. Benfield G, Leib S, Vollman J: Grief response of parents to neonatal death and parent participation in deciding care. *Pediatrics* 1978;62:171–177.
2. Hutti M: An examination of perinatal death literature: Implications for nursing practice and research. *Health Care Wom Int* 1984;5:387–400.
3. Zeanah C: Adaptation following perinatal loss: A critical review. *J Am Acad Child Adolesc Psychiatry* 1984;28:467–480.
4. Enriquez M: Dealing with neonatal death. *Neonat Net* 1982;Aug:24–28.
5. Kellner K, Donnelly W, Gould S: Parental behavior after perinatal death: Lack of predictive demographic and obstetric variables. *Obstet Gynecol* 1984;63:809–814.
6. Leon I: Psychodynamics of perinatal loss. *Psychiatry* 1986;49:312–323.
7. Bowlby J: *Loss*. New York, Basic Books, 1980.
8. Callahan E, Brasted W, Granados J: *Life Span Developmental Psychology*. New York, Academic Press, 1983.
9. Klaus M, Kennel J: *Parent-Infant Bonding*. St. Louis, CV Mosby, 1982.
10. Fletcher JC, Evans MI: Maternal bonding in early fetal ultrasound examinations. *N Engl J Med* 1983;308:392–393.
11. Lindeman E: Symptomatology and management of acute grief. *Am J Psychiatry* 1944;101:141–148.
12. Kennel J, Krause M: Helping parents cope with perinatal death. *Contemp OB/GYN* 1978;12:53–68.
13. Rowe J, Clyman R, Green C, Mikkelsen C, Haight J, Ataide L: Follow-up of families who experienced perinatal death. *Pediatrics* 1978;62:166–170.
14. Bruhn D, Bruhn P: Stillbirth: A humanistic response. *J Reprod Med* 1984;29:107–112.
15. Kubler-Ross E: *On Death and Dying*. New York, Macmillan, 1970.
16. Worden W: *Grief Counseling and Grief Therapy*. New York, Springer-Verlag, 1982.
17. Rando T (ed.): *Parental Loss of a Child*. Champaign, IL, Research Press, 1986.
18. Stierman E: Emotional aspects of perinatal death. *Clin Obstet Gynecol* 1987;30:352–361.
19. Schwiebert P, Kirk EP: *Still to be Born*. Portland, OR, Perinatal Loss Press, 1988.
20. Quirk T: Crisis theory, grief theory, and related psychological factors: The framework for intervention. *J Nurse Midwife* 1979;24:13–16.
21. Hutti M: Perinatal loss: Assisting parents cope. *J Emerg Nurs* 1988;14:338–346.
22. Bourne S: The psychological effects of a stillborn on women and their doctors. *J Coll Gen Pract* 1968;16:103–112.
23. Berger G, Goldsteinn M, Fuerst M: *The Couple's Guide to Fertility*. New York, Doubleday, 1989.
24. Schwiebert P, Kirk EP: *When Hello Means Goodbye*. Portland, OR, Perinatal Loss Press, 1985.
25. Gilson G: Care of the family who has lost a newborn. *Postgrad Med* 1976;60:67–70.
26. Segal S, Fletcher M, Meekison W: Survey of bereaved parents. *Can Med Assoc J* 1986;134:38–42.
27. Bryant M: Fathers grieve, too. *J Perinat Med* 1989;9:437–441.

28. Lieberman J, Hughes C: How fathers perceive perinatal death. *Matern Child Nurs J* 1990;15:320–323.

29. Hughes C, Page-Lieberman J: Fathers experiencing a perinatal loss. *Death Stud* 1989;13:537–556.

30. Arnold JH, Gemma PB: *A Child Dies: A Portrait of Family Grief.* Rockville, MD, Aspen Systems, 1983.

31. Berezin N: *After a Loss in Pregnancy.* New York, Simon and Schuster, 1982.

32. Lewis E, Page A: A failure to mourn a stillbirth: An overlooked catastrophe. *Br J Med Psychol* 1978;51:237–241.

33. Lewis E: Inhibition of mourning by pregnancy: Psychopathology and management. *Br Med J* 1979;2:27–28.

34. Lewis E, Bryan M: Management of perinatal loss of a twin. *Br J Med Psychol* 1988;297:1321–1323.

35. Glicken M: The child's view of death. *J Mar Fam Counsel* 1978;4:75–81.

36. Sahu S: Coping with perinatal death. *J Reprod Med* 1981;26:129–132.

37. Tripp-Reimer T: Cultural assessment: Content and process. *Nurs Outlook* 1984;32:78–82.

38. Lawson Lauren Valk: Culturally sensitive support for grieving parents. *Mat Child Nurs* 1990;15:76–79.

39. Craven C, Dempsey S, Carey J, Kochenour N: Evaluation of a perinatal autopsy protocol: Influence of the prenatal diagnosis conference team. *Obstet Gynecol* 1990;76:684–688.

40. Davidson G: *Understanding Mourning.* Minneapolis, Augsburg Publishing, 1984.

41. Edelstein L: *Maternal Bereavement.* New York, Prger, 1984.

42. Parkes CM: Bereavement counselling: Does it work? *Br Med J* 1980;2:3–6.

43. Parkes CM: Evaluation of a bereavement service. *J Prevent Psychiatr* 1981;1:179–187.

44. Gilbert K: Interactive grief and coping in the marital dyad. *Death Stud* 1989;13:605–626.

45. Herz E: Psychological repercussions of pregnancy loss. *Psychiatr Ann* 1984;14:454–457.

46. Rando T: *Grief, Dying and Death.* Champaign, IL, Research Press, 1984.

47. Kirk D: *Adoptive Kinship.* Port Angeles, Ben-Simon Publications, 1985.

48. Silverman P: *Helping Women Cope with Grief.* Sage Publications, 1981.

49. Wilson A, Lawrence J, Stevens D, Soule D: The death of a newborn twin: An analysis of parental bereavement. *Pediatrics* 1982;70:585–591.

50. Phipps S: The subsequent pregnancy after stillbirth: Anticipatory parenthood in the face of uncertainty. *Int J Psychiatry Med* 1985–86;15:243–264.

51. Poznanski E: The "replacement child": A saga of unresolved parental grief. *J Pediatr* 1972;81:1190–1193.

Appendix 17.1

Books for Parents to Read

Numerous books have been written in the past 5 years on the subject of perinatal bereavement. These books have a limited shelf life and are sometimes difficult to locate. Rather than list book titles that may no longer be available we offer a list of mail order bookstores and national organizations that carry current bereavement literature and referral information that may be helpful.

Centering Corporation
P.O. Box 3367
Omaha, Nebraska 68103-0367
(402) 533-1200

Birth and Life Bookstore
P.O. Box 70625
Seattle, Washington 98107
(206) 789-4444

Perinatal Loss
2116 NE 18th Ave.
Portland, Oregon 97212
(503) 284-7426

Resolve Through Sharing
LaCrosse Lutheran Hospital
1910 South Ave.
LaCross, Wisconsin 54601
(608) 785-0530 ext. 3696

Pregnancy and Infant Loss Center of Minnesota
1415 E. Wayzata Blvd.
Wayzata, Minnesota 55391
(612) 473-9372

National Maternal and Child Health Clearinghouse
38th and R Streets NW
Washington, DC 20057
(202) 625-8400

Chapter 18

Emesis and Hyperemesis Gravidarum

John P. O'Grady, MD and Lewis M. Cohen, MD

> They are as sick that surfeit with
> Too much, as they
> That starve with nothing
> —*The Merchant of Venice,* I,i,114
> William Shakespeare (1564–1616)

The earliest known references to nausea and vomiting during pregnancy are found in Egyptian papyri. Hippocrates recognized vomiting to be a sign of pregnancy and wrote, "If a woman's courses be suppressed, and neither rigor nor fever has followed, but she has been affected with nausea, you may reckon her to be with child."[1] The importance of repeated emesis in pregnancy and its potential complications were also discussed by the Roman author Soranus (c. AD 150) who was among the first to recognize jaundice as a potential complication and to hint that the sex of the fetus was related to the severity of the vomiting.[2]

In the 17th century, with the reawakening of interest in the physiology of pregnancy, morning sickness was recognized as a potential complication by Guillemeau, Mauriceau, and other major obstetrical writers.[3] However, minimal concern was given to gestational vomiting until the late 18th century when clinicians came slowly to the recognition that recurrent gestational emesis could be a serious and, occasionally, even a fatal disorder. By the mid-19th century there was increased appreciation of the risks of severe vomiting. The celebrated author Charlotte Brontë is believed to have died from complications of hyperemesis. Induced abortion was eventually recommended for intractable cases.

The late 19th century also saw the development of many theories of etiology for gestational emesis.[3] These same general ideas still influence modern therapeutics. Fairweather[4] divided these theories into three major categories: those implicating reflex irritation, those tying emesis to a manifestation of neurosis, and those relating the disorder to the pernicious effects of an unidentified absorbed toxin.

The *reflex* theory stated that some type of irritative focus arose from abnormal uterine positioning or cervical spasm. Not surprisingly, proponents of this theory believed that appropriate therapy should include cervical dilation, uterine suspension, or treatment of cervical inflammation.

The *neurotic* theory held that hysteria or a similar psychological/psychiatric mechanism was the etiology of the vomiting. This led to various suggestive or hypnotic treatments.

The *toxin* theory supposed that noxious substances arising from the gastrointestinal tract, liver, ovary, or fetus irritated the mother's stomach and/or central nervous system and was responsible for the emesis. Treatments proposed on the basis of this theory attempted to block, expel, dilute, or prevent the release of such toxins.

Clinical Presentation

Emesis gravidarum, or the morning sickness of pregnancy, is usually a transitory and minor first-trimester condition that occurs in 40% to 70% of normal gestations.[4-7] *Hyperemesis gravidarum*, or intractable gestational vomiting, is a more pernicious syndrome of the first trimester and occurs in approximately 3 of 1000 pregnancies. Hyperemesis gravidarum is characterized by weight loss, electrolyte imbalance, and disturbed nutrition.[4,8-10] Vomiting is of sufficient severity to require hospital admission and must be unassociated with medical conditions such as appendicitis or pyelonephritis.[4]

The clinical course of hyperemesis gravidarum is extremely variable. The onset of vomiting can precede the first missed menstrual cycle in up to 20% of cases and thus can be the initial symptom of pregnancy. The peak time for patient admission to the hospital is between 8 and 12 weeks[3] (Figure 18.1). The

Figure 18.1 Incidence of hospital admission for hyperemesis by weeks of gestational age (from LMP) (N=217). (From Fairweather DVI: Nausea and vomiting in pregnancy. *Am J Obstet Gynecol* 1968;102:148, with permission.)

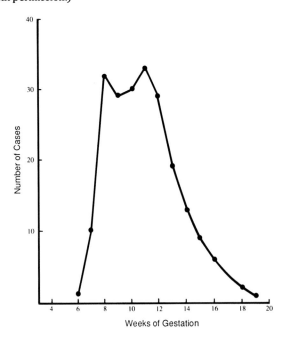

nausea initially begins in the morning, the classical "morning sickness," but there is a good deal of individual variation. As the disorder progresses, the vomiting becomes increasingly frequent and in advanced cases emesis may occur almost continuously. In severe cases, tachycardia occurs along with oliguria, a rising urinary specific gravity, and progressive ketosis. As the condition becomes increasingly worse, hemoconcentration develops accompanied by a rising blood urea nitrogen level and a falling serum sodium, chloride, and potassium.

Hypokalemic myopathy is responsible for much of the physical debility seen in such extreme cases.[8,11] Protein and bilirubin may also be found in the urine and patients often appear jaundiced. Nystagmus and other neurological signs such as drowsiness, mental confusion, peripheral neuropathy, blindness, and coma can progressively develop.[12–17]

Before the availability of antiemetic drugs and prior to an understanding of the fluid and electrolyte disturbances common to the advanced stages of this disorder, death would occasionally occur. In 1942, McGoogan[12] reviewed the literature concerning severe polyneuritis of pregnancy, a syndrome that is now rare but was once associated with prolonged hyperemesis. He identified a total of 154 cases, 40 (27.5%) of which had died.

More recently, adequate fluid and electrolyte replacement has been associated with the virtual disappearance of the most severe complications of hyperemesis gravidarum. Induced abortion is rarely required and the risk of maternal death has been eliminated. These advances are not attributable to any better understanding of the etiology of the disorder, but have resulted from improved management of fluid and electrolytes, adequate vitamin replacement, and carbohydrate supplementation, with or without central hyperalimentation.[4]

A review of fatal cases reported by Sheehan[18] in 1939 is helpful in understanding the pathology of hyperemesis. Cardiac atrophy, fatty hepatic and renal infiltrates, and petechial brain lesions were the primary findings. The characteristic observation in the central nervous system was tiny symmetrical hemorrhages occurring in the mammary bodies and along the walls of the third ventricle and on the floor of the fourth ventricle. These lesions are suggestive of the Wernicke-Korsakoff syndrome discussed below. Fatty infiltration of the liver occurred without evidence of liver cell destruction, suggesting fat mobilization rather than cellular necrosis as the etiology. These histologic changes in the liver were mild and it is likely that they were due to general debility, starvation, and vitamin deficiency rather than to any process unique to hyperemesis gravidarum.[17,19]

In general, in modern practice, if jaundice accompanies a case that clinically mimics hyperemesis, another diagnosis should be sought. However, jaundice may rarely recur accompanying hyperemesis in serial pregnancies.[20] Thus, at least in *some* individuals, an association exists between unknown abnormalities in bilirubin metabolism and hyperemesis

Unusual Complications

A number of disorders that are commonly associated with alcoholism can also appear in patients who have hyperemesis gravidarum. Prolonged retching can result in a *barogenic rupture of the esophagus*.[21,22] This uncommon condition results from a tear through all layers of the wall of the esophagus from violent, recurrent vomiting.[22] The *Mallory-Weiss syndrome* usually follows alcoholic bouts or retching and involves vertical laceration of the gastroesophageal junction. The clinical signs of eosphogeal rupture are chest pain, tachypnea, and subcutaneous emphysema and hematemesis. Pneumomediastinum documented by radiography suggests the correct diagnosis. Chest ascultation may also note a mediastinal "crunch" coincident with cardiac systole. This is thought to arise from the movement of air in the pericardium accompanying cardiac movement (Hamman's sign). Delay in surgical exploration/repair of this condition results in a high risk of mortality.

Wernicke-Korsakoff's encephalopathy is possible in unusually severe or prolonged cases.[23-33] This syndrome is caused by a deficiency in the enzyme cofactor thiamine, or vitamin B_1. Classically known as *beriberi*, thiamine deficiency is usually seen only in hospitalized patients in poor general health or among those who are seriously and chronically nutritionally deprived.[26] This condition complicates gastrointestinal disorders involving malabsorption, cases of prolonged starvation or anorexia nervosa, and alcoholism.

Mental confusion, ophthalmoplegia, nystagmus, and ataxia are the pathognomonic signs.[23,26] Peripheral neuropathy and retinal hemorrhages and hypotension may be present, while hypothermia, blindness, deafness, or fatal coma may occur.[28] Coma can be precipitated iatrogenically by providing carbohydrate intake without vitamin B_1 supplementation, presumably by rapid depletion of nearly exhausted thiamine stores.[30]

Vitamin B_1 is not stored in the body.[26] The deficiency syndrome occurs in hyperemetics due to their reduced oral intake of vitamin B_1 coupled with the normal increase in thiamine consumption during pregnancy.[23,26] In affected cases, an elevated level of serum pyruvate or reduced activity of the transketolase enzyme serves as a sensitive marker for the extent of the deficiency.[32]

When vitamin B_1 is deficient, the oxidation of α-keto acids is abnormal as thiamine pyrophosphate is a coenzyme in carbohydrate metabolism. It appears that development of the syndrome requires both the vitamin deficiency combined with a genetic predisposition to abnormal functioning of transketolase, a thiamine-dependent enzyme in the pentose phosphate pathway.[32,33] As a normal transketolase activity utilizes magnesium ion as a cofactor, adequate magnesium replacement is important as hypomagnesemia can occasionally be the cause of refractiveness to thiamine therapy.[34]

The Wernicke-Korsakoff disorder is a medical emergency whose recognition should be immediately followed by administration of thiamine. Prognosis is directly dependent upon the alacrity with which treatment is provided.

This condition is to be contrasted with *central pontine myelinolysis*, which is caused by overzealous hydration and correction of hyponatremia in severely and chronically depleted patients.[35] This is a condition of symmetrical pontine myelin destruction accompanied by unusual neurological signs. This usually avoidable complication is most common in malnourished alcoholics following rapid fluid infusion, but has also been reported among women with hyperemesis gravidarum.[36]

Table 18.1 Epidemiology of Hyperemesis Gravidarum: Statistically Significant (p ≤0.05) Associations*†

Primigravidas*†

< 12 years of education*

Younger women*†

Nonsmokers*

Obese

Recurrence in subsequent gestation*

Lower incidence of miscarriage*

Lower incidence of stillborn*

Female infant†

Twin gestation†

Congenital malformations†

* Klebanoff and Mills,[45] collaborative perinatal project study (N=9098).

† Kallen,[37] Swedish Medical Birth Registry (N=3068).

Incidence

If one accepts the definition of hyperemesis gravidarum as being vomiting associated with pregnancy that is severe enough to require hospitalization, then the prevalence in the United States and England is approximately 3 in 1000 live births.[4,37,38] The incidence varies due to differences between clinicians in the criteria used to establish diagnosis as well as spontaneous changes in prevalence.[37–39] Many experienced clinicians believe that clinically significant gestational vomiting is less common now than in past decades.

When studied carefully, it is apparent that hyperemesis gravidarum does exist in non-Western populations but is manifested in different ways.[39] The apparent absence of hyperemesis gravidarum in some groups is more an artifact of observation and reporting than a reflection of true occurrence.

Major historical and demographic factors affecting the incidence of hyperemesis gravidarum include: maternal age,[40] multiple pregnancy,[4,37,39] parity,[37,41] and a previous history of hyperemesis gravidarum[4] (Table 18.1). Of these, the most important factor is a prior history. The recurrence rate is 26% to 50%.[4,38,39] It is unclear whether a prior history of unsuccessful pregnancies is related to hyperemesis gravidarum. Fairweather[4] stated that 40% of his patients with hyperemesis gravidarum reported a history of abortion, stillbirth, or neonatal death. This claim has not been supported in other series.[5,37] Paradoxically, the occurrence of emesis and hyperemesis gravidarum in a specific gestation are important positive signs in prognosis. Pregnancies in which hyperemesis or emesis are *absent* have a higher likelihood of spontaneous miscarriage than those in which vomiting occurs.[5,40–42]

Certain abnormalities of pregnancy are commonly thought to be associated with a high incidence of vomiting. However, such data are often difficult to interpret. It has been both claimed [4,37,39] and refuted[43] that multiple pregnancies have a higher incidence of hyperemesis gravidarum. The consensus of opinion remains that hyperemesis gravidarum is more common when additional fetuses are present. Similarly, pregnancies complicated by gestational trophoblastic disease (hydatidiform mole) are generally held to be associated with an increased risk of hyperemesis gravidarum.

The influence of parity is unclear. The literature suggests that in Caucasian populations at least, the incidence of hyperemesis gravidarum is greatest in the first pregnancy.[5,37,40] If non-Caucasian populations are also considered, there are no significant differences between the first and later gestations.

In terms of the outcome of pregnancy, both low birth weight and fetal deformities are weakly associated with hyperemesis.[40] Kallen[37] also reports an increased incidence of hyperemesis gravidarum when the fetus is female, possibly due to a higher maternal level of human chorionic gonadotropin (HCG).

Weight loss associated with hyperemesis gravidarum is an interesting issue and emphasizes the possible dangers of prolonged vomiting.[44,45] Hyperemesis associated with a 5% or greater loss of maternal prepregnancy weight correlates with low birth weight and a higher incidence of intrauterine growth retardation ($p<0.025$).[46] Paradoxically, women with hyperemesis who retain their weight or gain throughout pregnancy, have an *increased* incidence of fetal macrosomia (ie, weight $\geq$4000 g).[46] These data focus attention on maternal weight gain as an important prognostic sign in the clinical course of hyperemesis—a point made by Fairweather more than 20 years ago.[3]

There is also an interesting negative correlation between hyperemesis and cigarette smoking. Smokers are less likely than nonsmokers to develop the disorder.[40,47] The etiology of the protective effect of smoking is speculative but is likely related to depressed estrogen levels in women who smoke.

Differential Diagnosis

The distinction between normal nausea and vomiting of gestation (emesis gravidarum) and the pernicious form of vomiting (hyperemesis gravidarum) is one of degree only. Clinically, no sharp distinction between the two conditions is possible. The separation of these patients into separate groups is artificial, and may obscure the similarities between cases while emphasizing the differences. Most authors apply the term hyperemesis gravidarum to those patients requiring hospitalization. This is a reasonable clinical distinction, as it permits identification of particularly difficult cases. However, it is important to be aware that the criteria used to decide upon hospital admission are by no means standard. Admission is greatly dependent upon economic barriers to hospital entry, clinical course, and the response to medications and other outpatient therapies. Thus, even hospitalized patients represent a heterogenous group of women with emesis of varying severity.

The timing of symptoms during gestation is important in establishing the correct diagnosis. True hyperemesis is a condition restricted to the first trimester. Only in rare cases does the emesis continue beyond 12 to 14 weeks. Further, if nausea/vomiting does persist it is unlikely to continue with the same intensity. Patients who begin to vomit only late in the second or third trimester are usually found to have some other disorder (Table 18.2).

The basic difficulty in evaluating emesis/hyperemesis is that the clinical condition is a *syndrome*. There are multiple causes for vomiting mimicking "classic" hyperemesis including various gastrointestinal disorders, endocrine

Table 18.2 Syndromes Associated with Nausea and Vomiting During Pregnancy*

I. Conditions unique to pregnancy
a. Well defined disorders
i. Pregnancy-induced hypertension
ii. Abruptio placentae
iii. Degenerating leiomyoma
iv. Gestational trophoblastic disease
v. Hydramnios
vi. Labor
b. Idiopathic disorders
i. Emesis gravidarum, "morning sickness"
ii. Hyperemesis gravidarum
iii. Ptyalism
iv. Acute fatty degeneration of the liver
II. Conditions not unique to pregnancy*
a. Hyperthyroidism
b. Hyperparathyroidism
c. Pyelonephritis
d. Hiatal hernia
e. Gastritis/gastroenteritis/peptic ulcer
f. Appendicitis and other bowel lesions
g. Hepatitis, cholestatic jaundice
h. Other infections (pneumonia, otitis media, etc)
i. Pancreatitis
j. Anorexia nervosa / bulimia

* See Refs. 3–6, 48–52, 109.

abnormalities, pyelonephritis, or unusual conditions such as ptyalism.[34,38] These and other specific diagnoses must be excluded before a diagnosis of emesis or hyperemesis gravidarum can be confidently established.

Ptyalism

Ptyalism, or the sialorrhea of pregnancy, is a fascinating and unusual disorder of undetermined etiology which can be confused with hyperemesis.[48–51] In ptyalism there is idiopathic and copious production of saliva that can exceed a liter a day. In the attempt to swallow secretions, women develop anorexia, nausea, or vomiting. Patients are considerably uncomfortable and sleeping is often particularly difficult. The women experience considerable embarrassment as their copious oral fluid production requires them to continuously expectorate. Not surprisingly, some individuals become homebound due to this unpleasant condition.

Ptyalism may begin soon after the onset of pregnancy and persist until virtually the moment of delivery. It rapidly resolves after delivery. In some instances, as with hyperemesis, it is the initial symptom of pregnancy. The etiology is unknown and there is little useful literature to guide the clinician. Ptyalism tends to be recurrent in subsequent gestation and repetitive episodes can be progressively severe.[51] Some patients will respond to treatment with belladonna alkaloids with a reduction in salivary production, but in many cases no specific therapy is effective. Administration of oxyphenomium bromide (*Antrenyl*, 20 to 80 mg every 24 hours in divided doses) can be attempted. Using this therapy Bernstine[51] reported control of symptoms without significant side effects in 7 of 24 cases (29%). However, in 67% of his cases the ptyalism was only partially relieved, or the patients experienced undesirable side effects from the medication.

The principle physiological change in ptyalism is an increase in saliva production with no change in its chemical constitution. Despite that the fact the volume of saliva production can approach 500 cc/hr, no distinct abnormality of the salivary gland has been identified.

The relationship between ptyalism and hyperemesis is unclear. Bernstine[51] reported that sialorrhea persisted in his patients even after the nausea/vomiting of early pregnancy had abated, suggesting a clinical separation between the disorders. The incidence of ptyalism is unknown but it clearly is uncommon. The author has seen three cases of ptyalism in 15 years of a high-risk obstetrical practice, testifying to its rarity in comparison to emesis and hyperemesis gravidarum.

Although ptyalism is uncommon, it is important that the clinician correctly identify this disorder. In contrast to hyperemesis, ptyalism usually persists throughout pregnancy at the same intensity. Thus, in ptyalism, neither the physician nor the patient can confidently expect improvement as the gestation proceeds, in marked distinction to classical hyperemesis. Also, ptyalism does not lead to true pernicious nausea/vomiting. Hospital admission for dehydration and/or electrolyte abnormalities is distinctly less likely with ptyalism than with hyperemesis.

Hyperparathyroidism

Endocrine abnormalities may produce a clinical picture that is indistinguishable from hyperemesis. *Primary hyperparathyroidism* can present with a hypercalcemic crisis (serum calcium ≥15 mg/dL) that can confuse the clinician.[52-54] This condition is characterized by weakness, fatigue, nausea and vomiting, anorexia, weight loss, dehydration, and confusion.[52,53] Coma and/or death can ensue. The correct diagnosis is established by noting an elevated serum calcium, accompanied by depressed concentration of magnesium and phosphorus in a patient with acute symptoms. Management consists of reducing the abnormally elevated calcium levels, restoring vascular volume, and replenishing potassium and magnesium.

Surgical exploration may be required to extricate the tumor(s). This condition is important to recognize as the accompanying fetal complications including neonatal tetany can be severe. Hyperparathyroidism is also associated with an increased risk of spontaneous abortion, stillbirth, and premature delivery. Associated clinical findings include bone pain, renal colic, muscular weakness, polyuria, polydipsia, pancreatitis, and peptic ulcer. While hyperparathyroidism is rare, diagnosis is easy and treatment highly successful if the correct initial evaluations are performed.

Pathophysiology

Chorionic Gonadotropin

It has long been suspected that a link exists between the nausea/vomiting of pregnancy and the serum concentration of human chorionic gonadotropin (HCG).[55-62] The relationship has proven difficult to establish and data on this point has been and remains controversial. The virtual disappearance of hyperemesis gravidarum closely parallels the physiological decline of HCG in the first trimester. Further, many observers have noted the association between the peak incidence of emesis with maximum maternal serum HCG levels [3] (Figure 18.1).

The advent of HCG immunoassays has not entirely settled this controversy but it has provided more consistent data for comparative study. Soules and co-workers[56] found no clear relationship between HCG or 17-hydroxy-progesterone levels and the incidence or severity of nausea/vomiting in either normally pregnant patients or women with molar pregnancies. However, in other studies,[57-60] Kauppila and co-workers[59,61] have reported a statistically significant relationship between elevated serum HCG concentrations and pregnancy nausea and vomiting. Similar findings have also been reported by Masson and co-workers.[60]

At least some of the discrepancies between these studies are due to differences in assay technique, patient population, and the timing of sampling. There is some evidence that HCG levels are affected by hydration, ambulation, and even sex of the fetus.[62] Yet, it is hard to credit these effects as entirely adequate explanations for the variations between the findings of these studies.

Other hormonal substances known to be altered by pregnancy have also been studied as possible contributors to gestational nausea. Investigations of serum concentrations of adrenocorticotropic hormone (ACTH), cortisol, follicle-stimulating hormone (FSH), thyroid-stimulating hormone (TSH), and growth hormone have failed to demonstrate any clear relationship to hyperemesis and, not surprisingly, intravenous therapy with ACTH is ineffective.[58,59,61-63] Measurements of serum prolactin and thyroxine have also been inconsistent and conflicting.[58]

Based on the available data, most investigators believe that there is reasonable data linking early pregnancy concentrations of HCG and hyperemesis. While it is likely that HCG is not the only substance present in early gestation causing emesis, it certainly is among the most important. The major difficulty lies in establishing the nauseogenic mechanism for HCG and other pregnancy-related hormones. Substantial data indicates that this connection is found in the dynamics of thyroid function.

Thyroid Dysfunction

There is an interesting body of data concerning the association between abnormal thyroid function and hyperemesis gravidarum.[64-69] It is unusual to diagnose frank hyperthyroidism or classic Graves' disease during pregnancy.[65,66,70] This condition is important to recognize as it places the pregnancy at risk for fetal growth retardation and/or preterm labor. Possible maternal complications of undiagnosed or incompletely treated hyperthyroidism in pregnancy can include delirium, hypertension, convulsions, and high-output cardiac failure.[71] The nausea, tachycardia, and restlessness of thyrotoxicosis mimic hyperemesis and confusion between the two disorders is easy. Routine thyroid function tests do not adequately distinguish between these conditions as the FT_4I and often the FT_3 are elevated, and the TSH low (Table 18.3). Likewise, the TRH stimulation test is unreliable in separating these disorders as most but not all hyperemetics have a blunted TSH response, resembling hyperthyroidism.[72]

Rosenthal[73] has reported that vomiting plays an important role in the presentation of true thyrotoxicosis in nonpregnant patients and is usually abolished by carbimazole treatment, implying a direct relationship between elevated thyroid hormone levels and stimulation of the vomiting center. This relationship is not simple. In a striking case of intractable hyperemesis and related thyroid dysfunction reported by Kirshon and co-workers,[74] nausea and vomiting persisted until delivery, despite normalization of thyroid function. Only in the postpartum period did the gastrointestinal symptoms disappear and the true etiology identified.

New data indicate that there is a physiologic activation of the thyroid gland in normal early pregnancy. This is documented by increased T_4 levels accompanied by decreased TSH concentration.[68] Some of the thyroid stimulation is believed due to the release of a placental-derived thyrotropin. However, there is also data that support a correlation between serum concentrations of HCG and free T_4.[68]

While the exact physiology remains unclear, 40% to 70% of women hospitalized with hyperemesis gravidarum have abnormalities of thyroid function[75–77] (Table 18.3). In these women, test indices are consistent with at least mild thyrotoxicosis.[64,65,69,72,77] In certain cases, specific antithyroid treatment has been administered including methimazole,[74] carbimazole,[71,78] or propylthiouracil.[65] It remains unclear whether such treatment is necessary as therapy does not invariably control the associated emesis, even when thyroid indices are returned to the normal range.[74]

Table 18.3 Differential Diagnosis Between Hyperthyroidism and Hyperemesis Gravidarum*

	Hyperemesis gravidarum	Hyperthyroidism
Weight loss	+ + + +	+ +
Vomiting	+ + + +	Occasionally
TT_4	↑	↑
FT_4I	↑	↑
FT_4 by dialysis	N or ↑	↑
TT_3	N or ↑	↑
FT_3I	N or ↑	↑
TRH test	N or – – –	– – –
Sensitive TSH	Suppressed	Suppressed
TSHRAb	Negative	Positive

TT_4, total thyroxine; FT_4I, free thyroxine index; TT_3, total triiodothyronine; FT_3I; free triiodothyronine index; ↑, increase; N, normal; – – –, no response; TRH test, thyrotropin-releasing hormone test; + + + +, very severe; + +, less severe.

*Reprinted from Mestman JH; Endocrine diseases in pregnancy, in Sciarra JJ (ed.): *Gynecology and Obstetrics.* Philadelphia, JB Lippincott, 1990;23(3):13, with permission.

Jeffcoate and Bain[78] described a woman in her middle 20s with hyperemesis gravidarum and biochemical evidence of thyrotoxicosis, a condition repeated in two consecutive pregnancies. Remarkably, when not pregnant, this woman was clinically normal and had normal laboratory studies. In this case, while a clinical association between pregnancy and recurrent thyroid hyperfunction was clear, it was uncertain whether antithyroid treatment had helped control this woman's emesis or whether therapy occurred during a spontaneous remission.

Hydatidiform molar pregnancy is an experiment of nature that helps us understand this problem. The characteristic finding in gestational trophoblastic disease (GTD) is markedly elevated serum concentrations of HCG.[79-81] There is good clinical evidence that many, but not all, patients with this disorder develop striking abnormalities in thyroid function and many of these patients experience gestational emesis of varying severity.

In GTD, it is theorized that a thyroid-stimulating substance derived from trophoblastic tissue is responsible for both TSH suppression and thyroid stimulation.[82] It is likely that the culprit is chorionic gonadotropin, a substance with intrinsic thyrotropic activity.[82-86] In GTD, the thyrotropic stimulation can be sufficient to produce a clinical picture that is indistinquishable from classical hyperthyroidism.

As mentioned previously, there is continued controversy about the levels of various thyroid hormones during pregnancy and among patients with hyperemesis.[69] A good deal of this reported variation is technical and due to differences in test techniques or assay methods. Maternal free thyroid hormone, for example, has been reported to be decreased, increased, or unchanged during normal pregnancy.[69] An important study for review is that of Mori and co-workers.[68] He and his co-workers used an immunoradiometric assay that was not influenced by gestational alterations in either thyroxine-binding globulin or albumin. In a study of 132 normal pregnant women and 20 nonpregnant control patients, a statistically significant increase in free T_4 and HCG and decreased TSH was observed during pregnancy. These changes correlated with the severity of morning sickness. Further, as emesis symptoms resolved in the mid-trimester, the values of both TSH and free T_4 spontaneously returned to the normal range.

How are these complex and sometimes conflicting data to be interpreted? A substantial percentage of hyperemetics have, as Bober and co-workers[69] put it, a form of transient "biochemical thyrotoxicosis." In the first trimester the rise of HCG (or a related substance) serves both as a thyroid stimulator and in some patients, but by no means all, as an emetic. As pregnancy advances, the normal decline in HCG concentration is followed by the disappearance of both the vomiting and the thyroid dysfunction.

While the implications for treatment remain unclear, a screen for thyroid function (TSH, T_4, T_3, free T4, and thyroid index) should accompany a hospital admission for the presumed diagnosis of hyperemesis. Testing for TSH receptor antibodies separates hyperemesis with thyroid dysfunction from thyrotoxicosis. Such antibodies are only found in women with Graves' disease.[72]

Obviously, if a clear diagnosis of thyrotoxicosis is possible, standard antithyroid medication is indicated. However, in the vast majority of cases of hyperemesis, abnormalities in thyroid function will prove transitory and require no treatment. Unfortunately, it remains unclear which patients do require therapy. We concur with Mestman's[72] suggestion that if thyroid tests remain abnormal for 2 to 4 weeks, if TSH receptor antibody test is positive, or if other clinical signs and symptoms of thyrotoxicosis are present, treatment with antithyroid drugs is indicated.

Hepatic Dysfunction

There is a strong association between emesis/hyperemesis gravidarum and abnormalities in liver metabolism.[87-91] A large percentage of women who experience nausea while using oral contraceptives also experience nausea/vomiting in early pregnancy.[89] In addition, among multiparas with surgically confirmed gallbladder disease, 98% develop nausea/vomiting in early pregnancy and 41% are similarly intolerant of oral contraceptives.[89] These findings imply that some patients with early pregnancy emesis have underlying hepatic disease, frequently, but not always manifested by gallstone formation. There may also be associated abnormalities in sex steroid metabolism, as suggested by the clinical association with intolerance to oral contraceptives.

There are other indications of underlying hepatic dysfunction.[87-91] Data on serum lipids and lipoproteins from women *with* early pregnancy nausea/vomiting document distinct differences in comparison to normal pregnant women.[89] Specifically, the lipid content of low-density lipoproteins is significantly higher in emetics while the lipid content of high-density lipoproteins is lower. Finally, third- trimester women whose pregnancies were complicated by early nausea/vomiting have higher serum values for total cholesterol and triglycerides than control patients ($p \leq 0.05$). This occurs despite the fact that the women are totally asymptomatic at the time of sampling. The etiology of these metabolic differences is uncertain. However, these data reinforce the hypothesis that an occult hepatic dysfunction exists in at least some women who develop gestational emesis.

An unusual hypothesis has been forwarded by Jarnfelt-Samsioe and coworkers,[89] based on an ultrasonographic study of 43 early pregnancies, 26 of which included a history of nausea/vomiting. In these patients, the corpus luteum was located on the *right side* in 69%. In unaffected pregnancies the corpus luteum was predominantly *left sided*. The speculative implication of these findings is that differences in ovarian-venous drainage are of importance in the etiology of hyperemesis gravidarum. This could occur by concentrating sex steroids in the portal venous circulation, leading to an enhanced metabolic load of such steroids directed to the liver.

These studies raise the possibility that some women have a propensity for nausea in response to a variety of conditions of hepatic dysfunction or when confronted with an increased demand to metabolize sex steroids.

Psychological Aspects

It has long appeared to clinicians that psychological factors play an etiologic role in hyperemesis gravidarum. There has been a recent shift from claiming that these factors are primarily responsible for the generation of the symptoms, to a more reasonable biopsychosocial perspective. This view holds that hyperemesis gravidarum is an end product of the complex interplay of biological, psychological, and sociological variables.[92]

Nausea and vomiting are symptoms that have prominent psychological components. Our common expressions, "It's enough to make me sick," or "To think about that makes me want to vomit," attest to the emotional aspect of the physiologic event of regurgitation. In susceptible individuals, specific sights or smells can evoke nausea or even emesis.

Anticipatory vomiting is a common problem in patients undergoing chemotherapy, and often occurs before drugs are administered. We are acquainted with an example of an anticipatory form of mal de mer. The unfortunate patient was a physician with severe seasickness who nonetheless would occasionally venture forth on small boats on social occasions. Quite often he would begin vomiting while still standing on the dock.

As discussed earlier in this book, in the *couvade syndrome* related to pseudocyesis, sympathetic nausea or vomiting occurs in the male partner, paralleling the condition in the pregnant woman. The couvade syndrome illustrates the influence of cultural and social factors on these symptoms.

Early psychoanalytic authors, such as Deutsch,[93] interpreted the vomiting in hyperemesis gravidarum as a symbolic rejection of the child. The women were assumed to be highly ambivalent about their pregnancies. The hyperemesis gravidarum was viewed as an attempt at abortion. The *choice* of the symptom of vomiting also reflected concerns engendered by primitive beliefs in "oral impregnation." This concept was similarly held to be of etiologic importance in anorexia nervosa.[94]

The theory of psychosomatic specificity held sway through the 1950s, and maintained that people who had disorders such as peptic ulcers or hyperemesis gravidarum would be found to have specific underlying personalities or intrapsychic conflicts. During this period, Grace and Graham[95] examined a sample of 11 women to delineate any common attitude. They theorized that women with hyperemesis gravidarum vomited as a way of undoing their *mistake*, and that the women wished to restore their nongravid state.

These earliest efforts at psychiatric research were followed by a number of case studies that used psychological testing, research criteria, and control groups. The endeavors of Guze and associates[96] is representative of this work, in that 48 patients were paired with normal controls and 80% were subsequently located and interviewed 42 months later. The only chronic psychiatric disorder identified among patients with hyperemesis gravidarum in higher proportion than controls was hysteria (15% versus 2%). They hypothesized that the histrionic nature of hysteria would lead to hospitalization. Purtel and co-workers[97] also found that 56% of a sample of women with hysteria complained of severe vomiting during the first trimester of pregnancy, compared to 5% of a control group. Fairweather[3,4] subjected 44 patients with hyperemesis gravidarum to psychiatric interviews and a battery of psychological tests. He found that the disorder was associated with a hysterical personality, below average intelligence, infantile or immature personalities, and marked maternal dependence. In seven of eight cases of clinical hysteria, the evidence suggested that the psychological disorder had been present long before the pregnancy. In the remaining case the onset of the disorder could not be determined. In 40% of the cases there was a prior history of gastric disorders, chiefly characterized by vomiting under stress.

Several recent studies have emphasized the presence of high stress and minimal social support in patients who have hyperemesis gravidarum.[98] It is not surprising that a majority of these women already live with or subsequently seek refuge with their parents.

A major problem of the psychiatric literature is that it lends itself to "blaming the victim." The term hysteria, although it has had a rich and varied history, has largely been abandoned in modern psychiatric nosology because of its pejorative connotations. The exaggerated claims of the "specificity" theory of psychosomatic medicine have fortunately been discounted, and the search for a single unifying clinical profile has proven to be a waste of time. Likewise, the doctor-patient relationship is undermined when the symptoms of hyperemesis gravidarum are interpreted as being "expressed to elicit care by physicians and family and to gain a 'time out' from stressful home environments."[92] While the hospitalization provides a haven and respite from some responsibilities and terrors, it is unhelpful for this to be viewed as somehow playing a role in the genesis of the disorder. The psychiatric concepts of primary and secondary gain have unfortunately mangled more than one treatment case.

A modern and sensitive view of hyperemesis gravidarum, such as the biopsychosocial perspective of Engel,[99] places it in a multifactorial framework,[92] in which there is an interplay between multiple etiologic and contributing variables. In our opinion, the underlying etiology of hyperemesis gravidarum is almost certainly primarily endocrinologic, but the clinical manifestations are heavily dependent upon the psychosocial characteristics of the women. Many of the women may warrant the diagnoses of histrionic personality disorder or somatization disorder, which are now used in place of hysteria. Others are merely "immature," or overly dependent on their mothers. A portion are probably of limited intelligence, while others are more limited in cultural or social spheres. Many of the women are experiencing overwhelming stress and have vomited under similar circumstances in the past. It is important to keep in mind that some of the women have no major psychiatric disorders. In all of these cases the biopsychosocial factors mutually interact, and successful treatment requires attention to the entire complex person.

Treatment

There are important medical interests in the treatment of hyperemesis. First, the weight loss, dehydration, and electrolyte abnormality associated with the severe forms of this disorder place the mother, and to a lesser degree the fetus, at risk. Second, the symptoms of recurrent nausea, retching, and related debility are generally distressing to patients, their families, and their physicians. Episodes of nausea/vomiting may lead to hospitalization, consuming a scarce and expensive resource. Finally, if in a particular case nausea/vomiting has important psychological overtones, routine medical therapy may not be efficacious, or succeed only partially. Nausea/vomiting is a symptom, not a disease, and the diagnosis of hyperemesis gravidarum should only be made after consideration of other alternatives.

There is another aspect of treatment that deserves discussion. Some practitioners and/or health care workers still retain a punitive approach to women with hyperemesis. A management program based on punishment misunderstands the complex interplay between psychology and physiology, increases the women's distress, confuses definitive therapy, and leads to unnecessary confrontations between patient, physician, and staff.[3,4]

Historically, many therapies have been reported to be successful in hyperemesis gravidarum.[4,31] Some of the therapies have little or no physiologic basis to explain their efficacy. Included among the long list of reportedly successful treatments are cervical dilation; administration of placental extract,[100] insulin,[3] or testosterone[3]; injection of husband's blood[101]; acupuncture/acupressure[102,103]; and hypnosis.[104,105] The reviewer is faced with substantial dilemmas in attempting to critique the reports. King[106] has observed that such treatments succeed only by virtue of being medicine administered by a concerned individual and not due to any intrinsic pharmacologic effect(s).

King[106] described a placebo control study of gestational emesis involving 102 patients who were given either meclizine, metamphetamine, or placebo. Fully 75% of these women improved or were cured of their nausea/vomiting by the placebo drug. While some of the volunteers in this study could distinguish between the effects of placebo or amphetamine when the drugs were changed during the crossover period, other participants could detect no difference. The importance of the psychological aspects of emesis are further emphasized by Semmens's experience. In a double-blind study of drug efficacy for nausea, 58% of 385 patients responded favorably to placebo treatment.[107]

Recent publications reviewing therapy for hyperemesis gravidarum still report long lists of agents used for the control of nausea[108] (Table 18.4). Continuing this tradition, most clinicians have their personal reserve of specific drugs or treatments for use in this disorder. It is difficult to make recommendations as to which agents to use, except to repeat the usual refrain of suggesting the least toxic agent(s), in the lowest possible dose, for the shortest possible time.

The mainstays of treatment of hyperemesis gravidarum remain hospital admission with fluid and electrolyte support for severe cases, in conjunction with psychological support. While antiemetic agents may be used, the most important aspect of therapy remains correction of dehydration and abnormalities in blood chemistry (Table 18.5).

There are no specific dietary rules to follow except to resume feeding slowly after the extreme retching has resolved. Oral dietary supplements of iron and vitamins should be omitted until bouts of nausea have entirely ceased. Dextrose in a balanced salt solution (eg, D_5W Ringers' Lactate-Hartman's solution) is given at 3 L every 24 hours or more rapidly if dehydration is present. Supplemental potassium (60 mEq every 24 hours) is provided by addition of concentrated KCl to the infusion solution. It is best to also administer 100 mg or more of thiamine as well as 1 g of magnesium sulfate ($MgSO_4$-7-H_2O) in the same infusion solution every 24 hours if vomiting has been severe and prolonged. Promethazine (50–100 mg q 4–6 hours) or prochlorperazine (Compazine, 10 mg IM/po q 6 or 25 mg suppository q 6) may be given acutely as antiemetics (see Table 18.4). In general, withholding oral feeding and maintenance of hydration intravenously are more effective than any specific antiemetics in gaining control of the vomiting. On occasion, patients experiencing recurrent bouts of severe nausea are managed by outpatient rehydration either by an indwelling peripheral venous line (changed every 48 hours or as needed) or, uncommonly, by an indwelling major venous access line (Hickman catheter or similar device). We have found that hospitalizations can be avoided by withholding feeding combined with out-of-hospital intravenous therapy if there is close telephone contact with these women or the close involvement of a visiting nurse. In unusually prolonged or severe cases, long-term intravenous hyperalimentation may be necessary.[17]

A careful patient interview is essential. In this discussion, the clinician seeks unusual symptoms and/or stressors that may suggest either a distinct disease process (eg, cholelithiasis) or the presence of discrete environmental stressors. When stress, anxiety, and complexing conditions such as anorexia nervosa or discrete psychopathology are believed to be major contributors to the problem, psychiatric consultation is indicated.[109]

The literature suggests that behavior modification, hypnosis, or brief psychotherapy are useful in this disorder (see Chapter 21). Zechnich and Hammer,[110] for example, describe a case in which the patient appeared to have responded to simple reassuring and educative interventions directed at her anxiety-laden belief that vomiting throughout pregnancy was inevitable. Behavioral therapists have successfully used techniques such as stimulus deprivation, relaxation training, self-monitoring and self-control models, and stimulus control and imagery in helping to control recurrent vomiting.[111,112]

Apfel and associates[113] found that patients with hyperemesis gravidarum (n = 17) were significantly more hypnotizable than those with milder symptoms (n = 13). They view hypnotherapy as being a readily available, non-

Table 18.4 Common Drug Therapies for Hyperemesis*

Generic name	Trade name	Dose/route/timing
Chlorpromazine hydrochloride	Thorazine	10–25 mg orally q 6 hr or 25 mg q 6 hr by rectal suppository
Dicyclomine hydrochloride	Bentyl, Antispas	10–20 mg orally q 4–6 hr
Dimenhydrinate	Dramamine	50–100 mg orally q 4 hr or 50 mg IM or IV q 4 hr
Diphenhydramine hydrochloride	Benadryl	25–50 mg orally q 4–6 hr or 25–50 mg IM or IV q 4–6 hr
Meclizine hydrochloride	Antivert, Bonine	12.5–50 mg orally q 12–24 hr
Metoclopramide hydrochloride	Reglan	10–15 mg orally q 8 hr or 10–20 mg IM or IV q 8 hr
Prochlorperazine edlsylate and maleate	Compazine	5–10 mg orally or IM q 6 hr or 25 mg by rectal suppository q 6–8 hr
Promethazine hydrochloride	Phenergan	12.5–50 mg IM or orally q 4–6 hr or 25 mg by rectal suppository q 4–6 hr
Triethylperazine maleate	Torecan	10–20 mg IM or orally 1–3 times qd
Trimethobenzamide hydrochloride	Tigan	250 mg orally q 6–8 hr or by rectal suppository 200 mg q 6–8 hr or 200 mg IM q 6–8 hr.

Modified from Buttino [108]

pharmacologic treatment that is a useful adjunct to basic psychological support. This has also been the finding of Fuchs and his co-workers, who treated 138 women with either individual or group hypnotherapy.[114] The women were seen after conventional medical treatment had failed. Out of 51 patients treated individually, 35 (69%) had an excellent response and two (4%) a good response to the hypnosis. Fourteen (26%) showed a poor response to the treatment. Out of 87 patients treated in groups (along with women preparing for natural childbirth), 61 (70%) had an excellent response and 24 (28%) had a good response to the hypnosis. In this sample, only two patients (2%) had a poor response. The authors were surprised to find that the results were substantially better with group hypnotherapy. Their impression was that the women apparently felt safer and less lonely with group treatment, and fewer hospitalizations were required.

Analysis of the psychotherapy literature is complicated by the fact that almost every patient studied has simultaneously received the physical treatments discussed earlier in this section. This is compounded by the high level of placebo response. There have been no studies of comparative efficacy of different psychotherapeutic modalities and it is safe to say that almost any type of psychotherapy can be safely offered.

Conclusions

What may we fairly conclude concerning the etiology of and therapy for hyperemesis and emesis gravidarum? First, newer studies utilizing various radioimmunoassay techniques have documented distinct abnormalities in thyroid function and HCG concentration in 50% or more of these women. The majority of these individuals have a transient type of thyroid hyperfunction characterized by exaggeratedly high levels of T_4 and markedly depressed concentrations of TSH (Table 18.3). There is a thread of evidence going back to early clinical observation of hyperemesis that links these symptoms to eleva-

Table 18.5 Basic Treatment for Hyperemesis Gravidarum*

1. Hospital admission for observation and vital sign recording.

2. Serial determinations of hemoglobin/hematocrit, renal function tests.

3. Daily weights, testing of urines for ketones and specific gravity. Calculation of intake and output.

4. Exclusion of specific medical conditions by appropriate evaluation; ie, urine culture, thyroid panel, liver function tests.

5. Intravenous therapy including magnesium and B vitamins to correct dehydration electrolyte imbalance and partially offset carbohydrate deficiencies; in unusual cases, central hyperalimentation.

6. Use of antiemetic agents, as required (see Table 18.4).

7. Psychological support, as necessary.

8. Abdominal or transvaginal ultrasonography to establish the gestational age and normality of pregnancy.

See Refs. 3, 4, 106, 108.

tions in HCG, which accompany normal early gestation. Thus, in at least some instances of pernicious vomiting, relatively high HCG concentrations either directly or indirectly induce thyroid hyperfunction, and result in nausea and vomiting in susceptible individuals. Although not all authors agree, the association between elevated HCG levels and emesis appears secure.

Studies of HCG levels, experiments of nature provided by multiple gestation and gestational trophoblastic disease, and the experience of nausea and vomiting following birth control pill administration provide evidence for an endocrine origin for pregnancy-related nausea. Presumably, this effect is mediated directly via the vomiting center in the medulla oblongata.

In our opinion, hyperemesis gravidarum can best be appreciated if viewed from a biopsychosocial perspective. The literature reveals that the symptoms of hyperemesis gravidarum are responsive to a variety of psychotherapeutic modalities. Removal from home, encouragement, compassionate nursing care, and attention to fluid and electrolyte disturbances are all necessary ingredients in the successful management of this disorder.

References

1. Hippocrates: *Hippocratic Writings.* Aphorisms no. 61. Chicago, Encyclopaedia Britannica, 1982.
2. Soranus: Temkin O, trans. *Gynecology.* Baltimore, The Johns Hopkins Press, 1956.
3. Fairweather DVI: Nausea and vomiting in pregnancy. *Am J Obstet Gynecol* 1968;102:135–175.
4. Fairweather DVI: Nausea and vomiting during pregnancy. *Obstet Gynecol Ann* 1978;7:91–105.
5. Klebanoff MA, Koslowe PA, Kaslow R, Rhoads GG: Epidemiology of vomiting in early pregnancy. *Obstet Gynecol* 1985;66L:612–614.
6. Fitzgerald JPB: Epidemiology of hyperemesis gravidarum. *Lancet* 1956;1:660–662.
7. Macy C: Psychological factors in nausea and vomiting in pregnancy: A review. *J Reprod Inf Psychol* 1986;4:23–55.
8. Riggs JE, Griggs RC, Gutmann L: Hypokalemic myopathy in hyperemesis gravidarum: Its historical significance. *W Va Med J* 1983;79:95–97.
9. Bergqvist N: Potassium deficiency in hyperemesis gravidarum. *Acta Obstet Gynecol Scand* 1951;30:428–438.
10. Rivière M, Chastrusse L, Dubecq JP, Maleviale G: Considerations sur la biologie des vomissements graves du début de la grossesse. *Gynécol Obstet* 1960;59:18–46.
11. Fitzgerald JPB: Potassium depletion and replacement in hyperemesis. *NZ Med J* 1955;54:36–50.
12. McGoogan LS: Severe polyneuritis due to vitamin B deficiency in pregnancy. *Am J Obstet Gynecol* 1942;43:752–762.
13. Bandstrup E: Some problems concerning the aetiology and treatment of hyperemesis. *J Obstet Gynaecol Br Emp* 1939;46:700–710.
14. Iber FL: Jaundice in pregnancy—a review. *Am J Obstet Gynecol* 1965;91:721–753.
15. Hammerli UP: Jaundice during pregnancy: With special emphasis on recurrent jaundice during pregnancy and its differential diagnosis. *Acta Med Scand* 1966;179(suppl)444:9–111.
16. Peckham CH: Observations on sixty cases of hyperemesis gravidarum. *Am J Obstet Gynecol* 1929;17:776–788.
17. Stellato TA, Danziger LH, Burkons D: Fetal salvage with maternal total parenteral

nutrition: The pregnant mother as her own control. *J Parenter Enteral Nutr* 1988;12:412–413.

18. Sheehan HL: The pathology of hyperemesis and vomiting of late pregnancy. *J Obstet Gynaecol Br Emp* 1939;46:685–699.

19. Campbell ACP, Biggart JH: Wernicke's encephalopathy (polioencephalitis haemorrhagica superior): Its alcoholic and non- alcoholic incidence. *J Path Bacteriol* 1939;48:245–262.

20. Larrey D, Rueff B, Feldmann B, Degott C, Danan G, Benhamou JP: Recurrent jaundice caused by recurrent hyperemesis gravidarum. *Gut* 1984;25:1414–1415.

21. Chirino O, Kovac R, Bale D, Blythe JG: Barogenic rupture of the esophagus associated with hyperemesis gravidarum. *Obstet Gynecol* 1978;52(suppl 1):51s–53s.

22. Bruno MS, Grier WRN, Ober WB: Spontaneous laceration and rupture of esophagus and stomach. *Arch Intern Med* 1963;112:170–179.

23. Lavin PJM, Smith D, Kori SH, Ellenberger C: Wernicke's encephalopathy: A predictable complication of hyperemesis gravidarum. *Obstet Gynecol* 1983;62:13s–15s.

24. Nightingale S, Bates D, Heath PD, Barron SL: Wernicke's encephalopathy in hyperemesis gravidarum. *Postgrad Med J* 1982;58:558–559.

25. Wood P, Murray A, Sinha B, Godley M, Goldsmith HJ: Wernicke's encephalopathy induced by hyperemesis gravidarum. Case reports. *Br J Obstet Gynaecol* 1983;90:583–586.

26. Reuler JB, Girard DE, Cooney TG: Wernicke's encephalopathy. *N Engl J Med* 1985;312:1035–1038.

27. Ebels EJ: How common is Wernicke-Korsakoff syndrome? *Lancet* 1978;2:781–782.

28. Wallis WE, Willoughby E, Baker P: Coma in the Wernicke- Korsakoff syndrome. *Lancet* 1978;2:400–401.

29. Chaturachinda K, McGregor EM: Wernicke's encephalopathy and pregnancy. *J Obstet Gynaecol Br Commonw* 1968;75:969–971.

30. Watson AJS, Walker JF, Tomkin GH, Finn MMR, Koegh JAB: Acute Wernicke's encephalopathy precipitated by glucose loading. *Ir J Med Sci* 1981;150:301–303.

31. Reinken L, Gant H: Vitamin B6 nutrition in women with hyperemesis gravidarum during the first trimester of pregnancy. *Clin Chim Acta* 1974;55:101–102.

32. Lu GD: Studies on the metabolism of pyruvic acid in normal and vitamin B1-deficient states. *Biochem J* 1939;33:249–254.

33. Blass JP, Gibson GI: Abnormality of a thiamine-requiring enzyme in patients with Wernicke-Korsakoff syndrome. *N Engl J Med* 1977;297:1367–1370.

34. Traviesa DC: Magnesium deficiency: A possible cause of thiamine refractoriness in Wernicke-Korsakoff encephalopathy. *J Neurol Neurosurg Psychiatry* 1974;37:959–962.

35. Fraser D: Central pontine myelinolysis as a result of treatment of hyperemesis gravidarum. Case report. *Br J Obstet Gynaecol* 1988;95:621–623.

36. Sterns RH, Riggs JE, Schochet SS: Osmotic demyelination syndrome following correction of hyponatremia. *N Engl J Med* 1986;314:1535–1542.

37. Kallen B: Hyperemesis during pregnancy and delivery outcome: A registry study. *Eur J Obstet Gynecol Reprod Biol* 1987;26:291–302.

38. FitzGerald CM: Nausea and vomiting in pregnancy. *Br J Med Psychol* 1984;57:159–165.

39. Chin RKH, Lao TTH, Kong AMY: Hyperemesis gravidarum in Chinese women. *Asia Oceania J Obstet Gynaecol* 1987;13:261–264.

40. Depue RH, Bernstein L, Ross RK, Judd HL, Henderson BE: Hyperemesis gravidarum in relation to estradiol levels, pregnancy outcome, and other maternal factors: A seroepidemiologic study. *Am J Obstet Gynecol* 1987;156:1137–1141.

41. Tierson FD, Olsen CL, Hook EB: Nausea and vomiting of pregnancy and association with pregnancy outcome. *Am J Obstet Gynecol* 1986;155:1017–1022.

42. Brandes JM: First-trimester nausea and vomiting as related to outcome of preg-

nancy. *Obstet Gynecol* 1967;30:427–431.

43. Bender: Twin pregnancy: A review of 472 cases. *J Obstet Gynaecol Br Emp* 1952;59:510–517.

44. Chin RKH, Lao TT: Low birth weight and hyperemesis gravidarum. *Eur J Obstet Gynecol Reprod Biol* 1988;28:179–183.

45. Klebanoff MA, Mills JL: Is vomiting during pregnancy teratogenic? *Br Med J* 1986;292:724–726.

46. Gross S, Librach C, Cecutti MD: Maternal weight loss associated with hyperemesis gravidarum: A predictor of fetal outcome. *Am J Obstet Gynecol* 1989;160:906–909.

47. Little RE, Hook EB: Maternal alcohol and tobacco consumption and their association with nausea and vomiting during pregnancy. *Acta Obstet Gynecol Scand* 1979;58:15–17.

48. Barnes CG: Disorders of the alimentary tract. *Medical Disorders in Obstetric Practice*, ed. 4. Oxford, Blackwell Scientific, 1974, pp 146–147.

49. Queries and minor notes: Ptyalism during pregnancy. *JAMA* 1951;146:1545–1546.

50. Queries and minor notes: Ptyalism during pregnancy. *JAMA* 1955;157:1457.

51. Bernstine RL: Salivation in pregnant and nonpregnant women. *Obstet Gynecol* 1957;10:184–189.

52. Pedersen NT, Permin H: Hyperparathyroidism and pregnancy. *Acta Obstet Gynecol Scand* 1975;54:281–283.

53. Soyannwo MAO, McGeown MG, Bell M, Milliken TG: A case of acute hyperparathyroidism, with thyrotoxicosis and pancreatitis, presenting as hyperemesis gravidarum. *Postgrad Med J* 1968;44:861–868.

54. Budd DC, Kumka MME, Suda AK, Fink DL: Hyperparathyroidism masquerading as hyperemesis gravidarum. *N Engl J Med* 1988;85:811–813.

55. Schoeneck FJ: Gonadotropic hormone concentrations in emesis gravidarum. *Am J Obstet Gynecol* 1942;43:308–312.

56. Soules MR, Hughes CL, Garcia JA, et al: Nausea and vomiting of pregnancy: Role of human chorionic gonadotropin and 17- hydroxyprogesterone. *Obstet Gynecol* 1980;55:696–700.

57. Kauppila A, Heikinheimo M, Lohela H, Ylikorkala O: Human chorionic gonadotrophin and pregnancy-specific beta-1-glycoprotein in predicting pregnancy outcome and in association with early pregnancy vomiting. *Gynecol Obstet Invest* 1984;18:49–53.

58. Jarnfelt-Samsioe A: Nausea and vomiting in pregnancy: A review. *Obstet Gynecol Surv* 1987;41:422–427.

59. Kauppila A, Huhtaniemi I, Ylikorkala O: Raised serum human chorionic gonadotrophin concentrations in hyperemesis gravidarum. *Br Med J* 1979;1:1670–1671.

60. Masson GM, Anthony F, Chau E: Serum chorionic gonadotrophin (hCH), schwangerschaftsprotein 1 (SP1), progesterone and estradiol levels in patients with nausea and vomiting in early pregnancy. *Br J Obstet Gynaecol* 1985;92:211–215.

61. Kauppila A, Ylikorkala O, Jarvinen PJA, Haapalahti J: The function of the anterior pituitary-adrenal cortex axis in hyperemesis gravidarum. *Br J Obstet Gynaecol* 1976;83:11–16.

62. Brody S, Carlstrom G: Human chorionic gonadotropin pattern in serum and its relation to the sex of the fetus. *J Clin Endocrinol Metab* 1965;25:792–797.

63. Ylikorkala O, Kauppila A, Ollanketo ML: Intramuscular ACTH or placebo in the treatment of hyperemesis gravidarum. *Acta Obstet Gynecol Scand* 1979;58:453–455.

64. Bouillon R, Maesens M, Van Assche FA, et al: Thyroid function in patients with hyperemesis gravidarum. *Am J Obstet Gynecol* 1982;143:922–926.

65. Dozeman R, Kaiser FE, Cass O, Pries J: Hyperthyroidism appearing as hyperemesis

gravidarum. *Arch Intern Med* 1983;143:2202–2203.

66. Valentine BH, Jones C, Tyack AJ: Hyperemesis gravidarum due to thyrotoxicosis. *Postgrad Med J* 1980;56:746–747.

67. Juras N, Banovac K, Sekso M: Increased serum reverse triiodothyronine in patients with hyperemesis gravidarum. *Acta Endocrinol* 1983;102:284–287.

68. Mori M, Amino N, Tamaki H, Miyai K, Tanizawa O: Morning sickness and thyroid function in normal pregnancy. *Obstet Gynecol* 1988;72:355–359.

69. Bober SA, McGill AC, Tunbridge WMG: Thyroid function in hyperemesis gravidarum. *Acta Endocrinol* 1986;111:404–410.

70. Sugrue D, Drury MI: Hyperthyroidism complicating pregnancy: Results of treatment by antithyroid drugs in 77 pregnancies. *Br J Obstet Gynaecol* 1980;87:970–975.

71. Menon V, McDougall WW, Leatherdale BA: Thyrotoxic crisis following eclampsia and induction of labour. *Postgrad Med J* 82;58:286–287.

72. Mestman JH: Endocrine diseases in pregnancy, in Depp R, Eschenbach DA, Sciarra JJ (eds.): *Gynecology and Obstetrics*, vol. 3. Philadelphia, JB Lippincott, 1990, 23: pp 1–37.

73. Rosenthal FD, Jones C, Lewis SI: Thyrotoxic vomiting. *Br Med J* 1976;2:209–211.

74. Kirshon B, Lee W, Cotton DB: Prompt resolution of hyperthyroidism and hyperemesis gravidarum after delivery. *Obstet Gynecol* 1988;71:1032–1034.

75. Lao TT, Chin RKH, Chang AMZ: The outcome of hyperemetic pregnancies complicated by transient hyperthyroidism. *Aust NZ J Obstet Gynaecol* 1987;27:99–101.

76. Lao TTH, Chin RKH, Cockram CS, Panesar NS: Transient hyperthyroidism in hyperemesis gravidarum. *Roy Soc Med* 1986;79:613–615.

77. Chin RKH, Lao TTH: Throxine concentration and outcome of hyperemetic pregnancies. *Br J Obstet Gynaecol* 1988;95:507–509.

78. Jeffcoate WJ, Bain C: Recurrent pregnancy-induced thyrotoxicosis presenting as hyperemesis gravidarum. Case report. *Br J Obstet Gynaecol* 1985;92:413–415.

79. Amir SM, Osathanondh R, Berkowitz RS, Goldstein DP: Human chorionic gonadotropin and thyroid function in patients with hydatidiform mole. *Am J Obstet Gynecol* 1984;150:723–728.

80. Hershman JM, Higgins HP: Hydatidiform mole—a cause of clinical hyperthyroidism. *N Engl J Med* 1971;284:573–577.

81. Brunn T, Kristoffersen K: Thyroid function during pregnancy with special reference to hydatidiform mole and hyperemesis. *Acta Endocrinol* 1978;88:383–389.

82. Miyai K, Tanizawa O, Yamamoti T, et al: Pituitary-thyroid function in trophoblastic disease. *J Clin Endocrinol Metab* 1976;42:254–259.

83. Davies TF, Platzer M: TSH receptor activation and growth acceleration in FRTL–5 thyroid cells. *Endocrinology* 1986;11:2149–2151.

84. Kenimer JG, Hershman JM, Higgins HP: The thyrotropin in hydatidiform moles is human chorionic gonadotropin. *J Clin Endocrinol Metab* 1975;40:482–491.

85. Davies TF, Taliadouros GS, Catt KJ, Nisula BC: Assessment of urinary thyrotropin-competing activity in choriocarcinoma and thyroid disease: Further evidence for human chorionic gonadotropin interacting at the thyroid cell membrane. *J Clin Endocrinol Metab* 1979;49:353–357.

86. Cave WT: Choriocarcinoma with hyperthyroidism: Probable identity of the thyrotropin with human chorionic gonadotropin. *Ann Int Med* 1976;85:60–63.

87. Adams RH, Gordon J, Combes B: Hyperemesis gravidarum: I. Evidence of hepatic dysfunction. *Obstet Gynecol* 1968;31:659–664.

88. Jarnfelt-Samsioe A, Eriksson B, Waldenstrom J, Samsioe G: Some new aspects on emesis gravidarum. *Gynecol Obstet Invest* 1985;19:174–186.

89. Jarnfelt-Samsioe A, Eriksson B, Mattsson A, Samsioe G: Serum lipids and lipoproteins in pregnancies associated with emesis gravidarum. *Gynecol Endocrinol* 1987;1:51–60.

90. Jarnfelt-Samsioe A, Samsioe G, Velinder GM: Nausea and vomiting in pregnancy—a contribution to its epidemiology. *Gynecol Obstet Invest* 1983;16:221–229.

91. Combes B, Adams RH, Gordon J, Trammell V, Shibata H: Hyperemesis gravidarum: II. Alterations in sulfobromophthalein sodium-removal mechanisms from blood. *Obstet Gynecol* 1968;31:665–673.

92. Katon WJ, Ries RK, Bokan JA, Kleinman A: Hyperemesis gravidarum: A biopsychosocial perspective. *Int J Psychiatry Med* 1980–81;10:151–162.

93. Deutsch H: *The Psychology of Women.* New York, Grune and Stratton, 1945.

94. Weiss E, English OS: *Psychosomatic Medicine*, Philadelphia, WB Saunders, 1943.

95. Grace WJ, Graham DT: Relationship of specific attitudes and emotions to certain bodily diseases. *Psychosom Med* 1952;14:243–251.

96. Guze SB, Delong WB, Majerus PW, Robins E: Association of clinical psychiatric disease with hyperemesis gravidarum. *N Engl J Med* 1959;261:1363–1368.

97. Purtel JJ, Robins E, Cohen ME: Observations on clinical aspects of hysteria: Quantitative study of 50 hysteria patients and control subjects. *JAMA* 1951;146:902–909.

98. Wolkind S, Zajicek E: Psycho-social correlates of nausea and vomiting of pregnancy. *J Psychosom Res* 1978;22:1–5.

99. Engel GL: The need for a new medical model: A challenge for biomedicine. *Science* 1977;196:129–136.

100. Cary E: The use of desiccated placenta: With special reference to the vomiting of pregnancy. *Surg Gynecol Obstet* 1917;25:206–208.

101. Hughes WL, Martin AC: Treatment of hyperemesis gravidarum with intramuscular injections of husband's blood. *Am J Obstet Gynecol* 1942;44:103–108.

102. Rongjun A: Thirty-nine cases of morning sickness treated with acupuncture. *J Trad Chin Med* 1987;7:25–26.

103. Dundee JW, Sourial FBR, Ghaly RG, Bell PF: P6 acupressure reduces morning sickness. *J Roy Soc Med* 1988:81:456–457.

104. Fuchs K, Paldi E, Abramovici H, Peretz BA: Treatment of hyperemesis gravidarum by hypnosis. *Int J Clin Exp Hypn* 1980:28;313–323.

105. Giorlando SW, Mascola RF: The treatment of hyperemesis gravidarum with hypnotherapy. *Am J Obstet Gynecol* 1957;73:444–447.

106. King AG: The treatment of pregnancy nausea with a pill. *Obstet Gynecol* 1955;6:332–337.

107. Semmens JP: Hyperemesis gravidarum: Evaluation and treatment. *Obstet Gynecol* 1957;9:586–594.

108. Buttino L Jr: Nausea and vomiting in pregnancy: It's enough to make you sick, in Cefalo RC (ed.): *Clinical Decisions in Obstetrics and Gynecology.* Rockville, MD, Aspen Publishers, 1990, p 6.

109. Silber TJ, D'Angelo LJ: The role of the primary case physician in the diagnosis and management of anorexia nervosa. *Psychosomatics* 1991;32:221–225.

110. Zechnich R, Hammer T: Brief psychotherapy for hyperemesis gravidarum. *Am Fam Prac* 1982;26:179–181.

111. Long MA, Simone S, Tucher JJ: Outpatient treatment of hyperemesis gravidarum with stimulus control and imagery procedures. *J Behav Ther Exp Psychiatry.*1986;17:105–109.

112. Simone SS, Long MA: The behavioral treatment of hyperemesis gravidarum. *Behav Ther* 1985;8:128–129.

113. Apfel RJ, Kelley SF, Frankel FH: The role of hypnotizability in the pathogenesis and treatment of nausea and vomiting of pregnancy. *J Psychosom Obstet Gynaecol* 1986;5:179–186.

114. Fuchs K, Paldi E, Abramovici H, Peretz BA: Treatment of hyperemesis gravidarum by hypnosis. *Int J Clin Exp Hypn* 1980;28:313–323.

Chapter 19

Elective Abortion

Miriam Rosenthal, MD

> In my view, every woman has the right to achieve
> motherhood and to renounce motherhood, and every
> normal woman seems to assume this right emotionally,
> whether it is legal or not.
> —*The Psychology of Women,* 1945
> H. Deutsch

Abortion, the induced termination of pregnancy prior to viability, is an extremely emotionally charged subject. An unwanted pregnancy is a crisis for a woman, her partner, her family, and, increasingly, for society. Although induced abortion has been practiced since the beginning of recorded history, it remains a controversial issue with major social, legal, and political overtones.[1-8] Perhaps not surprisingly, much of the literature concerning termination of pregnancy is far from impartial, reflecting the biases of the original authors. In recent years, new legal interpretations and continued social pressures have reopened the abortion issue. Current trends predict the possibility of new restrictions on pregnancy terminations, which may vary from state to state. This chapter reviews the demographics of abortion and discusses the psychological risks for women undergoing these procedures. Also discussed are the dilemmas and reactions among health care practitioners who care for the women facing the problem of unwanted pregnancy.

Following the liberalization of abortion with the *Roe v Wade* decision in 1973, the number of recorded induced abortions in the United States increased, but thereafter has remained relatively constant at approximately 1.6 million procedures per year. The number of pregnancy terminations performed annually prior to 1973 is not accurately known. At that time, most abortions were illegal and thus never recorded or reported.[1] Data from 1987 reveal that 60% of the women having abortions are less than 25 years of age, 82% are unmarried, 50% are primigravida, and 69% are white. Most terminations are first-trimester procedures, performed at a gestation of 9.2 weeks. Fully 97% are completed by "instrumental evacuation," primarily suction curettage. Most of these procedures are now performed in specialized clinics, and not in hospitals.[2]

Background

Prior to the 19th century, a woman with an unwanted pregnancy would turn to other women in her community. These individuals would know what to do and how to go about performing or obtaining a termination. There were usually practitioners of abortion in and out of the medical profession, some safer than others. When access to experienced operators was limited or impossible, many women died of infections and hemorrhage at the hands of unscrupulous operators or from self-induced efforts at termination. The medicalization of abortion procedures is a relatively recent event, occurring in the latter half of the 19th century aided by organized medicine. The goals of this program were mixed. There was clearly an attempt to provide better health care for women and to decrease maternal mortality and morbidity by raising the standards of practice. Other aims were to train professionals, as well as to control where and under what circumstances abortions could be performed. This move toward "professionalism" required increased knowledge and skills and restricted the performance of pregnancy terminations to physicians. Most of the recorded abortions during this early time period were performed by middle- and upper-class male physicians who provided these services for women of their own class who were "in trouble."[3] These practitioners employed arbitrary criteria, often dictated by their own morality and attitudes, for determining who they would accept for care. Some clinicians would only do procedures on women whose lives were threatened by certain medical conditions, while other physicians were more influenced by "quality of life issues" relating to social and economic conditions.[3] Abortions not performed by medical doctors were considered "criminal." These procedures were illegal and were described as being done by "abortionists." Such nonprofessional abortions generally came to medical attention only when complications such as infection or hemorrhage occurred. The number of procedures performed and morbidity/mortality rates for nonphysician abortions could not be accurately estimated due to the secrecy surrounding such practice. Despite the availability of safer procedures, criminal abortion persisted because terminations done by physicians were costly, difficult to obtain, and limited by the number of interested practitioners. Social ideas concerning sexual practices and fertility were also at work. In general, fertility control and sexual activity were considered private matters, not for open discussion. Also, marriage was viewed as the answer for unwanted pregnancies in single women. These beliefs and others long muted public discussion of both contraception and abortion.

The recurrent severe adverse complications of illegal abortion were a major factor in stimulating reform of American abortion law.[4] A combination of public health, legal, and medical experts lobbied legislatures for abortion reform for years. With the rise of human rights demands in the 1960s and early 1970s, pressures for liberalized laws grew, resulting in the *Roe v Wade* decision liberalizing the widespread practice of abortion in the United States.

Psychological Aspects for Patients

There is no painless way to go through an unwanted pregnancy. However, there is no firm evidence that there are any *unique* serious psychiatric sequelae or psychological syndromes resulting from induced abortion in women who did not have a psychiatric or psychological disorder prior to the pregnancy.[2]

The medical literature in this area needs critical review. In many cases, there has been a lack of appropriate controls and long-term follow-up. Some reports involve small numbers of individuals. Data on individuals whose abortions are performed in private practice settings are underrepresented in most samples. Frequently there is inattention to the pretermination psychological condition of the women undergoing abortions. Despite these and other limitations, the available studies are consistent in reporting a general decrease in stress following abortion and "relatively rare" instances of severe negative reactions, particularly for first- trimester procedures.[2,5]

Psychological reactions after induced abortion commonly include some degree of sadness, guilt, and regret. Basically, the problem is one of experiencing and resolving a pregnancy that is unwanted, or that cannot be continued for a variety of reasons. Following abortion, the major reaction for most women is relief with an accompanying decrease of stress, despite their sense of loss. In understanding the psychological response following induced abortion it is important to consider: (1) the decision process; (2) perceived social supports from partner, friends, and/or family; (3) coping styles and expectancies; and (4) past psychiatric history.

Women who experience ambivalence about the decision of whether or not to terminate their pregnancies may have more stress.[2] For example, women who decide to terminate a wanted pregnancy because of a fetal genetic or structural abnormality, or due to a severe medical condition in themselves, have more difficulty with the abortion than women seeking a termination who lack these problems. Not surprisingly, women who seek second-trimester terminations generally have more ambivalence and difficulty with their decision than those requesting first-trimester procedures.

Social support is of considerable importance in reactions to abortion. Women who have the approval and presence of the partners and family are more positive about their decision to terminate the pregnancy. Also, adolescents whose mothers agree with their choice are more likely to do well and less likely to develop adverse psychological reactions.[6]

Women who have positive coping styles and are more hopeful of a positive outcome have less depression and anxiety postabortion than those who do not. Women who use denial as a major defense mechanism have more difficulty with abortion, presumably due to their problems in facing and resolving their internal conflicts.

A past history of poor psychological functioning or prior psychiatric disorders are strongly predictive of pregnancy-related problems both postpartum as well as postabortion.[2,7] Specifically, more emotional difficulties are encountered when a prior psychiatric illness, a history of immature relationships with other people, severe conflicts with mother, a history of ambivalence and feelings of helplessness with regard to abortion, or religious or cultural ties that prohibit abortion are present.

Counseling

All women considering abortion should discuss their decision with an experienced counselor. Individuals with chronic social or psychiatric problems are particularly important to counsel in order to help resolve, or at least outline, their concerns.

None of the choices facing a woman with an unwanted pregnancy are happy ones. At times it is unclear whether abortion or continuing an unwanted pregnancy and either keeping a child or having the child adopted is best (Table 19.1). This is one of those complex social and personal issues where there is not necessarily a best answer, but instead a series of possible alternatives of variable desirability.

If possible, the counselor should be someone other than the person who will actually perform the termination procedure. This removes the woman's possible anxiety that the procedure will not be performed if the physician does not like what she says. The woman should be seen both alone as well as with her partner or family, if possible. She should clearly understand and be able to outline her options. Ideally, she should then take each option in turn, and work it through with all the possible details just as if that were her actual choice. During this process, the counselor asks relevant questions and provides information. The woman should be seen as many times as she needs to make up her mind. Adolescents; older women; women who are divorced, separated or widowed; and women whose fetuses have genetic defects are more vulnerable and should be counseled both before and after the procedure. In such difficult cases, it is helpful for the counselor to telephone the woman after the procedure and let her know of his or her availability. It is helpful, though often not possible, for the counseling to take place a few days before the actual procedure. However, just as it is desirable to perform abortions within the first trimester, due to the demands of scheduling in busy services, there may not be sufficient time available to allow counseling to occur separately from the day of the termination and reasonable compromises will need to be made.

Attitudes and Reactions of Staff

Physicians

Practitioners most involved in the termination of pregnancy are obstetricians/ gynecologists. An immediate conflict for many of these practitioners is that many, if not most, entered the field because of their desire to preserve maternal and fetal life. Abortion obviously conflicts with this stated goal. Thus, when

Table 19.1 Factors that Increase Emotional Difficulty with Abortion

Ambivalence

Fetus with genetic abnormality

Restrictive laws

Social disapproval

Religious prohibitions

Past psychiatric problems

Age less than 16 years or greater than 35 years

abortion is seen as "therapeutic" and part of the overall care of mothers and infants, it is better accepted by physicians than if it is perceived purely as an elective procedure performed for socioeconomic reasons.[8] Other factors affecting doctors' practices are the social acceptability of abortion and its legality. The practice of individual physicians is also influenced by their religion, education, and family situation. Most important are their personal experiences with fertility and with anomalous children. While a minority of physicians have basic moral objections to abortion, others simply find the procedures emotionally distasteful or are repelled by the idea of personally performing terminations. To these latter individuals, abortion is acceptable as a procedure, especially if "therapeutic" and, most importantly, if performed by others.

Resident physicians in obstetrics and gynecology training are expected to know the surgical techniques for the performance of abortion. They can refer patients to facilities where pregnancy terminations are performed if they are not willing to do these procedures themselves. The manual *Educational Objectives for Residents in Obstetrics and Gynecology* (1984),[9] published by the Committee on Residency Education in Obstetrics and Gynecology, states that an educational objective for those in training as practitioners is the ability to arrange contact between a woman seeking abortion and a facility that provides education, counseling, and legal pregnancy termination, *or* to be prepared to provide these assistances and to perform the procedure. Whether or not the trainee is prepared to perform the actual abortion, the resident must know the surgical procedures for termination of pregnancy, acceptable alternatives, and potential complications, as well as the legal facts concerning abortion in his or her legal jurisdiction.

Kane and co-workers[10] make a number of suggestions for obstetricians/gynecologists and hospitals who participate in abortion, which are generally followed in most programs. First, the participation of all staff is voluntary, and the hospital medical leadership should be supportive of the program. Frequent group meetings are desirable to discuss problems and procedures. If possible, hospitalized abortion patients are separated from general obstetrical patients. Kane also recommends specialized training in counseling and psychosocial issues for resident physicians to improve their skills in working with patients confronting such reproductive decisions.

In general, obstetricians/gynecologists believe that they are the physicians who should perform abortions due to their experience and training. While the preponderance of abortions are easy operative procedures, complications of pregnancy terminations do occur, especially in midtrimester operations and can sometimes be severe and, rarely, even life-threatening. Therefore, obstetricians/gynecologists are the appropriate professionals because their training includes extensive experience with the diagnosis of early pregnancy, uterine surgery, and treatment of potential complications of hemorrhage or infection related to retained products of conception or inadvertent pelvic organ injury.

Modern practitioners believe, as did their predecessors, that while they should retain control over abortion technology, no one should be forced to perform abortions who does not wish to do so. This occasionally leads to difficulties in residency programs with large abortion services due to a shifting of the responsibility for terminations to a small number of individuals. Uncommonly, some training programs have forbidden their residents to perform abortions, usually for religious or moral reasons.

Religion remains the most powerful predictor of whether or not obstetricians/gynecologists in general practice provide abortion services. In a study by Nathanson and Becker,[11] 85% of Catholic physicians, 28% of Protestant doctors, and 9% of Jewish doctors did not perform abortions. Most doctors who did abortions believed the procedure should be available, but with certain restrictions. In general, these restrictions included where such procedures should be done, by whom, and at what duration of gestation. In this study, most clinicians had fewer problems with first-trimester abortions in contrast to second-trimester procedures which were found to be more objectionable.

Resident physicians in training in obstetrics and gynecology and family medicine often admit they are in conflict about abortion. Like some of their faculty supervisors, while they support reproductive choice, they dislike performing certain procedures, especially operative second-trimester abortions. They also have difficulty with women who request repeat abortions. Unlike the private practitioner who may know his or her patients well, residents frequently know little about the psychosocial situation of the women they see and have limited or no ability to choose their own patients. They feel resentment toward women who appear to take abortion lightly and have more sympathy for the woman who appears either sad or serious.[12] Residents feel considerably empathetic to women requesting abortion for conditions that threaten the mother's physical or psychological life, such as rape or incest, or for serious fetal genetic defects. They have correspondingly less sympathy for women who request abortion for the stated reasons of economic hardship, loss of a partner, or who are overburdened with other children. Abortion practices also lead to dissension between the residents in a given program. If a substantial number do not perform terminations, the burden falls on a relatively small group of physicians who can easily become overburdened and progressively angry.

Although physicians often believe that their attitudes and values about abortion are not apparent to their patients, especially in a general hospital setting, the nurses who observe them do not always agree. Practitioners consciously and unconsciously conceal their internal conflicts and use rationalization and intellectual defenses to explain their abortion practices. Physicians performing pregnancy terminations commonly believe that they are working for the greater societal good and helping individuals. In general, doctors' views toward abortion become more moderate as they develop experience and have assisted during termination procedures.[8] This contact with reality has a peculiar leveling effect in physician attitudes; physicians with an initial strong opposition to abortion come to be more in favor of reproductive choice for women following actual experience with terminations while those who initially are strong proponents of abortion rights become less enthusiastic.

Different issues arise for physicians whose practice requires them to actually perform pregnancy terminations versus those who are limited to counseling or to referring women for abortion. When the question was asked of a wide range of practitioners: "Should abortion be available to any woman capable to giving legal consent upon her own request to a competent physician?" the highest number of yes answers came from psychiatrists and allergists, and the lowest number from general practitioners, obstetricians, and general surgeons.[8] An obvious problem in the interpretation of such surveys is the fact that the way the questions are asked strongly influences the reply. Thus, those who answered yes may or may not approve of abortion under all conditions—opinions that are lost when only the broader question of general acceptability is asked.[13-16]

In addition to differences between medical specialties in abortion attitudes, doctors are also sensitive to their communities and cultures in their pattern of practices. Doctors in urban areas are more likely to perform abortions than those in rural areas where abortions are generally less well accepted. Practitioners in the Eastern United States, in New England, and the Pacific West have more liberal attitudes than those in the Midwest or South. Not surprisingly, those who disapprove of abortion tend to be more politically conservative and have more conservative views about such issues as sex, homosexuality, and women's place in society.

Since doctors are the chief limiting factor regarding the number of abortions performed in the hospitals where they practice, their overall reticence to perform terminations, the high costs of hospital operations, and the political problems of an abortion service have caused a gradual shift of abortion procedures to specialized freestanding clinics. There have also been shifts in the funding of abortions. In general, Medicaid will not pay for abortions unless it is done to protect the life of a mother. This constitutes a financial barrier to abortion for poor women who receive most of their medical care in federally subsidized hospitals. Nonetheless, it is estimated that approximately 94% of women on Medicaid requesting abortions eventually do obtain them largely outside of the system of public health care financing.[17]

Doctors working in abortion clinics see themselves as performing a valuable service. They do not face the same peer pressures as those in hospital settings, where they can become objects of disapproval from other workers or, at times, the hospital administration. In contrast, the pressures for clinic workers come from pickets and opponents of abortion who organize other forms of social disapproval.

The increasingly strident presence of pickets from antiabortion groups is stressful for those who work in abortion clinics. In some cases, these workers and the women attending the clinics have not only been harassed but potentially endangered by some of the violence surrounding these protests. The belief of clinic personnel, in general, is that the men and women who have chosen to harass them have little knowledge or empathy for a woman with a troubled pregnancy. Increasingly, staff experiencing such strident and organized disapproval have in turn became angry, and are choosing to become more active in the prochoice movement.

Psychiatrists

Prior to 1973 and *Roe v Wade*, psychiatrists in many hospitals were required to write letters stating that in their opinion a given woman was at risk for committing suicide if she could not obtain an abortion. Many psychiatrists resented this role, yet felt deeply that women had the right to reproductive choice. Since then, mental health professionals have become more involved in counseling and in the study of the psychological aspects of abortion. They have not discovered any specific psychiatric or psychological complications related to abortion that are different in frequency than those associated with full-term birth.[18] However, psychiatrists remain concerned that if abortion becomes illegal again, they will be called upon anew to be gatekeepers, certifying that abortion is medically necessary to preserve the mental health of a specific woman.[19]

Nurses

The majority of nurses who go into maternity nursing do so because they enjoy working with pregnant women, caring for high- risk patients, or working in labor and delivery. When abortions are performed in hospital settings, nurses can feel directly or indirectly pressured into participating since these terminations are usually carried out in general obstetric or gynecologic services. In general, nurses consider themselves to be strong advocates for women's rights and are sensitive to the health issues of women. Many nurses voice pro-choice sentiments while others accept abortion only for special circumstances, such as rape, incest, or congenital defects of major severity, or maternal disease that is life threatening. A study of nurses in Michigan and New York suggested the "increased exposure to easily available abortion procedures tends to promote a more favorable general attitude to abortion."[20]

Participation of nurses in hospital-based abortions creates dilemmas. Nurses assisting in abortion procedures have rarely participated in the decision-making processes. They may feel conflicts between a woman's right to reproductive choice versus their sense of frustration about participating in an abortion that they perceive as being done for economic or convenience reasons. Nurses assisting with second-trimester abortions feel especially ambivalent about patients who seem to have very little understanding of the techniques and ask questions such as "What sex is it?" or "May I have a picture?" They may feel indignation when the physician is elsewhere and they are left alone with a woman undergoing a saline or prostaglandin second-trimester abortion. In many hospitals, high-risk pregnancy patients are on the same floor with patients undergoing second-trimester abortions and the same nurses are expected to care for both. Not surprisingly, the responsibility for helping to maintain one pregnancy while endeavoring to terminate another leads to cognitive and moral dissonance. The same is true for doctors who are involved in the care of abortion patients as well as women with high-risk pregnancies at the same time, and perhaps on the same floor.

The case of a head nurse who did not voice any objection to abortion, but "forgot" to look in each morning on abortion patients illustrates how attitudes and behavior may be discordant and how staff can deny their own feelings. Hospital-based nurses feel most supported by their peers who also participate, and find the mutual support therapeutic. Others report that they do not discuss the abortion aspect of their work with others, feeling either shame, guilt, or at least ambivalence about it.

In contrast, nurses working in freestanding abortion clinics have made the conscious choice to work in such settings and to participate in counseling and decision making. In general, they feel more in control, and less in conflict about their role than hospital nurses, despite the recent presence of strident pro-testers. The nurses in these clinics are nonjudgmental and are supportive of the women they care for. They are similar to the nurses in the 1950s and 1960s who chose to work in family planning clinics at a time when there was consid-erable public opposition to such services. Group support, as reflected in meet-ings and discussions, is helpful in such settings.

"Burn out" is a syndrome common to both nurses and physicians who assist in the performance of abortions, especially for second- trimester abor-tions. A feeling can grow among participating doctors and nurses of being over-whelmed. They begin to perceive that they are doing the work for others who lack any ideological objections to such terminations, but who fail to assist be-cause they are lazy, biased, uncaring, or lack a broader view of total health care for women. The staff grow tired, feel set upon, and become depressed. Mental health professionals should be part of such teams, and should attempt to offset these feelings by discussing cases and the feelings they engender with the staff.

Social Workers

Social workers tend to display the same range of attitudes as others in this field, with the important difference that they are not called on to participate in actual procedures. Social workers, by training, have more liberal attitudes than physicians or nurses.[20] Their training helps them to work with women trying to make difficult decisions. It is usual for social workers in maternity settings to have to deal with unwanted pregnancies in both adolescents and adults. They have a deep understanding of the effects of poverty, violence, disruption, and mental illness in people's lives. They can be extremely helpful to doctors and nurses in informing them about the psychosocial situation that has brought a woman to make a particular decision. By their interaction they lessen the anonymity of women in large urban hospitals. However, they often are frustrated by the effort to arrange abortions for women who are poor and have few economic resources. Social workers also struggle with their own conflicts concerning abortion in a similar fashion as do other health care workers.[21]

Conclusion

In summary, *there is no firm evidence for serious psychological problems follow-ing induced abortion for the overwhelming majority of women.* Abortion does represent a loss. For certain women this loss has more meaning or presents more of a problem than for others, especially if there is subsequent infertility, fetal abnormalities, or fetal loss. However, severe negative reactions are rare. While these conclusions are consistent in the literature and fit with our clinical experience, it is to be remembered that a good deal of the literature on this subject suffers from methodologic weaknesses, especially the absence of long-term follow-up, and some caution in all conclusions is prudent.

The political climate concerning abortion is currently in disarray. The legal trend is to progressively restrict access to abortions. The recent Supreme Court decision, *Webster v Reproductive Health Services*, is likely to result in states regulating abortion in ways that may not be medically sound and which may restrict obstetrical practice.[22] Despite this trend, the majority of clinicians continue to believe that in order to provide women with the best health care possible, abortion needs to be part of the wide spectrum of available health care services. Widespread experience since 1973 has documented abundantly that abortion is a safe procedure when performed by trained personnel in an appropriate environment. It is notable that while maternal mortality has declined 30% from 1970 to 1982, abortion-related mortality has declined 89% in the same interval and now approaches zero.[21] Despite the potential of these new restrictive trends, elective termination of pregnancy is likely to remain a choice for American women, although more effective means of contraception are an even greater goal.

References

1. Henshaw SK, VanVort J: Abortion services in the United States, 1987 and 1988. *Fam Plann Perspect* 1990;22:102–142.
2. Adler N, David H, Major B, et al: Psychological responses after abortion. *Science* 1990;248:41–44.
3. Luker K: *Abortion and the Politics of Motherhood.* Berkeley, University of California Press, 1984.
4. Rossi AS, Sitaraman B: Abortion in context: Historical trend and future changes. *Fam Plann Perspect* 1988;20:273–281.
5. Lazarus A: Psychiatric sequelae of legalized elective first trimester abortion. *J Psychsom Obstet Gynecol* 1985;4:141–150.
6. Rosenthal MB, Rothchild E: Some psychological considerations in adolescent pregnancy and abortion. *Adv Plan Parent* 1975;9:60–69.
7. Nadelson C: The emotional impact of abortion. *The Woman Patient*, vol. I. New York, Plenum Press, 1978, pp 173–179.
8. Imber J: *Abortion and the Private Practice of Medicine.* New Haven, CT, Yale University Press, 1986.
9. Committee on Resident Education in Obstetrics and Gynecology: *Educational Objectives for Residents in Obstetrics and Gynecology*, ed. 3. Washington, DC, CREOG Press, 1984.
10. Kane F, Feldman M, Jains S, Lipton M: Emotional reactions in abortion services personnel. *Arch Gen Psychiatry* 1973;28:409–411.
11. Nathanson C, Becker M: Obstetricians' attitudes and hospital abortion services. *Fam Plann Perspect* 1980;12:26.
12. Mascovich P, Behrstock B, Minor D, Colman A: Attitudes of obstetric and gynecologic residents toward abortion. *Calif Med* 1973;119:29–34.
13. Pratt G: Connecticut physicians' attitudes toward abortion. *Am J Public Health* 1976;66:288–290.
14. Sheehan M, Munro J, Ryan J: Attitudes of medical practitioners towards abortion: A Queensland study. *Aust Fam Physician* 1980;9:565–570.
15. Wolff J, Nielson P, Schiller P: Therapeutic abortion: Attitudes of medical personnel leading to complications in patient care. *Am J Obstet Gynecol* 1970;110:730–733.
16. Savage W, Francone C: Gynecologists' attitudes to abortion. *Lancet* 1989;2:1323–1324.
17. Cates W: Abortion myths and realities. Who is misleading whom? *Am J Obstet Gynecol* 1982;142:954–956.

18. David H, Rasmussen N, Holste E: Postpartum and postabortion psychotic reactions. *Fam Plann Perspect* 1981;13:88–92.
19. Stotland N: Psychiatrists fear abortion decision will put profession in gatekeeper role. *Psychiatric News* 1989; Aug. 4.
20. Allen D, Reichdt P, Shea FP: Two measures of nurses' attitudes toward abortion as modified by experience. *Med Care* 1977;15:849–857.
21. Hendershot G, Grimm J: Abortion attitudes among nurses and social workers. *Am J Public Health* 1974;64:438–441.
22. Chavkin W, Rosenfield A: A chill wind blows: Webster, obstetrics and the health of women. *Am J Obstet Gynecol* 1990;163:450–452.

Chapter 20

Conditions Mimicking Psychiatric Disease

Timothy Fitzpatrick, MD and John P. O'Grady, MD

Life is short, and Art long;
The crisis fleeting; experience perilous,
and decision difficult.
    —*Aphorisms*
    Hippocrates (c 460–375 BC)

Obstetricians have the unique responsibility of caring for healthy young women during the normal physiologic processes of pregnancy, delivery, and the puerperium. However, during the course of their pregnancies women remain susceptible to the same diseases or conditions affecting nongravid women of the same age. Pregnant women tend to identify their obstetrician as their primary physician, regardless of the nature of their medical problem. In their role as primary physicians, obstetricians are thus frequently forced to deal with medical conditions for which their original training as obstetricians provides limited guidance. Such disorders include problems as diverse as asthma to alopecia. While the obstetrician is not generally expected to have encyclopedic knowledge of medical or psychological disorders, there remains an obligation to develop a foundation of knowledge concerning many common disorders. The training of obstetricians reflects the varied demands of their practice yet remains inevitably incomplete. For example, given the wide range of possible complications, it is uncommon for the obstetrical specialist to have more than a cursory knowledge of psychiatric disorders unless he or she has individually pursued an interest in such problems. Yet, such difficulties are relatively frequent during pregnancy and the clinician needs to identify, and either treat or refer, these individuals.[1]

In this chapter the clinical problem of altered mental status and acute confusional states that mimic psychological and/or psychiatric conditions is discussed. Such problems fall somewhere among the specialties of general medicine, neurology, and psychiatry, yet the majority of women affected will be seen at least initially by obstetricians.

Alterations in Consciousness

An alteration in level of consciousness may be the initial presentation of illness. The potential causes are numerous and reflect etiologies as diverse as psychiatric disease to drug ingestion, or purely organic derangements such as electrolyte imbalance.[2–4]

The extensive differential diagnosis requires that the clinician approach such problems with a coherent plan of investigation. In general, the etiology of an acute change in mental status is related to one of three underlying causes: (1) *specific neurological lesions*, (2) *psychiatric disorders*, and (3) *delirium*. Our interest here is in developing a strategy to distinguish between these broad categories. Specifically, the evaluation of a pregnant woman found in a state of delirium is distinct from other causes for an alteration in mental status.

The word "delirium" is derived from the Latin term *delirare* which means "furrow," and is taken literally as "out of the furrow." Celsus introduced the term delirium into medical terminology in the first century AD. Until the 1800s the word was used as a general descriptive term for any alteration in mental function including disorders that today are considered clearly psychiatric in etiology. As used at present, delirium refers to a *transient, global alteration in attention, cognition, and perception that reflects some underlying cerebral process.*[5] Delirium is to be contrasted to conditions arising from a specific, anatomically isolated cerebral lesion such as a tumor or aneurysm.

Some authors described two types of delirium: a *depressant* variety caused by conditions that decrease reticular activating system cerebral arousal and an *excitatory* type caused by factors that increase central arousal and cerebral activity. For example, advanced hepatic failure commonly results in a depressant form of delirium while alcohol or barbiturate withdrawal is associated with an excitatory delirium.

Diagnostic Evaluation

The Medical History

The first step in the evaluation of patients with a change in mental status is to obtain a history. Frequently, because of the nature of the problem, sources of information other than the patient must be utilized. Family and friends may provide the most accurate account of recent events. The clinician should question the circumstances around the patient's change in mental status with particular emphasis on the time course over which the signs and symptoms developed.

If possible, a general medical history should be obtained as well. Particular attention is directed to evidence of chronic medical conditions such as diabetes or other endocrinopathies that predate pregnancy. A full listing of all medications that the patient might have ingested is important. This should include prescription as well as over-the-counter formulations.

For pregnant women, the prenatal medical record should provide a good review of current and past medical conditions, if available. Unfortunately, information about prior psychiatric treatment is often difficult to obtain, as the woman may not have volunteered such a history during initial questioning in the office or clinic. This information should be sought from persons close to the patient and should detail the nature of any psychiatric treatment such as whether hospitalization or drug therapies were needed. Specifically, it is important to determine if there is a history or prior peripartum mental disturbance. Similarly, accurate information regarding drug and alcohol usage and other personal habits is frequently best obtained or collaborated from sources close to the patient. It would be a mistake to assume that pregnancy is a period of abstinence from recreational drug use in any strata of society[6-8] (see Chapter 11).

In considering the problem of altered mental status, a complete history of the pregnant patient's medical and prenatal history is necessary. This practice would be routine in investigating any medical disorder. However, some assessment of the patient's premorbid personality is also needed. This includes biographical information such as education, hobbies, and employment as well as relationships and personal style. A woman with a healthy premorbid personality with good social relationships and reasonable educational and employment success who develops an acute mental disorder may well have an organic cause for her disturbance. In any event, under such circumstances the possibility of such a cause should be investigated.

Delirium as distinct from functional disorders may be suspected from features in the history. Rapid onset of symptoms with no antecedent alterations in personality and no prior psychiatric history strongly suggest delirium. Certain conditions such as postpartum psychosis or schizophrenic episode may present acutely; however, frequently an assessment of the premorbid personality gives useful diagnostic clues to the possibility of such disorders. The stability of symptoms over time may be helpful. For example, mental or personality symptoms that wax and wane and tend to exacerbate at night favor an organic cause.

Clinical Examination

The examination begins with a comprehensive physical assessment. Signs of trauma to head or torso are sought. Funduscopic examination may reveal retinal signs of raised intracranial pressure or other abnormalities and should never be omitted. The extremities are examined for signs of drug injection. The stigmata of alcoholism should be noted. However, the pregnant patient already may have palmar erythema and spider angiomas as a reflection of her hyperestrogenic state rather than as a marker for liver dysfunction. Particular attention is directed to the neurological exam. Abnormalities of the cranial nerves should be noted both for their help in confirming an organic process as well as for their assistance in anatomically localizing the suspected lesion. Nystagmus is frequently found in pharmacologically induced delirium or in certain deficiency states such as Wernicke's encephalopathy (see Chapter 18). Any asymmetry of sensation or deep tendon reflexes is carefully noted.

The diagnosis of delirium as distinct from pure psychiatric illness rests on the finding of multiple cognitive derangements. Therefore, the psychiatric portion of the examination focuses on relevant features. Typically, such individuals suffer from attention disturbances and the interview may be brief. The patient's orientation to person, place, and time should be established early in the interview. Typically, all three are disturbed in proportion to the severity of the delirium. Nonverbal behavior such as movements, habits, tics, and gestures are noted. Speech is carefully observed for the manner in which ideas are organized and their logical connection. Dysphasia where the content of the speech is disturbed may take two forms. In *motor dysphasia* the patient is unable to name an object spontaneously but can do so with some prompting. In *expressive dysphasia* there is a global failure to understand the meaning of words.

Specific tests of mental status can be performed at the bedside. Memory is tested by questions about both recent events, such as the details of hospitalization, and more distant events in the patient's life. Short-term memory can be tested by asking the patient to remember three objects and to recall them 5 minutes later. Attention disturbances are noted during the interview by the quality of the patient's responses and the degree of distractibility. Also, the test of serial sevens can be applied, where the patient is asked to subtract seven from 100 consecutively. Remembering numbers forward and backward has the same function. Most people are capable of remembering five or more forward and four or more backward. Abstract thinking may be tested by interpretation of proverbs or by asking the patient to define several words.

The obstetric status of the patient requires special consideration. An assessment of the well-being of the fetus is essential. This is especially important if the pregnancy has reached the point of potential infant survival (≥ 25 weeks, ≥ 650 grams). This is of particular importance since many of the organic disorders associated with delirium or acute mental status change may compromise fetal-placental function. The association between cocaine ingestion and placental abruption is an excellent example.[9] Nonstress testing, a biophysical profile, and general ultrasonography establish a healthy fetus free from major defects. Such tests are interpreted with consideration for the actual gestational age.

Laboratory Investigations

The use of ancillary laboratory studies is an essential element in the workup of the patient with an alteration in mental status. The tests ordered should be directed by the clinical situation and the results of the medical history and physical examination. However, a basic series of blood chemistries are easy to obtain and may promptly establish the true diagnosis and direct therapy. Studies performed should include blood studies for glucose concentration, electrolytes, BUN and creatinine, serum osmolarity, and a complete blood count (Table 20.1).

Drug dependency and abuse during pregnancy has become a widespread problem, cutting across social and class lines.[7] The clinician should consider

Table 20.1 Laboratory Evaluations of Delirium

Electrolytes

BUN, creatinine

Blood glucose

Arterial blood gases

Urinary and serum drug screens

Hemoglobin/hematocrit

this possibility in what is seemingly an unlikely situation. Drug screening using blood or urine is frequently helpful when the etiology of depressed affect, unusual behavior, or stupor is not immediately clear. A serum alcohol level is quickly obtained and helps to rapidly screen for ethanol, one of the most commonly abused drugs during pregnancy.[10] In addition to the illicit drugs, which have the potential to alter consciousness and induce delirium, a variety of drugs used for medical purposes can occasionally cause psychiatric or neurological symptoms[4,11] (Table 20.2). Serum and urine samples can be useful in screening for these pharmaceutical agents as well if a specific ingestion is suspected.

An electroencephalogram (EEG) is occasionally helpful, particularly in cases where the distinction between functional and organic disorders is difficult. Diffuse slowing or speeding of alpha waves is seen frequently in metabolic delirium.[12] Patients who do not have a readily explained cause for a mental status change are also candidates for a computed tomography (CT) scan or magnetic resonance imaging (MRI) scan. Both are safe diagnostic tests during pregnancy.

Early in the workup of this problem, a decision regarding a spinal tap is necessary. There are several important clinical considerations prior to performing this test. Patients with a platelet count $\leq 20,000$/cc or other evidence of a bleeding diathesis should be evaluated with other techniques, or the defect in coagulation corrected with platelet transfusion or by administration of fresh frozen plasma prior to performing the test. Similar concerns are present for patients receiving anticoagulants. Such situations do occasionally arise in pregnant patients; for example, the thrombocytopenia associated with pregnancy-induced hypertension (HELLP syndrome).[13] Raised intracranial pressure is another absolute contraindication to lumbar puncture due to the potential for herniation of the midbrain at the falx cerebri. The absence of papilledema on funduscopic examination and a normal CT or MRI scan are reassuring before a spinal tap is performed.

The finding of an altered mental status in a pregnant patient frequently qualifies as a medical emergency. The situation is given added urgency in that two lives are involved and that the patients are commonly healthy before the acute event. The diagnostic workup is conducted promptly to ensure that the time between evaluation and the initiation of appropriate therapy is brief. The approach to this clinical problem must therefore be directed efficiently. This may be done by moving from a search for general, systemic causes for delirium to specific, focal neurologic lesions (Table 20.3). A careful and complete neurological exam that excludes a focal defect should direct the clinician's attention toward systemic disorders. Apparent delirium associated with focal neurological signs requires careful assessment of the possibility of a specific lesion.

If one considers the causes of delirium in women in the childbearing years several possibilities are most likely. Drug and medication reactions should be strongly considered.[4,7,11] Table 20.2 lists a number of common medications with known psychological or psychiatric side effects. In this group of patients degenerative or metabolic diseases are rare and thus drug reactions and trauma should receive major attention as possible causes for disarrayed consciousness or behavior.

Table 20.2 Unusual Reactions to Drug Therapy*

Drug	Reactions	Comments
Amphetamines	Bizarre behavior, hallucinations, paranoia, agitation, anxiety, manic symptoms	Usually with overdose or abuse; can occur with inhaler abuse[20-27]
Anticonvulsants	Agitation, confusion, delirium, depression, psychosis, aggression, mania, toxic encephalopathy	Usually with high doses or high plasma concentrations[14-21]
Antihistamines	Anxiety, hallucinations, delirium	Especially with overdosage[28]
Anticholinergics and atropine	Confusion, memory loss, disorientation, depersonalization, delirium, auditory and visual hallucinations, fear, paranoia, agitation, bizarre behavior	More frequent in the elderly and children with high doses[29-30]; has occurred with transdermal scopolamine[31-32]
Barbiturates	Excitement, hyperactivity, visual hallucinations, depression, delirium tremens-like syndrome	Especially in children and the elderly, or on withdrawal[20-27]
Benzodiazepines	Rage, hostility, paranoia, hallucinations, depression, insomnia, nightmares, anterograde amnesia	During treatment or on withdrawal; may be more common in the elderly[33-47]
β-adrenergic blockers	Depression, confusion, nightmares, hallucinations, paranoia, delusions, mania, hyperactivity	With usual doses, including ophthalmic use[47-55]
Bromocriptine	Mania, delusions, hallucinations, paranoia, aggressive behavior, schizophrenic relapse, depression, anxiety	Not dose-related[56-58], may persist weeks after stopping the drug[59-62]
Caffeine	Anxiety, confusion, psychotic symptoms	With excessive doses[63-66]
Captopril	Severe anxiety, hallucinations, insomnia, mania	Especially in depressed patients[67-69]
Cephalosporins	Confusion, disorientation, paranoia, hallucinations	Several reports[70-71]
Clonidine	Delirium, hallucinations, depression	May resolve with continued use[72-74]
Cocaine	Anxiety, agitation, psychosis	Can occur with topical use[75]
Corticosteroids	Mania, depression, confusion, paranoia, hallucinations, catatonia	Especially with high doses[76]; can occur on withdrawal[77] or with inhalation treatment[78]
Digitalis glycosides	Nightmares, euphoria, confusion, amnesia, aggression, psychosis, depression	Especially with high doses or high plasma levels and in the elderly[79-81]
Fluoxetine	Mania, hypomania	Several reports[82-83]

Drug	Psychiatric symptoms	Comments
Gentamicin	Confusion, disorientation, hallucinations	Reported in three instances with IM administration[86]
Histamine H₂-receptor antagonists	Hallucinations, paranoia, bizarre behavior, delirium, disorientation, depression, mania	Usually with high doses; more common in the elderly or with renal dysfunction[87]
Isoniazid (INH)	Depression, agitation, hallucinations, paranoia	Several reports[88]
Isotretinoin	Depression	Noted in 6 of 110 patients[82,85]
Ketamine	Nightmares, hallucinations, crying, delirium	Common reaction with usual administered doses; reaction is acute[84,85]
Methyldopa	Depression, amnesia, nightmares, psychosis	Several reports[89]
Metroclopramide	Mania, severe depression, crying, delirium	Several reports[90-92]
Narcotics	Nightmares, anxiety, agitation, euphoria, dysphoria, depression, paranoia, hallucinations	Usually with high doses[94-105]
Nifedipine	Irritability, agitation, panic, belligerence, depression	Several reports[106-108]
Nonsteroidal anti-inflammatory agents	Paranoia, depression, inability to concentrate, anxiety, confusion, hallucinations, hostility	Not reported for all drugs of this class[108-114]
Phenelzine	Paranoia, delusions, fear, mania, rage	Mania or hypomania in about 10% of depressed patients[115-120]
Phenylephrine	Depression, hallucinations, paranoia	Overuse of nasal spray.[121]
Prazosin	Hallucinations, depression, paranoia	May be more common with renal failure[122,123]
Procaine derivatives	Terror, confusion, psychosis, agitation, bizarre behavior, depression, panic	Especially with penicillin G procaine treatment[124-134]
Pseudoephedrine	Hallucinations, paranoia	Reported in cases of overdosage[135,136]
Salicylates	Agitation, confusion, hallucinations, paranoia	Chronic intoxication[137]
Theophylline	Withdrawal, mutism, hyperactivity, anxiety, mania	Usually associated with high serum concentrations[138-140]
Thyroid hormone	Mania, depression, hallucinations, paranoia	Initial doses in susceptible individuals[141]
Tricyclic antidepressants	Mania or hypomania, delirium, hallucinations, paranoia	In about 10% of cases, or with drug withdrawal[116-120]
Trimethoprim-sulfamethoxazole	Psychosis, depression, disorientation	Occasional reports[142,143]
Verapamil	Auditory, visual, and tactile hallucinations	Single case report[144]

* Modified from Drugs that cause psychiatric symptoms. *Med Letter* 1989;31:113–118, by permission.

Table 20.3 Differential Diagnosis of Delirium

1.Metabolic	3. Infections
Fluid/electrolyte imbalance	Septicemia
Hepatic or renal failure	CNS infections
Hypoglycemia	4. Intracranial lesions
Hypoxia/asphyxia	Tumor
Vitamin deficiency (Wernicke-Korsakoff syndrome)	Hematoma, abscess
	Aneurysm
2. Drug Effects	Seizure disorders
Intoxication or overdose	Cerebral concussion
Reactions	Cerebral edema
Withdrawal (includes alcohol)	

Treatment options in pregnant patients present unique problems. Concern for fetal welfare, particularly with a potentially viable fetus (≥ 25 weeks), requires that treatments be considered for potential impact on both the patient and the fetus. The basic goal of therapy is directed at restoring normal physiology. In the case of drug or medication reactions, general supportive nursing care in a quiet room with adequate hydration may be all that is required. Delirious patients may require mild (or more than mild!) sedation for their own protection (eg haloperidol decanoate 2–10 mg IM q 4–6 prn). Recovery from delirium may take longer than resolution of the underlying cause. The course is often irregular with moments of clarity alternating with periods of confusion.

Treatment may involve neurosurgical consultation and surgery if focal neurological lesions such as tumor, hematoma, or abscess are found. On occasion, the clinician may face difficult decisions regarding the timing of delivery of the fetus to provide optimal care for the mother. Fortunately, such dilemmas are rare.

Conclusions

Acute mental dysfunction in a previously normal pregnant woman requires prompt evaluation. A careful examination for specific neurological signs suggesting a focal lesion, performance of screening tests for physiologic disturbance, and a careful review of substance ingestions are necessary for complete evaluation. Disordered thought processes, apparent mania, or severe depression in the face of an otherwise normal evaluation supports a psychological/psychiatric etiology for the dysfunction. Prompt, complete study is necessary to establish the appropriate diagnosis and thus guide therapy.

References

1. Bradley CF, King JF, Effer SB: Psychology in obstetrics: Extinct or extant? *J Psychosom Obstet Gynecol* 1987;6:49–57.
2. Rabins PV, Fulstein MF: Delirium and dementia: Diagnostic criteria and fatality rates. *Br J Psychiatry* 1982;140:149–153.

3. Engel G, Romano J: Delirium, a syndrome of cerebral insufficiency. *J Chronic Dis* 1954;9:260–277.

4. Drugs that cause psychiatric symptoms. *Med Letter* 1989;31:113–118.

5. American Psychiatric Association: *Diagnostic and Statistical Manual of Mental Disorders, Third Edition, Revised*. Washington, DC, American Psychiatric Association Press, 1987.

6. Chasnoff IJ, Burns WJ, Schnoll SH, Burns KA: Cocaine use in pregnancy. *N Engl J Med* 1985;313:666–669.

7. Chasnoff IJ, Landress HJ, Barrett ME: The prevalence of illicit drug or alcohol use during pregnancy and discrepancies in mandatory reporting in Pinellas County, Florida. *N Engl J Med* 1990;17:1202–1206.

8. Richards LG: *Demographic Trends and Drug Abuse*, 1980–1985. Washington, DC, U.S. Government Printing Office, 1981. NIDA Research Monograph 35, Department of Health and Human Services.

9. Acker D, Sachs BP, Tracey KJ, Wise WE: Abruptio placentae associated with cocaine use. *Am J Obstet Gynecol* 1983;146:220–221.

10. Abel EL, Sokol RS: Incidence of fetal alcohol syndrome and economic importance of FAS related anomalies. *Drug Alcohol Depend* 1987;19:51–70.

11. Pitts FN, Allen RE, Attiline O, Burgoyne RW: The dilemma of the toxic psychosis: Differential diagnosis and the PCP psychosis. *Psychiatr Ann* 1982;12:762–768.

12. Engel G, Romano J: Studies of delirium II: Reversibility of the encephalogram with experimental procedure. *Arch Neurol Psychiatr* 1944;51:378–392.

13. Weinstein L: Syndrome of hemolysis, elevated liver enzymes, and low platelet count. A severe consequence of hypertension in pregnancy. *Am J Obstet Gynecol* 1982;142:159–163.

14. Petursson H: Diethylpropion and paranoid psychosis. *Aust NZ J Psychiatry* 1979;13:67–68.

15. Schaffer CB, Pauli MW: Psychotic reaction caused by proprietary oral diet agents. *Am J Psychiatry* 1980;137:1256–1257.

16. Dietz AJ Jr: Amphetamine–like reactions to phenylpropanolamine. *JAMA* 1981;245:601–602.

17. Norvenius G, Widerlow E, Lonnerholm G: Phenylpropanolamine and mental disturbances. *Lancet* 1979;2:1367–1368. Letter to the editor.

18. Martin CA, Iwamoti ET: Diethylpropion-induced psychosis reprecipitated by an MAO inhibitor: Case report. *J Clin Psychiatry* 1984;45:130–131.

19. Ferrando RL, McCorvey E Jr, Simon WA, Stewart DM: Bizarre behavior following the ingestion of levo-desoxyephedrine. *Drug Intell Clin Pharm* 1988;22:214–217.

20. Franks RD, Richter AJ: Schizophrenia-like psychosis associated with anticonvulsant toxicity. *Am J Psychiatry* 1979:136:973–974.

21. Tollefson G: Psychiatric implications of anticonvulsant drugs. *J Clin Psychiatry* 1980;41:295–302.

22. Woodbury DM, et al (eds.): *Antiepileptic Drugs*. New York, Raven Press, 1972, pp 219, 377, 449.

23. Stores G: Behavioural effects of anti-epileptic drugs. *Dev Med Child Neurol* 1975;17:647–658.

24. Reynolds EH, Trimble MR: Adverse neuropsychiatric effects of anticonvulsant drugs. *Drugs* 1985;29:570–581.

25. Miller WI: Phenytoin chronic toxicity and associated psychosis. *Drug Intell Clin Pharm* 1988;22:1003–1004. Letter to the editor.

26. Gardner DL, Cowdry RW: Development of melancholia during carbamazepine treatment in borderline personality disorder. *J Clin Psychopharmacol* 1986;6:236–239.

27. Drake ME Jr, Peruzzi WT: Manic state with carbamazepine therapy of seizures. *J*

Natl Med Assoc 1986;78:1105–1107.

28. Hays DP, Johnson BF, Perry R: Prolonged hallucinations following a modest overdose of tripelennamine. *Clin Toxicol* 1980;16:331–333.

29. Greenblatt DJ, Shader RI: Drug therapy. Anticholinergics. *N Engl J Med* 1973;288:1215–1219.

30. Kellner U, Esser J: Acute psychosis caused by poisoning with cyclopentolate. *Klin Monatsbl Augenheilkd* 1989;194:458–461.

31. MacEwan GW, Remick RA, Noone JA: Psychosis due to transdermally administered scopolamine. *Can Med Assoc J* 1985;133:431.

32. Rozzini R, Inzoli M, Trabucchi M: Delirium from transdermal scopolamine in an elderly woman. *JAMA* 1988;260:478. Letter.

33. Strahan A, Rosenthal J, Kaswan M, Winston A: Three case reports of acute paroxysmal excitement associated with alprazolam treatment. *Am J Psychiatry* 1985;142:859–861.

34. Rapaport M, Braff DL: Alprazolam and hostility. *Am J Psychiatry* 1985;142:146. Letter.

35. Pfefferbaum B, Butler PM, Mullins D, Copeland DR: Two cases of benzodiazepine toxicity in children. *J Clin Psychiatry* 1987;48:450–452.

36. Lydiard RB, Laraia MT, Ballenger JC, Howell EF: Emergence of depressive symptoms in patients receiving alprazolam for panic disorder. *Am J Psychiatry* 1987;144:664–665.

37. Vital-Herne J, Brenner R, Lesser M: Another case of alprazolam withdrawal syndrome. *Am J Psychiatry* 1985;142:1515. Letter to the editor.

38. White MC, Silverman JJ, Harbison JW: Psychosis associated with clonazepam therapy for blepharospasm. *J Nerv Ment Dis* 1982;170:117–119.

39. Jaffe R, Gibson E: Clonazepam withdrawal psychosis. *J Clin Psychopharmacol* 1986;6:193. Letter to the editor.

40. Floyd JB Jr, Murphy CM: Hallucinations following withdrawal of Valium. *J Ky Med Assoc* 1976;74:549–550.

41. Karch FE: Rage reaction associated with clorazepate dipotassium. *Ann Intern Med* 1979;91:61–62.

42. Hall RCW, Joffe Jr: Aberrant response to diazepam: A new syndrome. *Am J Psychiatry* 1972;129:738–742.

43. van den Berg AA: Hallucinations after oral lorazepam in children. *Anaesthesia* 1986;41:330–331. Letter to the editor.

44. Burnakis TG, Berman DE: Hostility and hallucinations as a consequence of midazolam administration. *DICP* 1989;23:671–672.

45. Soldatos CR, Sakkas PN, Bergiannaki JD, Stefanis CN: Behavioral side effects of triazolam in psychiatric inpatients: Report of five cases. *Drug Intell Clin Pharm* 1986;20:294–297.

46. Patterson JF: Triazolam syndrome in the elderly. *South Med J* 1987;80:1425–1426.

47. Heritch AJ, Capwell R, Roy–Byrne PP: A case of psychosis and delirium following withdrawal from triazolam. *J Clin Psychiatry* 1987;48:168–169.

48. Viadero JJ, Wong SH, White WB: Acute psychotic behavior associated with atenolol. *Am J Psychiatry* 1983;140:1382. Letter to the editor.

49. Galicia Basart MA, Rodriguez Jornet A, Mate Benito G, Herranz-del-Rey S: Adverse effects of atenolol on the central nervous system. *Med Clin* 1988; 90:353. Letter to the editor.

50. Orlando RG: Clinical depression associated with betaxolol. *Am J Ophthalmol* 1986;102:275.

51. Lynch MG, Whitson JT, Brown RH, Nguyen H, Drake MM: A preliminary study comparing betaxolol and timolol. *Arch Ophthalmol* 1988;106:908–911.

52. Shader RI, Greenblatt DJ: Propranolol's psychiatric side effects. *J Clin Psychopharmacol* 1983;3:65. Editorial.

53. Parker WA: Propranolol-induced depression and psychosis. *Clin Pharm* 1985;4:214–218.

54. Patterson JF: Propranolol-induced mania. *South Med J* 1984;77:1603.

55. Shore JH, Fraunfelder FT, Meyer SM: Psychiatric side effects from topical ocular timolol, a beta-adrenergic blocker. *J Clin Psychopharmacol* 1987; 7:264–267.

56. Vlissides DN, Gill D, Castelow J: Bromocriptine-induced mania? *Br Med J* 1978;1:510. Letter to the editor.

57. Parkes D: Drug therapy: Bromocriptine. *N Engl J Med* 1979;301:874–878.

58. Turner TH, Cookson JC, Wass JA, Drury PL, Price PA, Besser GM: Psychotic reactions during treatment of pituitary tumours with dopamine agonists. *Br Med J* 1984;289:1101–1103.

59. Calne DB, Plotkin C, Williams AC, Nutt JG, Neophytides A, Teychenne PF: Long-term treatment of parkinsonism with bromocriptine. *Lancet* 1978; 1:735–738.

60. Pearson KC: Mental disorders from low-dose bromocriptine. *N Engl J Med* 1981;305:173. Letter to the editor.

61. Einarson TR, Turchet EN: Psychotic reaction to low-dose bromocriptine. *Clin Pharm* 1983;2:273–274.

62. Cabeza GA, Flores LF, Iniguez IE, Calarco ZE, Valencia PF: Acute psychosis secondary to bromocriptine treatment in a patient with a prolactinoma. *Rev Invest Clin* 1984;36:147–149.

63. Stillner V, Popkin MK, Pierce CM: Caffeine-induced delirium during prolonged competitive stress. *Am J Psychiatry* 1978;135:855–856.

64. Greden JF, Fontaine P, Lubetsky M, Chamberlin K: Anxiety and depression associated with caffeinism among psychiatric inpatients. *Am J Psychiatry* 1978;135:963–966.

65. Shaul PW, Farrell MK, Maloney MJ: Caffeine toxicity as a cause of acute psychosis in anorexia nervosa. *J Pediatr* 1984;105:493–495.

66. Parker WA: *Can J Hosp Pharm* 1986;39:13.

67. Gillman MA, Sandyk R: Reversal of Captopril-induced psychosis with naloxone. *Am J Psychiatry* 1985;142:270. Letter to the editor.

68. Cohen BM, Zubenko GS: Captopril in the treatment of recurrent major depression. *J Clin Psychopharmacol* 1988;8:143–144. Letter to the editor.

69. Germain L, Chouinard G: Captopril treatment of major depression with serial measurements of blood cortisol concentrations. *Biol Psychiatry* 1989; 25:489–493.

70. Saker BM, Musk AW, Haywood EF, Hurst PE: Reversible toxic psychosis after Cephalexin. *Med J Aust* 1973;1:497–498.

71. Al-Zahawi MF, Sprott MS, Hendrick DJ: Hallucinations in association with Ceftazidime. *Br Med J* 1988;297:858.

72. Brown MJ, Salmon D, Rendell M: Clonidine hallucinations. *Ann Intern Med* 1980;93:456–457.

73. Hoffman WF, Ladogana L: Delirium secondary to clonidine therapy. *NY State J Med* 1981;81:382–383.

74. Bodiou C, Bavoux F, Gavillon C, Krainik F: Hallucinatory syndromes regressing after withdrawal of clonidine. *Therapie* 1984:39:319–322.

75. Lesko LM, Fischman MW, Javaid JI, Davis JM: Iatrogenic cocaine psychosis. *N Engl J Med* 1982;307:1153. Letter to the editor.

76. Lewis DA, Smith RE: Steroid-induced psychiatric syndromes: A report of 14 cases and a review of the literature. *J Affective Disord* 1983;5:319–332.

77. Judd FK, Burrows GD, Norman TR: Psychosis after withdrawal of steroid therapy. *Med J Aust* 1983;2:350–351.

78. Meyboom RHB, de Graaf–Breederveld N: Budesonide and psychic side effect. *Ann Intern Med* 1988:109:683. Letter to the editor.

79. Closson RG: Visual hallucinations as the earliest symptom of digoxin intoxication. *Arch Neurol* 1983;40:386.

80. Carney MW, Rapp S, Pearce K: Digoxin toxicity presenting with psychosis in a patient with chronic phobic anxiety. *Clin Neuropharmacol* 1985;8:193–195.

81. Eisendrath SJ, Sweeney MA: Toxic neuropsychiatric effects of digoxin in therapeutic serum concentrations. *Am J Psychiatry* 1987;144:506–507.

82. Hazen PG, Carney JF, Walker AE, Stewart JJ: Depression—a side effect of 13-*cis*-retinoic acid therapy. *J Am Acad Dermatol* 1983;9:278–279. Letter to the editor.

83. Bruno NP, Beacham BE, Burnett JW: Adverse effects of isotretinoin therapy. *Cutis* 1984;33:484–486.

84. Hawks WN Jr, et al: *J Pediatr Ophthalmol* 1971;8:171.

85. Dundee JW, Know JW, Black GW, et al: Ketamine as an induction agent in anesthetics. *Lancet* 1970;1:1370–1371.

86. Byrd GJ: Acute organic brain syndrome associated with gentamicin therapy. *JAMA* 1977;238:53–54.

87. Ward WQ, Walter-Ryan WG, Shehi GM: Toxic psychosis: A complication of anti-malarial therapy. *J Am Acad Dermatol* 1985;12:863–865.

88. Ball R, Rosser R: Psychosis and anti-tuberculosis therapy. *Lancet* 1989;2:105. Letter to the editor.

89. Endo M, Hirai K, O'Hara M: Paranoid-hallucinatory state induced in a depressive patient by methyldopa: A case report. *Psychoneuroendocrinology* 1978;3:211–215.

90. Ritchie KS, Preskorn SH: Mania induced by metoclopramide: Case report. *J Clin Psychiatry* 1984;45:180–181.

91. Bottner RK, Tullio CJ: Metoclopramide and depression. *Ann Intern Med* 1985;103:482. Letter to the editor.

92. Adams CD: Metoclopramide and depression. *Ann Intern Med* 1985;103:960. Letter to the editor.

93. Fishbain DA, Rogers A: Delirium secondary to metoclopramide hydrochloride. *J Clin Psychopharmacol* 1987;7:281–282. Letter to the editor.

94. Paraskevaides EC: Near fatal auditory hallucinations after buprenorphine. *Br Med J* 1988;296:214. Letter to the editor.

95. MacEvilly M, O'Carroll C: Hallucinations after epidural buprenorphine. *Br Med J* 1989;298:928–929.

96. Eisendrath SJ, Goldman B, Douglas J, Dimatteo L, Van Dyke C: Meperidine-induced delirium. *Am J Psychiatry* 1987;144:1062–1065.

97. D'Souza M: Unusual reaction to morphine. *Lancet* 1987;2:98. Letter to the editor.

98. Waller SL, Bailey M: Hallucinations during morphine administration. *Lancet* 1987;2:801. Letter to the editor.

99. Kalso E, Vainio A: Hallucinations during morphine but not during oxycodone treatment. *Lancet* 1988;2:912. Letter to the editor.

100. Jellema JG: Hallucination during sustained-release morphine. *Lancet* 1987;2:392. Letter to the editor.

101. Kane FJ Jr, Polorny A: Mental and emotional disturbance with pentazocine (*Talwin*) use. *South Med J* 1975;68:808–811.

102. Wood AJ, Moir DC, Campbell C, Davidson JF, Gallon SC, Henney E, McAllion S: Medicines evaluation and monitoring group: Central nervous system effects of pentazocine. *Br Med J* 1974;1:305–307.

103. Miller RR: Clinical effects of pentazocine in hospitalized medical patients. *J Clin Pharmacol* 1975;15:198–205.

104. Hamilton RC, Dundee JW, Clarke RS, Loan WB, Morrison JD: Studies of drugs given

before anaesthesia. Pentazocine and other opiate antagonists. *Br J Anaesth* 1967;39:647–656.

105. Fraser HF, Isbell H: *Bull Narc* 1960;12:9.

106. Ahmad S: Nifedipine-induced acute psychosis. *J Am Geriatr Soc* 1984;32:408. Letter to the editor.

107. Sandyk R, Gillmlan MA: Nifedipine-induced psychosis. *J Am Geriatr Soc* 1985;33:154. Letter to the editor.

108. Hullett FJ, Potkin SG, Levy AB, Ciasca R: Depression associated with nifedipine-induced calcium channel blockade. *Am J Psychiatry* 1988;145:1277–1279.

109. Griffith JD, Smith CH, Smith RC: Paranoid psychosis in a patient receiving ibuprofen, a prostaglandin synthesis inhibitor: Case report. *J Clin Psychiatry* 1982;43:499–500.

110. Goodwin JS, Regan M: Cognitive dysfunction associated with naproxen and ibuprofen in the elderly. *Arthritis Rheum* 1982;25:1013–1015.

111. Gotz V: Paranoid psychosis with indomethacin. *Br Med J* 1978;1:49. Letter to the editor.

112. Schwartz JI, Moura RJ: Severe depersonalization and anxiety associated with indomethacin. *South Med J* 1983;76:679–680.

113. Thornton TL: Delirium associated with *Sulindac. JAMA* 1980;243:1630–1631. Letter to the editor.

114. Kruis R, Barger R: Paranoid psychosis with *Sulindac. JAMA* 1980;243:1420. Letter to the editor.

115. Sheehy LM, Maxmen JS: Phenelzine-induced psychosis. *Am J Psychiatry* 1978;135:1422–1423.

116. Bunney WE Jr: In Lipton MA, et al (eds.): *Psychopharmacology: A Generation of Progress.* New York, Raven Press, 1978, p 1249.

117. Dilsaver SC, Greden JF: Antidepressant withdrawal phenomena. *Biol Psychiatry* 1984;19:237–256.

118. Gupta R, Narang RL: Mania induced by gradual withdrawal from long-term treatment with imipramine. *Am J Psychiatry* 1986;143:260. Letter.

119. Jones BD, Steinbert S, Chouinard G: Fast-cycling bipolar disorder induced by withdrawal from long-term treatment with a tricyclic antidepressant. *Am J Psychiatry* 1984;141:108–109.

120. Gomolin IH, Melmed CA: Prolonged delirium without anticholinergic signs following amitriptyline overdose. *Can Med Assoc J* 1983;129:1203–1204.

121. Snow SS, Logan TP, Hollender MH: Nasal spray addiction and psychosis: A case report. *Br J Psychiatry* 1980;136:297–299.

122. Chin DK, Ho AK, Tse CY: Neuropsychiatric complications related to use of *Prazosin* in patients with renal failure. *Br Med J* 1986;293:1347.

123. Patterson JF: Auditory hallucinations induced by *Prazosin. J Clin Psychopharmacol* 1988;8:228. Letter to the editor.

124. Bjornberg A, Selstam J: Acute psychotic reaction after injection of procaine penicillin. A report of 33 cases. *Acta Psychiatr Neurol Scand* 1960;35:129–139.

125. Green RL, Lewis JE, Kraus SJ, Frederickson EL: Elevated plasma procaine concentrations after administration of procaine penicillin G. *N Engl J Med* 1974;291:223–226.

126. Silber TJ, D'Angelo L: Psychosis and seizures following the injection of penicillin G procaine. Hoigne's syndrome. *Am J Dis Child* 1985;139:335–337.

127. Biddle N, McCormack H: Panic disorder and the procaine in penicillin G. *Am J Psychiatry* 1988;145:1317. Letter to the editor.

128. Silber T, D'Angelo L: Doom anxiety and Hoigne's syndrome. *Am J Psychiatry* 1987;144:1365. Letter to the editor.

129. Ackerman WE, Phero JC, Juneja MM: Panic disorder following 2-chloroprocaine. *Am J Psychiatry* 1989;146:940–941. Letter to the editor.

130. Turner WM: Lidocaine and psychotic reactions. *Ann Intern Med* 1982;97:149–150. Letter to the editor.

131. McCrum ID, Guidry JR: Procainamide-induced psychosis. *JAMA* 1978;240:1265–1266.

132. Schubert DS, Gabinet L, Hershey LA: Psychosis induced by sustained-release procainamide. *Can Med Assoc J* 1984;131:1188,1190. Letter to the editor.

133. Currie P, Ramsdale DR: Paranoid psychosis induced by tocainide. *Br Med J* 1984;288:606–607.

134. Bikadoroff S: Mental changes associated with tocainide, a new antiarrhythmic. *Can J Psychiatry* 1987;32:219–221.

135. Leighton KM: Paranoid psychosis after abuse of *Actifed*. *Br Med J* 1982;284:789–790.

136. Sankey RJ, Nunn AJ; Sills JA: Visual hallucinations in children receiving decongestants. *Br Med J* 1984;288:1369.

137. Greer HD 3d, Ward HP, Corbin KB: Chronic salicylate intoxication in adults. *JAMA* 1965;193:555–558.

138. Wasser WG, Bronheim HE, Richardson BK: Theophylline madness. *Ann Intern Med* 1981;95:191.

139. De Pablo J, Garcia-Pagan JC, Picado C, Perez P: Anxiety attacks provoked by theophylline. *Med Clin* 1987;11;88:549–550.

140. Jounieaux V, Aubry P, Pedinielli JL, Levi-Velensi P: Hypomanic attack under slow-release theophylline. A case report. *Presse Méd* 1988;17:918. Letter to the editor.

141. Josephson AM, Mackenzie TB: Thyroid-induced mania in hypothyroid patients. *Br J Psychiatry* 1980;137:222–228.

142. Mermel LA, Doro JM, Kabadi UM: Acute psychosis in a patient receiving trimethoprim-sulfamethoxazole intravenously. *J Clin Psychiatry* 1986;47:269–270.

143. Saxe TG: Severe depression from TMP-SMX. *Drug Intell Clin Pharm* 1988;22:267. Letter to the editor.

144. Jacobsen FM, Sack DA, James SP: Delirium induced by verapamil. *Am J Psychiatry* 1987;144:248. Letter to the editor.

Chapter 21

Drug Treatment and the Use of Electroconvulsive Therapy

John P. O'Grady, MD and Lewis M. Cohen, MD

The sovereignest thing on earth
Was parmaceti for an inward bruise.
—*King Henry IV* Part 1, I,iii,53
William Shakespeare (1564–1616)

Heretofore, the discussion in this text has been focused primarily on issues of clinical description, differential diagnosis, and etiology of the various psychological and psychiatric conditions that arise during or coexist with pregnancy. A critical review of possible treatments is a difficult, yet important companion to these clinical descriptions. Therapeutics for psychiatric disorders were developed both as the result of careful study of the neuropharmacology of various psychiatric disorders, as well as through clinical experience and observation. This long-term effort has resulted in the successful treatment of numerous conditions, especially the depressions.

The issue of appropriate drug therapy for individuals pregnant at the time of the presentation of a psychiatric disorder, or those women who become pregnant during the course of treatment, is complex, with many uncertainties. The tendency of clinicians has been to stop many if not all medications once pregnancy is diagnosed. This is prompted by concerns of possible fetal damage or possible untoward effects of drugs on the mother due to the altered physiology of pregnancy. However, such discontinuations are not without risk, especially if severe maternal symptoms recur.

There are other problems. Many if not most agents given for psychiatric conditions have never been extensively tested nor approved for use during pregnancy. Of course, the same charge can be leveled against the majority of drugs available in our armamentarium, whether or not they are utilized principally for the treatment of psychiatric conditions.

Also, not all therapies for psychiatric disorders in or out of pregnancy consist of drug administration. There remains an important role for the various forms of behavior modification therapy (see Chapter 22) as well as for traditional psychotherapy. Electroconvulsive therapy (ECT) also retains a small but important position among potential treatments.

In this chapter, the use of drug therapy for various psychiatric conditions occurring during pregnancy is reviewed, and the possible applications of ECT for selected cases discussed. It is our intention to present a clinically oriented approach to therapeutics that will assist practitioners in their choice of pharmacologically active agents or ECT during pregnancy.

Electroconvulsive Therapy

The induction of seizures was introduced as a treatment for schizophrenia in 1934.[1] By 1938, patients with mania and depression were successfully responding to this form of therapy. The initial technology was extremely limited and seizures were induced by the administration of potentially dangerous substances such as insulin and metrazol, or with what are now considered to be unnecessarily high and prolonged jolts of electricity. Although electroconvulsive therapy was especially efficacious in treating patients with affective disorders, the procedure became notorious because of its widespread and often indiscriminate use, the frightening grand mal seizures, and the significant morbidity and mortality. Hollywood managed to graphically portray this early version of ECT and terrify a generation of moviegoers.

In the 1950s ECT was generally superseded by the development of psychoactive drugs. During the next two decades the use of ECT was largely limited to patients who had severe and unremitting psychotic disorders, and especially patients whose suicidal risk precluded waiting for antidepressant medications to take effect. Nevertheless, the treatment became progressively more refined and its side effects were lessened. After curare-like medications began to be used during the procedure to transiently paralyze patients' voluntary musculature, the morbidity became limited to a residual organic mental syndrome or amnesia. All complications have been reduced by such developments as minimal induction currents, unilateral and nondominant placement of electrodes, hyperoxygenation, and simultaneous electroencephalograms and electrocardiograms. The mortality risk associated with ECT has subsequently decreased to that of anesthesia alone.[1]

During the 1980s, as physicians became more aware of the immediate and delayed side effects of psychotropic medications, there has been an awakening of interest in the therapeutic value of ECT. It is now believed to be as effective and rapidly acting as many of the pharmacological agents, and is recognized to be the safest treatment for elderly, debilitated patients, or those who have severe medical illness, such as recent coronary occlusion or acute renal or hepatic decompensation.[1]

It has also been acknowledged to have particular value in the treatment of psychiatrically disturbed pregnant women, who cannot or should not be treated with psychotropic medications, most of which are known to either cross the placenta or enter breast milk.[2] Certain medications, such as lithium, have been demonstrated to be frankly teratogenic and affect the physical development of the fetus, while others may cause behavioral teratogenicity with sequelae that include temporary or permanent disturbances of adaptation, and/or acute withdrawal syndromes.[2]

The first instance of a pregnant woman treated with ECT was reported in 1941. The patient later successfully delivered a full-term, developmentally normal male child.[3] Developmental follow-up of other children who were in utero when their mothers underwent ECT also failed to reveal defects.[4] This appears to have been the situation even when the ECT employed the less sophisticated treatment techniques of the 1950s and 1960s. Currently available technology allows one to monitor the fetus, the mother, and the mother's seizure, and some authors maintain that this permits the comparatively safe use of ECT in even high-risk pregnancies.[5]

Although the prevailing attitude in society continues to favor the use of medication, the safety of ECT cannot be ignored.[6] Several authors have published guidelines for the use of ECT with pregnant patients,[7,8] or have strongly advocated it as an intervention.[9,10] The American Psychiatric Association has reviewed the literature in a monograph, and finds that case material supports the use of ECT in the management of affective episodes and psychoses during all three trimesters of pregnancy.[11] They advise monitoring fetal heart rate during treatments after 10 weeks gestation, and suggest that obstetrical resources be available to manage untoward effects. They note that preterm labor has not been reported with ECT, but it is advisable to have an obstetrician present in high-risk cases or those that are close to term. ECT is a low-risk and highly effective form of treatment, and it is important to recall that the absence of psychiatric therapy when there is significant mental dysfunction may adversely affect the welfare of both the woman and her fetus.

Drug Therapies

Risk-Benefit Considerations

Our knowledge of the effects of various pharmacologic agents during pregnancy is incomplete. While some data exists on the potential of certain agents to produce fetal structural abnormalities, very little information is available concerning the potential of these agents for long-term behavioral effects.[12] Of direct concern to the clinician are the primary risks associated with drug treatment to any patient during pregnancy which include[10,13–17,20,21]: (1) the *teratogenic potential* of the agent; (2) the *potential direct toxic effects* of a given drug on the fetus, or residual effects in the neonate; (3) the *effects of the drug on the process of labor and delivery*; (4) the *potential for long- term alterations in neonatal behavior* from in utero drug exposure; (5) the *drug concentration in breast milk* and its possible effects on the newborn; and (6) *alterations in drug absorption, distribution, or serum levels due to the physiologic changes in hepatic, renal, or vascular volume due to pregnancy.*

There are certain conditions and types of behavior where drug therapy is indicated despite real or potential risks.[13,15,17] For example, suicidal or psychotic behaviors demand drug treatment for the safety of the patient as well as those in her immediate area. There are other areas in which the need for therapy is less clear and the risk/benefit equation uncertain. In mentally dysfunctional women, the potential deleterious effects on pregnancy of chronic stress and the associated elevated catecholamine and steroid levels are uncertain, but require careful consideration.[18,19] There are other issues as well. Certain behaviors such as extreme anxiety states or panic disorders may prevent women from seeking antepartum care or severely interfere with their ability or willingness to comply with rest, dietary manipulations, or other treatments thought to be necessary during their pregnancies. For example, the acute withdrawal of medication for a woman at term with severe panic attacks could result in extreme symptoms, or precipitate obstetric complications. In these as in other conditions, the clinician must weigh the known risks, the alternative therapies available, the prior response of the individual woman, and the stage of gestation in deciding whether or not some drug therapy is in the best interests of both mother and fetus.

General Approach to Therapy

For the obstetrician, the primary goal in the initial evaluation of a woman with a preexisting psychiatric disorder is determining what drugs were administered during the periconception period and the conditions for which these agents were given. It is not at all uncommon to receive patient referrals from otherwise well-intentioned psychologists or psychiatrists with little indication as to the actual diagnosis or consideration of possible alternative therapies. Acute withdrawal of treatment in women who had previously been under reasonable control for bipolar disease, anxiety states, or endogenous depressions may present the obstetrician with the undesirable combination of *both* acute recurrent symptoms as well as early pregnancy exposure to drugs.

Clearly, a more desirable situation would be a planned pregnancy with consultation with both the psychiatrist and the patient *prior* to conception. Unfortunately, this is possible only in a minority of cases. When such preconceptual counseling occurs, the aim should be to titrate drug treatment to the lowest reasonable level, and discontinue the most potentially dangerous agents, if possible, or institute effective nondrug therapies.[15] It is always appropriate to attempt to institute nonpharmacologic treatments such as various types of behavioral modification or psychotherapy (see Chapter 22). Plans should be made and openly discussed with the individual and, hopefully, with her family and the father of the baby for actions to be taken if psychiatric symptoms increase during pregnancy and there is a need for additional control. Hospitalization with joint psychiatric/obstetric management for the tapering or withdrawal of medication should be used without hesitation.

Because of our difficult medicolegal climate, it is prudent to carefully note the various discussions and plans concerning treatment in the medical record. This notation should review the thinking of the clinicians, general plans for therapy, the options considered, and the concurrence of the patient and/or family with the proposed course of management. Both the psychiatrist and the obstetrician need to work in concert on such management issues and reach a consensus before presenting a treatment plan to the patient and family.

Because of the recognized sensitivity of the developing conceptus, it is desirable to minimize the exposure of the fetus to drugs during the first 60 days of gestation. Unfortunately, many pregnancies are not clinically recognized until after this period of time. Thus, early trimester drug exposures are common events, evoking anxiety in both the patient and the physician.

There is no single test for fetal condition that will assure normality. However, there are several investigations worth pursuing as they provide a level of reassurance for all concerned. The single best predictor of fetal condition is normal serial growth. As careful an anatomic survey by ultrasonic scanning as is possible given the period of gestation is a good first step. As last menstrual period dating can often be inaccurate, early ultrasound will also fix the true period of gestation, permitting retrospective analysis of whether or not a given drug exposure occurred at a potentially critical time of fetal development. By the use of abdominal and vaginal scanning, the conceptus can be easily visualized by 7 weeks of gestational age, and reasonable anatomic surveys of the major organ systems can usually be performed by 14 weeks, and often earlier.

When the pregnancy has reached 16 to 17 weeks, repeat ultrasound scans for fetal anatomy combined with serum alpha-fetoprotein (AFP), human chorionic gonadotrophin, and estriol levels—the "triple screen"—can collectively make a strong statement concerning fetal structural normality. Very little can be said about possible long-term behavioral effects of most drugs except to state that various animal studies suggest that such effects are possible but at present cannot be accurately quantitated.[10,12,20] The obstetrician must do his or her best to present accurate information concerning fetal condition when the patient and/or her family express their concerns. In many instances, the various fetal studies will prove normal, compounding the problem of possible pregnancy termination. The role of the clinician is to seek information and accurately and completely inform the patient and family. This is no easy task given the major uncertainties in this field.

In most instances in the absence of the identification of a specific fetal structural abnormality, there is little value in amniocentesis and chromosomal analysis. Such studies are indicated for the usual obstetric reasons, eg, when a pedigree review suggests the possibility of a hereditary risk for fetal malformation for which specific testing is possible, if advanced maternal age is present, or if there are abnormal values in the AFP or triple-screen screening tests.

Treatment for Acute Conditions

The most common acute psychiatric problems faced by clinicians are manic behavior and panic attacks. Such cases may present de novo through the emergency service of the hospital, be seen in previously normal postpartum and, occasionally, antepartum women, or occur in individuals with chronic conditions who were previously known to the physician in whom medications have been tapered or discontinued. There are a multitude of possible diagnoses that must be considered before an observed delirium or stupor can be confidently attributed to a psychological or psychiatric disorder (see Chapter 20). In brief, the clinician must consider organic brain lesions, manifestations of illicit drug ingestion, the unusual presentation of common medical diseases, and unusual side effects of prescribed or over-the-counter drugs in the differential diagnosis. In all instances, a reasonable effort must be made to immediately exclude easily treatable metabolic conditions such as electrolyte disturbances, hypoglycemia, or hyperthyroidism, among others, which can closely mimic psychiatric disease.

Once the evaluation indicates a primary psychiatric disorder, and maternal symptoms are acute, hospitalization is usually required. Drug therapy is often necessary for the safety of both patient and staff if the observed symptoms are severe. As previously discussed, ECT has a role to play in controlling mania and psychotic depression and its potential for acute treatment should not be overlooked. However, most clinicians will try a combination of hospitalization and drug therapy first. Haloperidol decanoate (2 to 10 mg IM_9 4-6 hrs prn) will often control acute agitation. Subsequent doses can be given as often as hourly, if required. Total daily oral maintenance doses vary from 1.5 to 15.0 mg administered in divided doses bid or tid, titrated against symptoms. Cohen and co- workers[17] recommend the use of a adjuvant benzodiazepine such as clonazepam to potentiate the effect of the major tranquilizer, reducing the dose required for symptom control.

The preferred antidepressants for use during pregnancy are the secondary amines such as nortriptyline or disipramine.[14] These drugs are of relatively rapid onset and are considered reasonably safe. Monamine oxidase inhibitors should be avoided. For the severely depressed with neurovegetative dysfunction and suicidal ideation, ECT is an additional treatment option. In general, physical restraint is not advisable in pregnant women, but is preferable to injury to staff or patient in extreme, short-term situations until a measure of pharmacologic control is possible (see Chapter 20).

Chronic Treatment

In the treatment of chronically psychotic women, the piperazine phenothiazines such as trifluoperazine or perphenazine are generally more desirable than the aliphatic phenothiazines such as chlorpromazine as the teratogenic risk may be lower.[14,17,21] Exposure of the fetus to antipsychotics may result in long-term neonatal extrapyramidal symptoms or transient jaundice. Thus, some attention should be given to the tapering of such drugs 2 weeks prior to delivery, if clinically possible. In general, there is no good evidence that these antipsychotic medications are either structural or behavioral teratogens.[14,21] However, given the limitations of our data, fetal exposure to such drugs in the first trimester should be avoided, if possible. If exposure does occur, an ultrasonic screen for fetal abnormalities is a reasonable measure for patient reassurance. Routine administration of antiparkinsonian agents is not recommended, especially in the first trimester. Such drugs should be used sparingly for specific symptoms only.

In many cases of chronically disturbed women maintained on low-dose medications, the possibility of drug tapering or discontinuation needs consideration. However, there is minimal solid evidence for adverse pregnancy effects of antipsychotic medications. Thus, if abrupt discontinuation of medication leads to decompensation and abnormal behavior, this is likely of greater risk to the pregnancy than continuation of the original dose. Reasonable choices need to be made in clinical management, but *misplaced zeal in avoiding all possible fetal exposures to drugs may result in other, less desirable events.* Acute maternal decompensation with the need to rebolus additional and larger concentrations of drug to achieve control increases rather than reduces maternal/fetal risks, to say nothing of the personal and family distress accompanying such events.

The best candidates for drug tapering or discontinuation are symptom-free individuals who have experienced a single depressive episode but are still maintained on tricyclic antidepressants. The tricyclic dose can usually be reduced at 25 mg/week with close clinical observation of symptoms.

As previously mentioned, monoamine oxidase inhibitors are contraindicated during pregnancy and if a pregnant patient is receiving these medications they should be promptly discontinued. Also, as the tricyclics can adversely effect neonates due to placental passage of the drug with subsequent newborn depression, tapering to the lowest possible maintenance dose prior to labor is desirable.

Bipolar Disorders

Individuals with bipolar disease represent a special and difficult group for drug therapy. For several years, the agent most commonly prescribed for this condition has been lithium. Unfortunately, lithium is a recognized teratogen due to its potential for placental transfer and has important side effects for the neonate.[14,21,22] Lithium exposure during early development is associated in the literature with an increased risk of fetal anomalies, especially to the cardiovascular system. The prevalence of Ebstein's anomaly in lithium-exposed pregnancies is controversial, and may be less than previously suspected, given the biases associated with registry recordings. Nonetheless, there is reasonable evidence that lithium has the potential to generate anomalies and thus should, if possible, be avoided in the first trimester of pregnancy.[14] Lithium also passes into the fetus through the placental circulation and lithium toxicity in the neonate consisting of cyanosis, hypotonia, bradycardia, and thyroid abnormalities is well described. These effects are transitory, however, reflecting the progressive excretion of the drug. The drug also passes into breast milk, and milk levels average some 40% of concomitant maternal concentrations. Thus, breast-feeding is contraindicated for lithium-ingesting mothers.[23] Clinicians must also recall that lithium is renally excreted, and thus maternal levels reflect the alterations in renal clearance characteristic of pregnancy and the puerperium. Therefore, lithium levels need close monitoring during pregnancy and immediately postpartum as changes in dose are necessary to avoid both undertreatment and overtreatment.[22] (See Tables 21.1 and 21.2.)

In clinical circumstances in which continuation of some medication is necessary but it has been decided to stop lithium, carbamazepine has been suggested as a possible replacement.[17] This drug, a tricyclic anticonvulsant, is probably also a teratogen but, as usual, the magnitude of the risk is unclear.[21,24,25] The principal abnormalities identified are midface hypoplasias similar to those previously described in association with the fetal hydantoin syndrome. This drug does cross the placenta, but at relatively low concentrations, and is thus compatible with breast-feeding.[23]

When a bipolar patient receiving lithium becomes pregnant there are several options: the pregnancy can be terminated; pregnancy may continue following discontinuation of the drug; lithium may be omitted in the remainder of the first trimester then reinstituted with careful observation of serum levels, or carbamazepine may be substituted; and finally, especially if the pregnancy is advanced at the time of diagnosis, lithium may simply be continued.[14,22] In some cases, control is possible with either an oral phenothiazine or a butyrophenone. If these agents are effective, they may be continued during

Table 21.1 Guidelines by Diagnosis for Psychotropic Drug Use and ECT During Pregnancy*

Psychosis

1. Recall that maintenance of low-dose antipsychotic therapy may offset the risk of relapse and the need for higher doses later for acute control
2. Review of medical differential diagnosis and a workup for new-onset psychotic states is essential (see Chapter 20)
3. High-potency neuroleptics may be safer than older agents and, in general, are preferred
4. No conclusive human evidence exists for teratogenicity of the standard neuroleptics, yet first trimester exposure is best avoided
5. Neuroleptic medications are present in breast milk

Mania

1. Review of medical differential diagnosis and a workup for new-onset manic symptoms is essential (see Chapter 20)
2. Critical evaluation for prophylaxis is required, especially if lithium has been administered
3. First trimester issues:
   i. Avoid lithium carbonate, if possible
   ii. If there is fetal exposure to lithium before week 12, consider ultrasound surveillance/fetal cardiac scanning/fetal echocardiography
   iii. Consider a trial of carbamazepine (CBZ) for bipolar patients with a clear need for antimanic prophylaxis early in pregnancy
   iv. Recall that termination of pregnancy remains an option
4. Second and third trimesters
   i. After week 12 and if treatment is necessary, lithium carbonate may be given with close maternal monitoring; CBZ may be an additional option
   ii. Administer lithium in small, divided doses; monitor serum levels every 2 weeks
   iii. Discontinue lithium or decrease the dose by 50% prior to delivery, if possible
   iv. Consider early, induced delivery in selected cases
   v. Give careful attention to postpartum lithium levels
5. Manic breaks during pregnancy
   i. Hospitization is required
   ii. Treat with neuroleptics or ECT for acute control
6. Recall that lithium treatment is contraindicated during breast-feeding

Depression

1. Review of medical differential diagnosis is essential (see Chapter 20)
2. Withhold medication in the first trimester, if possible
3. Clinical observation is mandatory. The inability to care for self or to provide prenatal care indicates the need for hospitalization
4. In therapeutics, favor secondary over tertiary amine tricyclics
5. Recall that ECT remains a reasonable alternative for delusional depression or for unusual, recalcitrant cases
6. Antidepressants pass into breast milk and attention to neonatal condition and avoidance of high-level dosing just prior to delivery is necessary

(continued)

Table 21.1 Guidelines by Diagnosis for Psychotropic Drug Use and ECT During Pregnancy (cont.)

Anxiety Disorders

1. Review of medical differential diagnosis, especially drug ingestion, is essential (see Chapter 20)

2. Withhold medication in the first trimester, if possible

3. In general, it is best to taper or discontinue benzodiazepine therapy prior to conception: slow taper vs change to a tricyclic antidepressant needs consideration

4. If the patient is on anxiolytics when pregnancy is confirmed, attempt taper to lowest effective dose

5. Avoid additional drug introduction, particularly in the first trimester

6. Adjunctive behavioral and supportive psychotherapy should be attempted and may avoid or minimize the need for drug therapy (see Chapter 20)

7. Benzodiazepines cross into breast milk and chronic use in lactating mothers is contraindicated

---

* Modified from Cohen LS, Heller VL, Rosenbaum JF: Treatment guidelines for psychotropic drug use in pregnancy. *Psychosomatics* 1989;30:25–33, with permission.
See Refs. 2, 3, 13–15, 17

pregnancy at the lowest effective dose. In all instances when continuation of pregnancy is decided upon, it is prudent to fully document all discussions in the medical record and perform ultrasonic surveillance of the fetus, as well as inform the pediatrician of the drug exposure and request their attendance at delivery. As usual in such settings there are no correct answers in therapeutics, only a series of alternatives of greater or lesser desirability.

Anxiety Disorders

For the treatment of nonpregnant women with chronic anxiety disorders, benzodiazepines and tricyclic antidepressants remain the drugs of choice.[26] However, there are important considerations of possible adverse drug effects on the fetus that need to be considered if these agents are continued or instituted during pregnancy.[13–17]

The potential risk associated with fetal exposure to the benzodiazepines is controversial.[14,21] There is a weak association between these agents and cleft lip/palate that may be potentiated by concomitant maternal smoking. In other studies, dysmorphic features, growth retardation, and central nervous system abnormalities have also been reported in association with chronic maternal ingestion of the benzodiazepines.[27] The level of risk for individual pregnancies, the importance of timing during gestation for the more severe effects, and if there is a dose-response curve for these drugs remains unknown. Avoidance of first-trimester dosing is desirable. Chronic maternal ingestion can also result in a substantial transfer of drug to the fetus, which can result in either a "floppy infant" syndrome due to a high neonatal concentration of drug or a withdrawal syndrome of tremors, irritability, and hypertonicity.[14,15,17] The use of these drugs is, in general, contraindicated during labor except as anticonvulsants. The benzodiazepines may also accumulate in breast-fed infants due to their impaired ability to excrete these agents and thus their use in lactating women is generally not recommended.[15,23] Occasional use after the first trimes-

Table 21.2 Special Considerations in Psychotropic Drugs Administration During Pregnancy and Lactation [13, 14, 21–23]

Drugs	Teratogenicity	Labor/Delivery	Effects on Newborn	Long Term Effects on Child	Lactation	Comments
I. Major Tranquilizers						
Alphatic Phenothiazines	Caution in first trimester due to a possible increase in malformed babies (congenital anomalies)	Reduce anxiety. No increase in duration of labor or operative deliveries.	Last trimester use of neuroleptics may cause extrapyramidal symptoms in infant: excessive crying, motion, hypertonia, hyperreflexia, and vasomotor instability. Jaundice possible especially in prematures.	Few studies. IQ at age 4 equal to control population.	Excreted in breast milk. No serious side effects reported as yet. Use with caution.	Potent antipsychotics should not be routinely used for gestational emesis. In active psychosis severity of symptoms may favor treatment. Benztropine should only be given for discrete symptoms, not routinely.
Butyrophenones	No evidence at present for teratogenicity (limited data)		Apparently minimal		Excreted in breast milk.	
II. Lithium Carbonate	Caution in first trimester. Drug is teratogenic with CV anomalies prominent.	Uncommonly, the fetus may develop a goiter. Woman's blood level of lithium may rise to toxic levels due to drop in G.F.R. after delivery. Use small divided doses; close monitoring of levels (q2 wks)	Third trimester use may cause fetal hypotonia, lethargy, cyanosis, poor sucking, shallow respiration, arrhythmias ("floppy baby syndrome"). This is reversible and self-limiting, disappearing with drug clearance.	Few studies. No different to siblings in physical or mental anomalies at age 5.	Excreted in breast milk; severe toxic reactions possible. Thus contraindicated during breast feeding.	Sodium restricted diets or diuretics should be avoided. U/S cardiac and thyroid studies of the fetus are advisable if drug is used chronically.
III. Anti-Depressants						
Tricyclics	No clear link with fetal deformity or limb dysgenesis. Use with caution in first trimester.	No reported problems.	Possible withdrawal symptoms in infant if used just prior to delivery. Heart failure, tachycardia myoclonus, respiratory distress, urinary retention, cyanosis, irritability, feeding difficulty.	Few studies.	Excreted in breast milk. Use with caution as effect on developing neurotransmitter systems unknown.	If discontinuation is desired, tapering is necessary to avoid a withdrawal syndrome

Drug						
MAOI	Phenelzine is teratogenic in animals. Avoid in first trimester.	Contraindicated during pregnancy				
Carbamazepine	Safety not established. Possible fetal malformations.					
IV. Anxiolytics Benzodiazepine	Safety in first trimester not established. Cleft lip/palate increased if used in first trimester.	Reduces anxiety. No association with labor complications.	Decreased sucking rate. Chronic use in pregnancy withdrawal: tremor, hypertonia, hyperreflexia. High doses prior to delivery result in low Apgars, hypothermia, neurological depression. Floppy infant syndrome. Possible increased jaundice.	Few studies	Excreted in breast milk; lethargy, jaundice, poor temperature regulation. Contraindicated during breast feeding	If possible, taper to lowest possible dose early in pregnancy and labor. Early teratogenic risk may be increased by smoking.
Meprobamates	Cleft lip/palate. Other severe congenital anomalies. Do not use in first trimester.	Reduces anxiety.		Few studies.		
Barbiturates	First trimester-growth retardation, facial dysmorphism, oral clefts. Skeletal anomalies. Dose related.	Reduces anxiety	Chronic use in pregnancy withdrawal in infant 10-14 days after birth, increased tone, tremor irritable.	Few studies.		Probably has a lower teratogenic potential than phentoins
Hydroxyzine	Teratogenic in animals when given in early development	Reduces anxiety	Jitteriness, myoclonic jerks, hypotonia after large doses prior to delivery.	Few studies.		Occasional use in labor is probably safe

Modified from Robinson by permission.[13]

ter and prior to the onset of labor is unlikely to be dangerous but the dose used should be kept as low as possible.

Tricyclic antidepressants are felt to have a low potential for teratogenicity, although neonatal withdrawal symptoms have been reported.[21] The American Academy of Pediatrics drug and breast-feeding report[23] lists imipramine, the most commonly used tricyclic, as an agent of possible concern whose effect on the neonate is unknown.

Alprazolam, a triazolo analogue of the benzodiazepines is among the most common drugs used to treat panic disorders. Unfortunately, there is little data on the use of this agent during pregnancy.[28] However, it is prudent to assume that this drug has fetal effects similar to other agents of the same type and thus represents at least a minimal teratogenic risk.[21]

Women receiving alprazolam or similar benzodiazepines chronically who wish to conceive should have the drug tapered or discontinued. For individuals who cannot tolerate discontinuation, administration of a tricyclic may alleviate emergent panic attacks. Concomitant behavioral therapy may reduce anticipatory anxiety and reduce the likelihood of attacks or result in less severe events. As Cohen and co-workers[17] point out, the aim of therapy is to reduce symptomatology to the lowest acceptable level permitting a balance between fetal drug exposure and maternal symptomatology. This balance is not necessarily the level of control acceptable for the nonpregnant individual but represents a reasonable compromise between maternal and fetal risks.

Breast-feeding for mothers receiving various potent drugs presents especial problems in management. The recognized benefits of breast milk and the psychological advantages of breast-feeding for both mother and child must be weighed against potential adverse effects on the neonate. Mothers receiving lithium or taking chronic doses of the benzodizepams should not breast-feed. The tricyclics and the phenothizides are probably safe for the neonate; however, as these medications have at least some passage into breast milk, careful evaluation of the baby is essential. If the infant is continuously drowsy or has poor tone or suck, then breast-feeding should be discontinued. In cases involving premature or ill neonates, individualization and consultation with the pediatrician or neonatologist will be necessary.

Conclusions

Drug therapy for psychiatric disorders during pregnancy is a complex issue with many uncertainties. General outlines of therapeutics are presented in Tables 21.1 and 21.2. Obstetricians need to coordinate treatment with psychiatrists. In all cases, reasonable compromises between control of symptoms and fetal/maternal risks need to be reached. The importance of the weighing of alternatives and flexibility are the essential components to successful management.

References

1. Fink M: Convulsive and drug therapies of depression. *Ann Rev Med* 1981;32:405–412.

2. Repke JT, Berger NG: Electroconvulsive therapy in pregnancy. *Obstet Gynecol* 1984;63(suppl):39S–41S.

3. Goldstein HH, Weinberg J, Sankstone MI: Shock therapy in psychosis complicating pregnancy: A case report. *Am J Psychiatry* 1941;98:201–202.

4. Forssman H: Follow-up study of sixteen children whose mothers were given electric convulsive therapy during gestation. *Acta Psychiatr Neurol Scand* 1955;30:437–441.

5. Wise MG, Ward SC, Townsend-Parchman W, Gilstrap LC, Hauth JC: Case report of ECT during high-risk pregnancy. *Am J Psychiatry* 1984;141:99–101.

6. Impastato DJ, Gabriel AR, Lardara HH: Electric and insulin shock therapy during pregnancy. *Dis Nerv Syst* 1964;25:542–546.

7. Nurnberg HG, Prudic J: Guidelines for treatment of psychosis during pregnancy. *Hosp Community Psychiatry* 1984;35:67–71.

8. Remick RA, Maurice WL: ECT in pregnancy. *Am J Psychiatry* 1978;135:761–762.

9. Kramer BA: Electroconvulsive therapy use during pregnancy. *West J Med* 1990;152:77, Letter to the editor.

10. Gelenberg AJ: Pregnancy, psychotropic drugs, and psychiatric disorders. *Psychosomatics* 1986;27:216–217.

11. Weyner RD, Fink M, Hammersley DW, Small IF, Moench LA, Sackheim H: *The Practice of Electroconvulsive Therapy: A Task Force Report of the American Psychiatric Association.* Washington, DC, American Psychiatric Association Press, 1990;16:72–73.

12. Kilata GB: Behavioral teratology: Birth defects of the mind. *Science* 1978;202:732–734.

13. Robinson GE, Stewart DE, Flak E: The rational use of psychotropic drugs in pregnancy and postpartum. *Can J Psychiatry* 1986;31(3):183–190.

14. Harding JJ: The use of psychotropic medication during pregnancy and lactation, in Zatuchni GI, Laferla JJ, Sciarra JJ (eds.): *Gynecology and Obstetrics,* vol. 6. Philadelphia, JB Lippincott, 1990:79:1–8.

15. Mortola J: The use of psychotropic agents in pregnancy and lactation. *Psychiatr Clin North Am* 1989;12:69–87.

16. Harding JJ: Psychopharmacologic treatment of anxiety and depressive disorders in the female patient, in Zatuchni GI, Laferla JJ, Sciarra JJ (eds.): *Gynecology and Obstetrics*, vol. 6. Philadelphia, JB Lippincott, 1990;73:1–15.

17. Cohen LS, Heller VL, Rosenbaum JF: Treatment guidelines for psychotropic drug use in pregnancy. *Psychosomatics* 1989;30:25–33.

18. Crandon AJ: Maternal anxiety and neonatal wellbeing. *J Psychosom Res* 1979;23:113–115.

19. Lederman RP, Lederman E, Work B, et al: Anxiety and epinephrine in multiparous women in labor; relationship to duration of labor and fetal heart rate pattern. *Am J Obstet Gynecol* 1985;153:870–877.

20. Vorhees CV, Brunner RL, Butcher RE: Psychotropic drugs as behavioral teratogens. *Science* 1979;205:1220–1225.

21. Briggs GG, Freeman RK, Yaffe SJ: *Drugs in Pregnancy and Lactation,* ed. 3. Baltimore, Williams and Wilkins, 1990.

22. Linden S, Rich CL: The use of lithium during pregnancy and lactation. *J Clin Psychiatry* 1983;44:358–361.

23. Committee on Drugs, American Academy of Pediatrics: Transfer of drugs and other chemicals into human milk. *Pediatrics* 1989;84:924–936.

24. Jones KL, Lacro RV, Johnson KA, Adams J: Pattern of malformations in the children of women treated with carbamazepine during pregnancy. *N Engl J Med* 1989;320:1661–1666.

25. Paulson GW, Paulson RB: Teratogenic effects of anticonvulsants. *Arch Neurol*

1981;38:140–143.
26. Rosenbaum JF: The drug treatment of anxiety. *N Engl J Med* 1982;306:401–404.
27. Laegreid L, Olegard R, Walstom J, Conradi N: Teratogenic effects of benzodiazepine use during pregnancy. *J Pediatr* 1989;114:126–131.
28. Barry WS, St. Clair SM: Exposure to benzodiazepines in utero. *Lancet* 1987;1:1436–1437. Letter to the editor.

Chapter 22

Behavioral Interventions

Zev S. Ashenberg, PhD and Shelley M. Falkin, PhD

Thou, like an exorcist, hast conjur'd up
My mortified spirit. Now bid me run,
And I will strive with things impossible;
Yea, get the better of them.
　—*Julius Caesar* II,i,323
　William Shakespeare (1564–1616)

Behavior therapy is an empirically derived treatment approach to maladaptive human behavior. Based on the principles of learning theory, behavior therapy assumes that abnormal human behavior is acquired and maintained by the same principles that affect normal behavior. Ross[1] suggests that behavior therapy not be defined in terms of a specific *technique* or theory, but rather as a scientific *approach* to the treatment of maladaptive behavior and psychological disorders.

Although the application of learning principles to the treatment of human disorders was reported as early as the 1920s,[2,3] it is generally agreed that contemporary behavior therapy has its origins in several major developments occurring during the 1950s. In B.F. Skinner's book, *Science and Human Behavior*,[4] he discussed the theories of operant conditioning and its application to human problems as a more empirical alternative to traditional psychoanalytic approaches. Hans Eysenck,[5] emphasizing both Hullian learning theory[6] and Pavlovian conditioning,[7] was also a strong proponent of these scientific approaches as the treatment of choice for a variety of psychological disorders. He pointed out that the major advantage of behavioral interventions over traditional psychotherapies is that it is an applied science that can be easily subjected to experimental investigation. Concurrently, Joseph Wolpe's *Psychotherapy by Reciprocal Inhibition*[8] discussed the application of learning principles to the treatment of anxiety and phobic disorders. Subsequent developments in the field over the next two decades emphasized the importance of cognitive factors in addition to purely behavioral phenomena in the acquisition of normal and abnormal behavior.[9–13]

The earliest applications of behavioral interventions were for the treatment of various psychological disorders, particularly phobic and obsessive-compulsive disorders.[8,14] By the late 1970s it became increasingly apparent, however, that the same learning principles involved in the development of maladaptive behaviors leading to psychological disorders could also lead to the

347

development of medical disorders. Indeed, some of the major leading causes of death in the United States could be attributed to nonadaptive human behaviors. For example, excessive eating, alcohol consumption, and cigarette smoking all contribute to an increase in disease and mortality rates. This recognition led to the burgeoning fields of health psychology and behavioral medicine. Currently, behavioral approaches have been found particularly effective in medical populations suffering from chronic disorders such as pain, diabetes, arthritis, chronic obstructive pulmonary disease, and cardiovascular disease.[15,16]

Unfortunately, professionals who are not well versed in the theoretical foundations of behavior therapy tend to view this treatment approach as a collection of "techniques" or procedures. This rather simplistic view often leads to inappropriate or indiscriminate application of behavioral interventions, the results of which are often less than satisfactory. Behavioral interventions are most effective when implemented in the context of a comprehensive psychotherapeutic relationship and are provided by a therapist trained in behavioral principles and their utilization.

The purpose of this chapter is to introduce obstetricians to a representative sample of different behavioral interventions and their applications to various medical and psychological disorders often seen during the course of pregnancy. Rather than providing practitioners with specific treatment recommendations, our intention is to sensitize readers to the important role that behavioral interventions play during the course of pregnancy, and assist them to identify cases in which behavioral consultation is warranted.

Components of Behavioral Interventions

Behavioral treatment approaches can be viewed as consisting of three major categories of intervention. *Physiological* interventions are those strategies that are designed to help individuals gain some voluntary control over their own physiological responses. *Behavioral* interventions, based on the principles of classical and operant conditioning, are designed to help individuals gain control over environmental contingencies that may influence their behavior. *Cognitive* interventions are those strategies that are designed to help individuals identify and manage those maladaptive thought processes that may exacerbate physical or psychological conditions.

It should be kept in mind that these three categories of behavioral interventions are not mutually exclusive, and simply serve as a useful conceptualization for the convenience of readers. It is not uncommon in behavioral therapy for the treatment of specific disorders to include a combination of physiological, behavioral, and cognitive interventions.

Physiological Interventions

Physiological interventions are designed to help individuals learn to obtain voluntary control over their own physical processes. It is assumed that by controlling such processes as muscle tension or autonomic arousal, individuals will be able to obtain an increased state of relaxation and will consequently decrease their physical and emotional discomfort. Relaxation techniques and biofeedback are representative of behaviorally based physiological interventions, and are described below.

Relaxation Strategies

Relaxation strategies are often the foundation for a number of behavior therapy and behavioral medicine interventions. Relaxation strategies can be traced back to the beginning of recorded times; however, it is only in the 20th century that Western civilization has begun to empirically explore the utility of these techniques.[17] Although there are numerous relaxation inductions reported in the research literature, for the purpose of this chapter we will focus on three major approaches to relaxation training: progressive muscle relaxation, autogenic training, and meditation.

Progressive muscle relaxation, as developed by Edmund Jacobson,[18] is perhaps the most popular and widely used relaxation technique. Although extensively researched by Jacobson, progressive muscle relaxation did not obtain notoriety until Wolpe[8] used this procedure in his famous work on systematic desensitization and reciprocal inhibition, discussed below.

Progressive muscle relaxation training is based on the assumption that excessive muscle tension is associated with increased anxiety and physical distress. By gaining voluntary control over the degree of muscle tension in the body, it is assumed that individuals can learn to better decrease their anxiety and physical discomfort. In this procedure, patients are taught to identify tension in a number of muscle groups throughout their body by systematically tensing and relaxing each successive muscle group. This systematic tensing and relaxing of different muscle groups enables individuals to better discriminate between feelings of tension and relaxation, thereby allowing them to gain control of these processes.

Jacobson's original procedure identified approximately 50 muscle groups throughout the body, and required months of training before the technique was mastered. Wolpe[8] utilized a simplified version of the technique which allowed all muscle groups to be covered within six sessions. The procedure underwent further refinement and evolved into approximately 15 muscle groups that could be learned within the course of a single session.

Autogenic training, developed by Schultz and Luthe,[19] is a passive relaxation procedure designed to decrease sympathetic activity and tension. It includes six standard "exercises": heaviness, warmth, cardiac regulation, respiration, abdominal warmth, and cooling of the forehead. These exercises are practiced in the context of a comfortable, quiet, and dimly lit environment in which the patient is instructed to imagine pleasant and peaceful scenery. By using this form of passive concentration, it is assumed that one can promote general muscle relaxation throughout the body.[20]

The roots of *meditation* techniques can be traced back approximately six thousand years to the Hindu religion. It evolved into the six primary schools of yoga, which have been a major influence on the development of meditation procedures in the Buddhist religion.[21] In this context, meditation was used to achieve relaxation, or altered states of consciousness, as well as for contemplation and to increase wisdom.[22]

Herbert Benson[23] introduced a nonsecular version of meditation procedures that has become widely popular and is frequently taught in clinical practice. He describes four major elements of a relaxation procedure.[24] These include: a quiet environment, a passive attitude, a comfortable position, and an object upon which to focus. Benson recommends the use of the word "one" as the point of focus, in order to clear one's mind and obtain a state of relaxation. The focus word is usually repeated silently, much in the same way that a mantra might be used in transcendental meditation.

All of the above relaxation procedures (meditation, autogenic training, and progressive muscle relaxation) have similar components and overlapping procedures. Relaxation procedures in general have been extremely well researched and have been found quite effective in addressing a variety of psychological and physiological problems.[17] As noted above, these procedures are the foundation upon which many behavior therapy and behavioral medicine interventions are based.

Biofeedback

Biofeedback is a relatively new treatment intervention that is second only to relaxation training in terms of its popularity and utility in behavioral medicine. Biofeedback is exactly what its name implies: individuals receive feedback that provides them with information concerning specific physiological processes in their bodies. Biofeedback can be used to help a person learn to gain some voluntary control over those physiological processes that are typically involuntary, such as heart rate and muscle tension. This procedure can also be used to help an individual regain voluntary control over a physiological process that has been diminished due to injury or disease, such as spinal cord injury or cerebral trauma-related spasticity.[25,26]

The types of physiological information commonly used in biofeedback training include electromyography (EMG), peripheral skin temperature, and heart rate. This type of informational feedback is used to treat a variety of disorders including: anxiety,[27] tension and migraine headaches,[28,29] Raynaud's disease,[30,31] back pain,[32] bruxism,[33] temporomandibular joint pain,[34] and essential hypertension.[35,36]

Biofeedback is often used in conjunction with some form of relaxation training. In general, biofeedback has not been found superior to relaxation training alone in the treatment of a number of disorders.[37-40] However, there is some recent evidence that using biofeedback for site-specific bilateral muscle equalization training is superior to relaxation training alone in the treatment of certain pain disorders.[41]

Behavioral Interventions

Behavioral interventions, founded on the principles of operant and classical conditioning, became widely used in the 1960s and have since become synonymous with the stereotyped interventions associated with "behavior modification." The following section presents a representative sample of several major interventions included in this category.

Reinforcement Procedures and Operant Interventions

Operant learning theory has provided a number of principles that affect the acquisition and extinction of normal and abnormal behaviors. A *positive reinforcer* is any event that, when presented, increases the probability that the preceding behavior will increase in frequency. Giving a child praise for earning a good grade on an exam is an example of positive reinforcement. Similarly, a *negative reinforcer* is any event that, when *removed*, increases the probability that the preceding behavior will recur. Picking up a child who is crying is an example of negative reinforcement; if the child stops crying when held by the parent, it increases the likelihood that the parent will again pick up the child under similar circumstances. Both positive and negative reinforcement are methods designed to strengthen or increase the probability of a given behavior. Conversely, *punishment* is the presentation of an aversive event (eg, spanking) or the removal of a positive event (eg, losing television privileges) that *decreases* the probability of the recurrence of the preceding behavior (eg, playing baseball in the living room). It is important to note that reinforcing and punishing stimuli are not necessarily consistent across individuals and must be defined empirically. For example, a teacher's admonishment may be punishing to a child who perceives the reprimand as an aversive event, but may be positively reinforcing to a child who craves attention.

Operant interventions attempt to modify behavior through the use of these reinforcement contingencies. The first step in these procedures typically involves identifying a "target behavior," which is the specific behavior requiring modification. If the target behavior is a desirable response, the therapist seeks to increase the frequency of this behavior through either positive or negative reinforcement. Conversely, if the target behavior is classified as undesirable, the therapist attempts to decrease the frequency of this behavior by the withholding of reinforcement and, less often, by the use of punishment. It is assumed that by controlling these environmental contingencies, one can eventually modify an individual's behavior.

Operant interventions have been widely utilized and well researched with psychiatric populations.[42,43] These procedures have been used successfully either to decrease such maladaptive behaviors as delusions, paranoid ideations, or irrational verbalizations,[44,45] or to increase appropriate social behaviors.[46] They have also been employed to increase appropriate self-care and independence in activities of daily living for psychiatric patients.[47] Similar interventions have been found useful with children in classroom settings to decrease disruptive and inattentive behavior[48] and to improve academic performance.[49]

Systematic Desensitization

Systematic desensitization was developed by Joseph Wolpe[8] for the treatment of anxiety associated with phobic responses. In this procedure, based on the principles of counter-conditioning and reciprocal inhibition, patients are gradually exposed to a graded or progressive hierarchy of fearful stimuli and learn to replace their initial feelings of fear and anxiety with feelings of calmness and relaxation. It is postulated that the feelings associated with relaxation and anxiety are incompatible; therefore, individuals can extinguish fearful responses to specific events using this procedure. Systematic desensitization, which can be employed during both in vivo and imagined situations, has proven effective in treating a variety of phobic and obsessive-compulsive disorders.[50,51]

Aversion Therapy

Aversion therapy attempts to diminish the attractiveness of a specific object or event by pairing that stimulus with an extremely noxious or uncomfortable sensation. It is assumed that by repeatedly pairing negative consequences (eg, electric shock) with an undesirable behavior (eg, cigarette smoking), the individual will become aversively conditioned and will consequently decrease the frequency of this behavior.

One of the most well-known clinical applications of aversive procedures is the use of disulfiram (Antabuse) in the treatment of alcohol addiction.[52] The ingestion of disulfiram followed by alcohol consumption will result in an extremely noxious, but temporary, physical reaction. It has been assumed that the severe illness produced by the disulfiram will be associated with the alcohol ingestion and will lead to a decrease in its future desirability. Although some case studies have reported the benefits of these types of procedures, there is no conclusive evidence that aversive techniques are effective[53] and, in fact, there has been some research suggesting that some aversive procedures may impose health risks.[54] This type of treatment is definitely contraindicated during pregnancy.

Cognitive Interventions

Cognitive interventions are based on the assumption that an individual's reaction to a particular event is determined primarily by her *perception* of the situation rather than by the reality of the actual event. It is further assumed that a number of emotional and physical disorders are a result of dysfunctional or maladaptive thought processes in response to stressful situations.

Cognitive therapies are designed to modify or alter these maladaptive thoughts and replace them with more adaptive cognitive processes. Most cognitive therapies are based on the work of Beck,[11,55] Meichenbaum,[12] and Ellis.[13] These therapies have become extremely popular over the past two decades, and the following section will briefly describe some of the major cognitive interventions.

Cognitive Restructuring

Cognitive restructuring is the most well known of the cognitive interventions and assumes that emotional disorders and maladaptive behaviors are a result of dysfunctional thinking (ie, irrational beliefs, maladaptive thought patterns). Cognitive restructuring procedures attempt to modify and "restructure" these faulty cognitions. Patients are taught to (1) identify maladaptive thoughts, (2) recognize the negative emotions resulting from these dysfunctional thoughts, (3) replace these maladaptive cognitions with more adaptive thoughts, and (4) practice this procedure in vivo during stress-provoking situations.

Stress Inoculation Training

The primary goal of stress inoculation training[56] is to help individuals develop and practice the necessary coping skills to confront a specific potential stressor. After the individual identifies a stressor, she is taught a number of self-instructional coping statements in hopes of "inoculating" her against the future occurrence of that stressor. She is then encouraged to practice these newly acquired skills during actual or simulated stress-provoking situations. It should be noted that the coping skills utilized during stress inoculation training include a variety of different strategies, such as relaxation techniques, cognitive restructuring, and coping self-statements.

Problem-Solving Training

Problem-solving training is a procedure in which individuals are taught a *general* strategy for identifying and coping with any problem or stressor they might face, as opposed to stress inoculation training, which addresses a *specific* stressor. During problem-solving training, individuals are taught how to (1) identify specific problems, (2) generate a variety of hypothetical coping strategies, (3) select the most appropriate coping strategies for a particular situation, and (4) systematically apply each selected strategy until the problem is resolved.

Obstetric Applications of Behavioral Interventions

As noted above, while behavioral interventions traditionally have been used to address psychological problems, recently these interventions have also been found to be beneficial for individuals with various medical disorders. Some common disorders amenable to behavioral interventions include headache,[28,57] chronic pain,[58,59] anticipatory nausea and vomiting related to chemotherapy,[60] diabetes compliance,[61] and preparation for invasive medical and dental procedures.[62] Most recently, attention has been focused on the specific application of behavior therapy to the fields of obstetrics and gynecology.[63,64] The following section will discuss the application of behavioral interventions to the lifestyle changes necessitated by pregnancy, as well as to various medical and psychological problems seen in both normal and complicated pregnancy.

Lifestyle Changes Associated with Pregnancy

During the course of normal pregnancy, women are often required to make dramatic alterations in their lifestyles. It is not uncommon for pregnant women to be instructed to make dietary changes and to abstain from cigarettes, alcohol, and a variety of prescription and nonprescription drugs. Ideally, these interventions should occur prior to the onset of pregnancy; unfortunately, most patients do not seek preconceptual care. Thus, many of these changes do not take place until pregnancy is well under way.[65] In addition, patient adherence to and compliance with these and similar recommendations remains a serious problem, occurring in only 30% to 60% of patients.[66,67]

Typically, there are three components to nonadherence including: (1)

medication errors (eg, failure to fill prescription, taking nonprescribed medication); (2) *poor treatment attendance* (eg, delay in seeking care, not keeping appointments); and (3) *failure to make appropriate behavioral changes* (eg, not taking recommended preventive measures, not controlling smoking, nonparticipation in prescribed health programs).[68] Recently, behavioral interventions have been successful in increasing adherence to and compliance with various medical regimens.[69]

Dietary Changes and Nutrition

Nutritional choices have a profound effect on long-term health and well-being. In fact, nutrition has been cited as a factor in such major health problems as coronary heart disease, hypertension, and diabetes.[70] It has been well documented that adequate nutrition during the course of pregnancy is imperative.[71] Good nutrition is particularly important during the first trimester, as well as during lactation, when increased nutritional demands are placed upon the mother.[73] In addition, nutritional deficiencies such as anemia are also frequently a problem in pregnant women, increasing the risks for premature labor or spontaneous abortion.[72]

Behavioral interventions have been successfully utilized in many preventive health programs designed to increase nutritional awareness. For example, these interventions have been effective in improving eating habits among employees at various work sites as well as in reducing the cholesterol and triglyceride levels of these individuals.[73,74] Similarly, during pregnancy, behavioral principles and interventions can be used to assist patients in improving their eating patterns and nutritional intake.

Alcohol and Drug Abuse

It has been estimated that approximately 13 million Americans either abuse or are dependent on alcohol and other drugs, with 55% to 60% of the drinkers being female.[75] Alcoholics are 12 times as likely as nonalcoholics to die of cirrhosis of the liver and two times as likely to die of coronary heart disease.[76] Research has provided evidence that alcohol consumed during pregnancy crosses the placenta and has a strong association with fetal structural and mental abnormalities as well as spontaneous abortion.[77-79]

Early behavioral treatments for alcohol abuse included aversive conditioning procedures such as the administration of disulfiram (*Antabuse*).[52,80] However, as detailed above, these procedures may be dangerous and inappropriate for pregnant women. More recent approaches to alcohol treatment include alternate skills training[81] and contingency management.[82] Behavioral treatment outcome studies have reported modest success with these interventions, but maintenance of treatment gains has been problematic. Recently, Marlatt and Gordon[83] have developed a relapse prevention program to increase treatment efficacy and to enhance long-term outcome.

Smoking Cessation

Cigarette smoking is considered the leading preventable cause of death in the

United States and is a major risk factor for heart disease, cancer, and emphysema.[84] Yet, despite increasing awareness of the deleterious consequences of cigarette smoking,[85] it is estimated that more than 54 million Americans, 23 million of which are women, continue to smoke.[86] Only 25% to 30% of women smokers quit during pregnancy and an additional one third reduce their cigarette intake. Research has indicated that cigarette smoking during pregnancy increases the incidence of low-birth-weight infants and developmental delays in children.[87,88] Unfortunately, research has also indicated that the recidivism rate of smoking is high.[81]

Behavioral interventions for smoking cessation have been effectively utilized for a number of years.[89] Most recent behavioral treatments have been multidimensional, incorporating a variety of interventions including aversive conditioning, operant techniques, stress management strategies, and cognitive and behavioral coping techniques.[90-92] In addition, Lichtenstein and Brown[93] have developed a relapse prevention/maintenance program for smokers designed to increase long-term abstinence rates. Although many studies have included aversive conditioning techniques for smoking reduction,[94,95] this method of cessation has come under criticism[54] and may be inappropriate for use with pregnant women.

Stress

For many women, the lifestyle changes associated with pregnancy are sources of increased stress and depression.[96] Stress has long been implicated in the onset of a variety of physical and psychological problems.[97] Major life stressors have been associated with myocardial infarctions,[98] severity of chronic illness,[99] schizophrenic symptomatology,[100-102] and neurotic illness.[103,104] Similarly, stress has been associated with complications of pregnancy and delivery[105] as well as with duration of labor.[96]

While everyone may experience stress in their daily lives, it appears that not everyone is equally prone to experience the deleterious physical and psychological consequences stress may induce.[106,107] Increasingly, research suggests that the way people *cope* with stress is more important to overall morale, social functioning, and somatic health than the frequency and severity of the stress episodes themselves.[108,109]

Behavioral approaches have been found extremely useful in helping individuals acquire the necessary coping skills to deal with physical and psychosocial stressors. These interventions typically consist of a combination of the physiological, behavioral, and cognitive strategies described in the previous section of this chapter. Given the apparent harmful effects of stress on pregnancy, it should not be surprising that stress management training is a major component of most prepared childbirth programs.[110,111]

Depression

It has been estimated that between 10% and 25% of all women will experience a depressive episode at least once in their lifetime, with approximately 4% to 9% affected at any one time.[112] The incidence of depression is greater following childbirth than during pregnancy[113,114]; nevertheless, the major lifestyle changes associated with childbearing may lead to the development of depressive symptomatology.

There is growing evidence that suggests that biochemical processes and heredity may play an important role in many types of depression.[115-117] Although pharmacological treatment is the most often used intervention for depression, cognitive-behavioral treatments have also shown promise as an alternate treatment for this disorder.

Beck's cognitive theory,[11] as previously mentioned, proposes that depression is a result of an individual's predisposition to view the self, the future, and the world in a dysfunctional and overly negative manner. Beck developed a detailed therapy manual designed to provide a systematic and structured method for the use of cognitive interventions with depressed patients.[55] Reviews of a number of well-controlled research studies suggest that cognitive therapy may be at least as effective as tricyclic antidepressant pharmacotherapy, with the combination of these two treatments being superior to either intervention alone.[118] Although the use of cognitive therapy for depression associated with pregnancy has not been well researched, it is reasonable to assume that this treatment approach can be beneficial for this population as well.

Medical Complications Associated with Pregnancy

Medical complications in pregnancy pose added problems over and above the modifications and lifestyle changes necessary during normal pregnancy. Some of these complications include: nausea and vomiting, pain, hypertension, and gestational diabetes.

Nausea and Vomiting

Nausea and vomiting are common symptoms of first-trimester pregnancies, occurring in approximately 50% of women.[86] In most cases, the symptoms are relatively mild and treatment may consist of soft food and frequent small meals. However, in severe cases of protracted vomiting (hyperemesis gravidarum), both hospitalization and the administration of various drugs may be required. Since the use of antiemetics in the treatment of nausea and vomiting associated with pregnancy raises concerns about possible adverse effects, they are usually avoided except in the more severe cases.[86] Therefore, treating such symptoms with nonpharmacologic measures is warranted whenever possible.

Behavioral interventions have only recently been utilized for nausea and vomiting associated with pregnancy.[63] However, behavioral treatment of anticipatory nausea and vomiting has been shown to be effective in patients undergoing chemotherapy.[60] In particular, progressive muscle relaxation, EMG biofeedback combined with relaxation training, and systematic desensitization have been utilized with this population. Results of treatment studies consistently indicate that patients provided with therapist-directed relaxation and biofeedback successfully reduce their pulse rate, blood pressure, anxiety, and their nausea.[119]

Pain

Pain is the most frequent complaint made by patients to their physicians, yet it remains a very poorly understood phenomenon. It has been estimated that the financial cost of acute and chronic pain disorders, calculated from health care expenses and lost workdays, may equal 10% of the U.S. annual budget.[120] In recent years, it has been increasingly recognized that pain is a subjective experience affected by physical and psychological factors, both of which must be taken into account for successful management.[121]

Labor pain is considered among the most intense forms of pain an individual may ever endure.[122] This has made prepared childbirth training[110,111] one of the most popular and widely used psychological approaches to pain management.[123,124] The techniques typically included in prepared childbirth training involve: (1) providing the patient with detailed information about pregnancy and labor to decrease anxiety and increase feelings of self-control, (2) training in relaxation and breathing exercises designed to decrease pain and anxiety, and (3) training in cognitive coping strategies designed to distract the patient from pain.

A number of studies have reported many positive effects associated with antenatal training such as reduced use of analgesic and anesthetic medications,[125,126] decreased perception of pain,[127,128] and enhanced health benefits for the child.[129, 130] However, other studies have failed to support many of these findings.[131,132] Consequently, it has been suggested that prepared childbirth training be used as an adjunct to, rather than a replacement for, regional anesthesia during parturition.[133,134]

In addition to the acute pain associated with childbearing, obstetricians will undoubtedly encounter numerous pregnant women with various chronic pain-related disorders. Unfortunately, many of the medications that can adequately manage chronic pain (eg, nonsteroidal anti-inflammatory drugs) may be inappropriate for use during pregnancy due to their possible teratogenic effects or concern over other, unknown adverse effects. Behavioral interventions for pain management may prove to be a viable alternative to pharmacological treatment for many pregnant women. These interventions have been proven effective in the treatment of a number of chronic pain disorders including low back pain,[59,135,136] tension and migraine headaches,[137,138] Raynaud's syndrome,[30,31] and arthritis.[139]

Hypertension

Hypertension is a serious health problem in the United States and is a leading cause of cardiovascular disease, renal failure, and cerebrovascular disease.[140,141] Pregnancy-induced hypertension occurs in about 5% to 10% of all pregnant Caucasian women in the United States; estimates for black women are somewhat higher.[142] Such pregnancy-related hypertension often occurs after 20 weeks gestation and occasionally as late as 48 hours postpartum.[143] Although pharmacological intervention is the most common method of treatment for hypertension, relaxation and biofeedback have also been shown to be effective.

Numerous researchers have investigated the use of behavioral interventions with essential hypertensives[144–147]; they found significant reductions in blood pressure following relaxation procedures. Biofeedback has also been used as a technique to reduce blood pressure both directly and as an adjunct to general relaxation training.[148-151] Similarly, stress management and cognitive-behavioral strategies have also been shown to be effective in reducing hypertension during pregnancy.[152]

Diabetes Mellitus

It has been reported that over 10 million Americans have diabetes mellitus, with about 80% to 90% classified as non-insulin- dependent, or type II, diabetics.[153] Gestational diabetes occurs in 5% to 9% of pregnancies and results in increased fetal and maternal complications.[154] It has been estimated that 60,000 to 90,000 babies are born to women with gestational diabetes each year, and 10,000 are born to women with type I or type II diabetes.[155]

Behavioral interventions for type I, or insulin-dependent, diabetes have been found to be effective in increasing compliance with glucose-monitoring regimens.[156] In addition, recent behavioral weight loss and exercise programs developed specifically for obese type II diabetics have also been successful.[157,158] Only a few studies have investigated behavioral interventions designed to increase diabetes control in pregnant women. One study, which developed a preconception education program, found that only one birth defect occurred in 128 deliveries compared to 7.5% born to women who did not participate in the total program. This was due, presumably, to improved metabolic control and lower blood glucose levels in the program participants.[159]

Summary

Behavioral treatment approaches may prove effective in addressing many of the lifestyle changes as well as the psychological factors and medical complications that may be encountered during pregnancy. Given the potential utility of behavioral interventions, it is surprising that a recent study found that psychology services are typically underutilized in obstetric departments. In fact, only 35% of obstetric departments make referrals to psychology services, and only 10% of these departments have routine involvement with psychology programs.[160] Behavioral factors play an important role in pregnancy and childbirth, and behavioral health professionals can make a valuable contribution to the management of selected patients.

References

1. Ross AO: Behavior therapy with children, in Garfield SL, Bergin AE (eds.): *Handbook of Psychotherapy and Behavior Change: An Empirical Analysis*, ed. 2. New York, Wiley, 1978.
2. Jones MC: The elimination of children's fears. *J Exp Psychol* 1924;7:383–390.
3. Watson JB, Rayner R: Conditioned emotional reaction. *J Exp Psychol* 1920;3:1–4.
4. Skinner BF: *Science and Human Behavior*. New York, Macmillan, 1953.
5. Eysenck HJ: *Behavior Therapy and the Neuroses*. New York, Pergamon, 1960.
6. Hull CL: *Principles of Behavior*. New York, Appleton- Century-Crofts, 1943.

7. Pavlov IP: *Conditioned Reflexes*. London, Oxford University Press, 1927.

8. Wolpe J: *Psychotherapy by Reciprocal Inhibition*. Stanford, CA, Stanford University Press, 1958.

9. Rotter JB: *Social Learning and Clinical Psychology*. Englewood Cliffs, NJ, Prentice-Hall, 1954.

10. Bandura A: *Principles of Behavior Modification*. New York, Holt, Rinehart and Winston, 1969.

11. Beck AT: *Depression: Clinical, Experimental, and Theoretical Aspects*. New York, Harper and Row, 1967.

12. Meichenbaum DH: *Cognitive Behavior Modification*. Morristown, NJ, General Learning Press, 1977.

13. Ellis A: *Reason and Emotion in Psychotherapy*. New York, Lyle Stuart, 1962.

14. Marks IM: Behavioral treatment of phobic and obsessive-compulsive disorders: A critical appraisal, in Hersen R, Eisler RM, Miller PM (eds.): *Progress in Behavior Modification*, vol. 1. New York, Academic Press, 1975.

15. Doleys DM, Meredith RL, Ciminero AR (eds.): *Behavioral Medicine: Assessment and Treatment Strategies*. New York, Plenum Press, 1975.

16. Gatchel RJ, Baum A: *An Introduction to Health Psychology*. Reading, MA, Addison-Wesley, 1983.

17. Lichstein KL: *Clinical Relaxation Strategies*. New York, Wiley, 1988.

18. Jacobson E: *Progressive Relaxation*. Chicago, University of Chicago Press, 1929.

19. Schultz JH, Luthe W: *Autogenic Training: A Psychophysiological Approach in Psychotherapy*. New York, Grune and Stratton, 1959.

20. Luthe W: *Autogenic Therapy*, vol. 4. New York, Grune and Stratton, 1970.

21. Feuerstein G: *Textbook of Yoga*. London, Rider, 1975.

22. Shapiro DH: *Meditation: Self-regulation Strategy and Altered State of Consciousness*. Hawthorne, NY, Aldine, 1980.

23. Benson H: *The Relaxation Response*. New York, Morrow, 1975.

24. Benson H: Systemic hypertension and the relaxation response. *N Engl J Med* 1977;296:1152–1156.

25. Blanchard EB, Epstien LH: *A Biofeedback Primer*. Reading, MA, Addison-Wesley, 1978.

26. Ince LP, Brucker BS, Alba A: Behavioral techniques applied to the care of patients with spinal cord injuries. *Behav Eng* 1976;3:87–95.

27. Townsend RE, House JF, Addario D: A comparison of biofeedback-mediated relaxation and group therapy in the treatment of chronic anxiety. *Am J Psychiatry* 1975;132:33–38.

28. Blanchard EB, Andrasik F: Psychological assessment and treatment of headache: Recent developments and emerging issues. *J Consult Clin Psychol* 1982;50:859–879.

29. Chapman S: A review and clinical perspective on the use of EMG and thermal biofeedback for chronic headaches. *Pain* 1986;23:1241–1247.

30. Surwit RS, Pilon RN, Fenton CH: Behavioral treatment of Raynaud's disease. *J Behav Med* 1978;1:323–335.

31. Surwit RS: Behavioral treatment of Raynaud's syndrome in peripheral vascular disease. *J Consult Clin Psychol* 1982;50:922–932.

32. Dolce J, Raczynski J: Neuromuscular activity and electromyography in painful backs: Psychological and biomechanical models in assessment and treatment. *Psychol Bull* 1985;97:502–520.

33. Mulhall DJ, Todd RW: Deconditioning by the use of EMG signals. *Behav Ther* 1975;6:125–127.

34. Gessel AH: Electromyographic biofeedback and tricyclic antidepressants in myofascial pain-dysfunction syndrome: Psychological predictors of outcome. *J Am*

Dent Assoc 1975;91:1048–1052.

35. McCaffery RJ, Blanchard EB: Stress management approaches to the treatment of essential hypertension. *Ann Behav Med* 1985;7:5–12.

36. Shapiro D, Goldstein IB: Biobehavioral perspectives on hypertension. *J Consult Clin Psychol* 1982;50:841–858.

37. Tarler-Benlolo L: The role of relaxation in biofeedback training: A critical review of the literature. *Psychol Bull* 1978;85:727–755.

38. Turk DC, Meichenbaum DH, Berman WH: Application of biofeedback for the regulation of pain: A critical review. *Psychol Bull* 1979;86:1322–1338.

39. Linton SJ: Behavioral remediation of chronic pain: A status report. *Pain* 1986;24:125–141.

40. Cox DJ: Nonpharmacological integrated treatment approach to headache. *Behav Med Up* 1979;1:14–19.

41. Klonoff EA, Janata JW: The use of bilateral EMG equalization training in the treatment of temporomandibular joint dysfunction—a case report. *J Rehabil* 1986;13:273–277.

42. Gripp RF, Magaro PA: The token economy program in the psychiatric hospital: A review and analysis. *Behav Res Ther* 1974;12:205–228.

43. Kazdin AE: Recent advances in token economy research, in Hersen M, Eisler RM, Miller PM: *Progress in Behavior Modification*, vol. 1. New York, Academic Press, 1975.

44. Patterson R, Teigen J: Conditioning and post-hospital generalization of nondelusional responses in a chronic psychotic patient. *J Appl Behav Anal* 1973;6:65–70.

45. Kazdin AE: The effect of response cost in suppressing behavior in a pre-psychotic retardate. *J Behav Ther Exp Psychiatry* 1971;2:137–140.

46. Bennet PS, Maley RS: Modification of interactive behaviors in chronic mental patients. *J Appl Behav Anal* 1973;6:609–620.

47. Kazdin AE: *The Token Economy: A Review and Evaluation*. New York, Plenum Press, 1977.

48. Drabman RS: Behavior modification in the classroom, in Craighead WE, Kazdin AE, Mahoney MJ (eds.): *Behavior Modification: Principles, Issues and Applications*. Boston, Houghton Mifflin, 1976.

49. Ayllon T, Layman D, Burke E: Disruptive behavior and reinforcement of academic performance. *Psychological Record* 1972;22:315–323.

50. Emmelkamp PMG: *Phobic and Obsessive Compulsive Disorders: Theory, Research and Practice*. New York, Plenum Press, 1982.

51. Wolpe JP, Brady J, Brady JP, Serber M, Agras WS, Lieberman RP: The current status of systematic desensitization. *Am J Psychiatry* 1973;130,961–965.

52. Davidson RS: Alcoholism: Experimental analysis of etiology and modification, in Calhoun KS, Adams HE, Mitchell KM (eds.): *Innovations in Treatment Methods in Psychopathology*. New York, Wiley, 1974.

53. Wilson GT, Brownell KD: Behavior therapy for obesity: An evaluation of treatment outcome. *Adv Behav Res Ther* 1980;3:49–86.

54. Horan JJ, Linberg SE, Hackett G: Rapid smoking: A cautionary note. *J Consult Clin Psychol* 1977;45:344–347.

55. Beck AT, Rush AJ, Shaw BF, Emery G: *Cognitive Therapy of Depression: A Treatment Manual*. New York, Guilford Press, 1979.

56. Meichenbaum D, Cameron R: Stress inoculation training: Toward a general paradigm for training coping skills, in Meichenbaum D, Jaremko ME (eds.): *Stress Reduction and Prevention*. New York, Plenum Press, 1983.

57. Williamson DA, Ruggiero L, Davis CJ: Headache, in Blechman EA, Brownell KD (eds.): *Handbook of Behavioral Medicine for Women*. New York, Pergamon Press, 1984.

58. Keefe FJ: Behavioral assessment and treatment of chronic pain: Current status and future directions. *J Consult Clin Psychol* 1982;50:896–911.

59. Turk DC, Meichenbaum DH, Genest M: *Pain and Behavioral Medicine: A Cognitive Behavioral Perspective*. New York, Guilford Press, 1983.

60. Redd WH, Andrykowski MA: Behavioral intervention in cancer treatment: Controlling aversion reactions to chemotherapy. *J Consult Clin Psychol* 1982;50:1018–1029.

61. Fisher EB, Delamater AM, Bertelson AD, Kirkley BG: Psychological factors in diabetes and its treatment. *J Consult Clin Psychol* 1982;50:993–1003.

62. Anderson KO, Masur FT: Psychological preparation for invasive medical and dental procedures. *J Behav Med* 1983;6:1–40.

63. Callahan EJ, Disiderato L: Disorders in pregnancy, in Blechman EA, Brownell KD (eds.): *Handbook of Behavioral Medicine for Women*. New York, Pergamon Press, 1984.

64. Klonoff EA, Janata JW: Use of behavior therapy in obstetrics and gynecology, in Wise TN (ed.): *Advances in Psychosomatic Medicine*, vol. 12. New York, Karger,1985.

65. Taylor CM, Pernoll ML: Normal pregnancy and prenatal care, in Pernoll ML, Benson RC (eds.): *Current Obstetric and Gynecologic Diagnosis and Treatment*. Norwalk, CT, Appleton and Lange, 1987.

66. Masek BE: Compliance and medicine, in Doleys DM, Meredith RL, Ciminero AR (eds.): *Behavioral Medicine: Assessment and Treatment Strategies*. New York, Plenum Press, 1982.

67. Steele DJ, Jackson TC, Gutmann MC: Have you been taking your pills? The adherence-monitoring sequence in the medical interview. *J Fam Pract* 1990;30:294–299.

68. Meichenbaum D, Turk DC: *Facilitating Treatment Adherence: A Practitioner's Guidebook*. New York, Plenum Press, 1987.

69. Epstein LH, Cluss PA: A behavioral medicine perspective on adherence to long-term medical regimens. *J Consult Clin Psychol* 1982;50:950–971.

70. Hastedt P: Nutrition guidelines in health promotion, in Blumenthal JA, Mckee DC (eds.): *Applications in Behavioral Medicine and Health Psychology: A Clinician's Source Book*. Florida, Professional Resource Exchange, 1987.

71. Moore PJ: Maternal physiology during pregnancy, in Pernoll ML, Benson RC (eds.): *Current Obstetric and Gynecologic Diagnosis and Treatment*. Norwalk, CT, Appleton and Lange, 1987.

72. St. Jeor ST, Sutnick MR, Scott BJ: Nutrition, in Blechman EA, Brownell KD (eds.): *Handbook of Behavioral Medicine for Women*. New York, Pergamon Press, 1982.

73. Ziffenblatt SM, Wilbur CS, Pinky J: Changing cafeteria eating habits. *J Am Diet Assoc* 1980;76:15–23.

74. Foreyt JP, Scott LW, Mitchell RE, Giotto AM: Plasma lipid changes in the normal population following behavioral treatment. *J Consult Clin Psychol* 1979;47:440–452.

75. Brandsma JM, Maultsby MC, Welsh RJ: *Outpatient Treatment of Alcoholism: A Review and a Comparative Study*. Baltimore, University Park Press, 1980.

76. Davidson RA: Addictive behaviors: Alcohol, drugs, and smoking, in Doleys DM, Meridith Rl, Ciminero AR (eds.): *Behavioral Medicine: Assessment and Treatment Strategies*. New York, Plenum Press, 1982.

77. Low JA: Maternal smoking in human reproduction. *Can J Public Health* 1981;72:390–393.

78. Morrissey ER, Schuckit MA: Stressful life events and alcohol problems among women seen at a detoxification center. *J Stud Alcohol* 1978;39:1559–1576.

79. U.S. Department of Health and Human Services: Women and Health, United States, in Moore E (ed.): *Public Health Reports Supplement*. Washington, DC, U.S. Government Printing Office, 1980.

80. Wiens AN, Menustik CE: Treatment outcome and patient characteristics in an aversion therapy program for alcoholism. *Am Psychol* 1983;38:1096–1098.

81. Marlatt A, Gordon JR: Determinants of relapse: Implications for maintenance of behavior change, in Davidson OP (ed.): *Behavioral Medicine: Changing Health Lifestyles*. New York, Brunner/Mazel, 1978.

82. Lawson DM, Boudin HM: Alcohol and drug abuse, in Hersen M, Bellack AS (eds.): *Handbook of Clinical Behavior Therapy with Adults*. New York, Plenum Press, 1985, pp 293–318.

83. Marlatt GA, Gordon JR: *Relapse Prevention: Maintenance Strategies in the Treatment of Addictive Behaviors*. New York, Guilford Press, 1985.

84. Department of Health, Education and Welfare: *Smoking and Health: A Report of the Surgeon General*. Washington, DC, DHEW Publication no. (PHS) 79-5066, 1979.

85. *Gallup Opinion Index*. June 1974. Report no. 108, pp 20–21. Comment.

86. American Cancer Society: *Cancer Facts and Figures*. New York, American Cancer Society, 1982.

87. U.S. Department of Health and Human Services: *A Report of the Surgeon General*. Washington, DC, U.S. Government Printing Office, 1980.

88. Taylor CM, Pernoll ML: Normal pregnancy and prenatal care, in Pernoll ML, Benson RC (eds.): *Current Obstetric and Gynecologic Diagnosis and Treatment*. Norwalk, CT, Appleton and Lange, 1987.

89. Lichtenstein E: The smoking problem: A behavioral perspective. *J Consult Clin Psychol* 1982;50:804–819.

90. Pomerleau OF, Adkins D, Pertschuk M: Predictors of outcome and recidivism in smoking cessation treatment. *Addict Behav* 1978;3:65–70.

91. Glasgow RE: Effects of a self-control manual, rapid smoking, and amount of therapist contact on smoking reduction. *J Consult Clin Psychol* 1978;46:1439–1447.

92. Spring FL, Sipich JF, Trimble RW, Goeckner DJ: Effects of contingency and non-contingency contracts in the context of a self- control-oriented smoking modification program. *Behav Ther* 1978;9:967–968.

93. Lichtenstein E, Brown RA: Current trends in the modification of cigarette dependence, in Bellack AS, Hersen M, Kazdin AE (eds.): *International Handbook of Behavior Modification and Therapy*. New York, Plenum Press, 1982, pp 575–612.

94. Lando HA: Successful treatment of smokers with a broad- spectrum behavioral approach. *J Consult Clin Psychol* 1977;45:361–366.

95. Lando HA: Effects of preparation, experimenter contact, and a maintained reduction alternative on a broad-spectrum program for eliminating smoking. *Addict Behav* 1981;6:123–133.

96. Beck N, Siegel LJ, Davidson NP, Kormeier S, Breitenstein A, Hall D: The prediction of pregnancy outcome: Maternal preparation, anxiety and attitudinal sets. *J Psychosom Res* 1980;24:343–351.

97. Zung WWK, Cavenar JO: Assessment scales and techniques, in Kutsch IL, Schlesinger LB (eds.): *Handbook of Stress and Anxiety*. San Francisco, Jossey-Bass, 1980.

98. Theorell T, Rahe RH: Psychosocial factors and myocardial infarction. I. An inpatient study in Sweden. *J Psychosom Res* 1971;15:25–31.

99. Wyler AR, Mesuda M, Holmes TH: Magnitude of life events and seriousness of illness. *Psychosom Med* 1971;33:115–122.

100. Brown GW, Birley JLT: Crises and life changes and the onset of schizophrenia. *J Health Soc Behav* 1968;9:203–214.

101. Jacobs SC, Myers JK: Recent life events and acute schizophrenic psychosis: A controlled study. *J Nerv Mental Dis* 1976;162:75–87.

102. Jacobs SC, Prusoff BA, Paykel ES: Recent life events in schizophrenia and depression. *Psychol Med* 1974;4:444–453.

103. Cooper JE, Sylph J: Life events and onset of neurotic illness: An investigation in

general practice. *Psychol Med* 1973;3:421–435.

104. Tennant C, Andrews G: The pathogenic quality of life event stress in neurotic impairment. *Arch Gen Psychiatry* 1978;35:859–863.

105. Gorusch RL, Key MK: Abnormality of pregnancy as a function of anxiety and life stress. *Psychosom Med* 1974;36:352–361.

106. Andrews G, Tennant C, Hewson D, Vaillant G: Life event stress, social support, coping style, and risk of psychological impairment. *J Nerv Ment Dis* 1978;116:307–316.

107. Cassel J: The contribution of the social environment to host resistance. *Am J Epidemiol* 1976;104:107–123.

108. Roskies E, Lazarus RS: Coping theory and the teaching of coping skills, in Davidson P (ed.): *Behavioral Medicine: Changing Health Lifestyles.* New York, Brunner/Mazel, 1979.

109. Cobb S: Social support as a moderator of life stress. *Psychosom Med* 1976;35:375–389.

110. Dick-Reid G: *Natural Childbirth.* London, W. Heinemann, 1933.

111. Lamaze F: *Painless Childbirth: Psychoprophylactic Method.* Chicago, Regnery, 1970.

112. Boyd J, Weissman M: Epidemiology of affective disorders. *Arch Gen Psychiatry* 1981;38:1039–1046.

113. Noll KM, Davis JM, DeLeon-Jones F: Medication and somatic therapies in the treatment of depression, in Beckham EE, Leber WR (eds.): *Handbook of Depression: Treatment, Assessment and Research.* Homewood, IL, Dorsey Press, 1985.

114. O'Hara M, Neunabar D, Zekoski E: Prospective study of postpartum depression: Prevalence, course and predictive factors. *J Abnorm Psychol* 1984;93:158–171.

115. Mendlewicz K: Genetic research in depressive disorders, in Beckham EE, Leber WR (eds.): *Handbook of Depression: Treatment, Assessment and Research.* Homewood, IL, Dorsey Press, 1985.

116. Kupfer DJ, Reynolds CF: Neurophysiologic studies of depression: State of the art, in Angst J (ed.): *The Origins of Depression: Current Concepts and Approaches.* New York, Springer- Verlag, 1983.

117. Charney DS, Menkes DB, Heninger GR: Receptor sensitivity and the mechanism of action of antidepressant treatment. *Arch Gen Psychiatry* 1981;38:1160–1180.

118. Hollon SD, Beck AT: Cognitive and cognitive behavioral therapies, in Garfield Sl, Bergin AE (eds.): *Handbook of Psychotherapy and Behavior Change,* ed. 3. New York, Wiley, 1986.

119. Burish TG, Lyles JN: Effectiveness of relaxation training in reducing adverse reactions to cancer chemotherapy. *J Behav Med* 1981;4:65–78.

120. Bonica JJ: Pain research and therapy: Past and current status and future needs, in Ng LKY, Bonica JJ (eds.): *Pain, Discomfort and Humanitarian Care.* New York, Elsevier, 1980.

121. International Association for the Study of Pain: Classification of Chronic Pain. Supplement 3. 1986.

122. Melzack R, Wall PD: *The Challenge of Pain.* New York, Basic Books, 1983.

123. Genest M: Preparation for childbirth: A selected review of evidence for efficacy. *J Obstet Gynecol Neonatal Nurs* 1981;10:82–85.

124. Beck N, Hall D: Natural childbirth: A review and analysis. *Obstet Gynecol* 1978;52:371–379.

125. Scott JR, Rose NB: Effect of psychoprophylaxis (Lamaze preparation) on labor and delivery in primiparas. *N Engl J Med* 1976;294:1205–1207.

126. Klusman LE: Reduction of pain in childbirth by the alleviation of anxiety during pregnancy. *J Consult Clin Psychol* 1975;43:162–165.

127. Worthington EL: Labor room and laboratory: Clinical validation of the cold pres-

sor as a means of testing preparation for childbirth strategies. *J Psychosom Res* 1982;26:223–231.

128. Bergstrom-Whalen M: Efficacy of education for childbirth. *J Psychosom Res* 1963;7:131–146.

129. Stahler F, Stahler E, Gutanian R: Perinatal mortality of the child lowered by psychoprophylaxis, in Morris N (ed.): *Psychosomatic Medicine in Obstetrics and Gynecology.* New York, Karger, 1972.

130. Petrov-Maskakov MA: Physiopsychoprophylactic preparation for labor in pathology of pregnancy, in Morris N (ed.): *Psychosomatic Medicine in Obstetrics and Gynecology.* New York, Karger, 1972.

131. Cogan R, Henneborn W, Klopfer F: Predictors of pain during prepared childbirth. *J Psychosom Res* 1976;20:523–533.

132. Davenport-Slack B, Boylan CH: Psychological correlates of childbirth pain. *Psychosom Med* 1974;36:215–223.

133. Bonica JJ, Chadwick HS: Labour pain, in Wall PD, Melzack R (eds.): *Textbook of Pain,* ed. 2. New York, Churchill Livingstone, 1989.

134. Melzack R, Taenzer P, Feldman P, Kinch RA: Labour is still painful after prepared childbirth training. *Can Med Assoc J* 1981;125:357–363.

135. Fordyce WE: *Behavioral Methods for Chronic Pain and Illness.* St. Louis, CV Mosby, 1976.

136. Kriegler JS, Ashenberg ZS: Management of chronic low back pain: A comprehensive approach. *Semin Neurol* 1988;7:303–312.

137. Blanchard EB, Andrasik F, Ahles TA, Teders SJ, O'Keefe D: Migraine and tension headache: A meta-analytic review. *Behav Ther* 1980;11:613–631.

138. Holroyd KA, Andrasik F, Westbrook T: Cognitive control of tension headache. *Cognit Ther Res* 1977;1:121–133.

139. Achterberg-Lawlis J: The psychological dimensions of arthritis. *J Consult Clin Psychol* 1982;50:984–992.

140. McCann BS: The behavioral management of hypertension, in Hersen M, Eisler RM, Miller PM (eds.): *Progress in Behavior Modification.* New York, Academic Press, 1987, pp 191–230.

141. Rose RJ, Chesney MA: Cardiovascular stress reactivity: A behavior-genetic perspective. *Behav Ther* 1986;17:314–323.

142. Chesley L, Lindheimer MD (eds.): *Pregnancy, Report of the Hypertension Task Force,* vol. 9. Washington, DC, U.S. Public Health Service, 1979. NIH Publication no. 79-1631.

143. Doan-Wiggins L: Pregnancy-induced hypertension: Combating the dangers. *Emerg Med* 1990;3:29–35.

144. Agras WS: Relaxation therapy in hypertension. *Hosp Pract* 1983;5:129–137.

145. Agras WS, Taylor CB, Kraemer HC, Allen RA, Schneider JA: Relaxation training: Twenty-four-hour blood pressure reductions. *Arch Gen Psychiatry* 1980;37:859–863.

146. Crowther JH: Stress management training and relaxation imagery in the treatment of essential hypertension. *J Behav Med* 1983;6:169–187.

147. Southam MA, Agras WS, Taylor CB, Kraemer HC: Relaxation training: Blood pressure lowering during the working day. *Arch Gen Psychiatry* 1982:39:715–717.

148. Benson H, Shapiro D, Tursky B, Schwartz GE: Decreased systolic blood pressure through operant conditioning techniques in patients with essential hypertension. *Science* 1971;173:740–742.

149. Blanchard EB, McCoy GC, Wittrock D, Musso A, Gerardi RJ, Pangburn L: A controlled comparison of thermal biofeedback and relaxation training in the treatment of essential hypertension: II. Effects on cardiovascular reactivity. *Health*

Psychol 1988;7:19–33.

150. Engel BT, Gaarder KR, Glasgow MS: Behavioral treatment of high blood pressure. I: Analysis of intra- and interdaily variations of blood pressure during a one month baseline period. *Psychosom Med* 1981;43:255–270.

151. Engel BT, Glasgow MS, Gaardner KR: Behavioral treatment of high blood pressure. III: Follow-up results and treatment recommendations. *Psychosom Med* 1983;45:23–29.

152. Bloom LJ, Cantrell D: Anxiety management training for essential hypertension in pregnancy. *Behav Ther* 1978;9:377–382.

153. Wing RR, Nowalk MP, Guare JC: Diabetes mellitus, in Blechman EA, Brownell KD (eds.): *Handbook of Behavioral Medicine for Women*. New York, Pergamon Press, 1988.

154. Lorber D: Diagnosing type II diabetes: Don't wait for the crisis. *Emerg Med* 1990; 45–50.

155. National Diabetes Data Group: Classification and diagnosis of diabetes mellitus and other categories of glucose intolerance. *Diabetes* 1979;28:1039–1057.

156. Epstein LH, Beck S, Figueroa J, Farkas G, Kazdin AE, Daneman D, Becker D: The effects of targeting improvements in urine glucose on metabolic control in children with insulin-dependent diabetes. *J Appl Behav Annal* 1981;14:365–375.

157. Wing RR: Improving dietary adherence in patients with diabetes, in Jovanovic L, Peterson CM (eds.): *Nutrition and Diabetes*. New York, Alan Liss, 1985.

158. Wing RR, Koeske R, Epstein LH, et al: Long-term effects of modest weight loss in type II diabetic patients. *Arch Intern Med* 1987;147:749–753.

159. Furhmann K, Reiher H, Semmler K, Fischer F, Fischer M, Glockner E: Prevention of congenital malformation in infants of insulin-dependent diabetic mothers. *Diabetes Care* 1983;6:219–223.

160. Bradley CF, King JF, Effer SB: Psychology in obstetrics: Extinct or extant? *J Psychosom Obstet Gynecol* 1987;6:49–57.

Index

Muscle relaxation, progressive, 349
Mutual support organizations, for perinatal
loss, 257
Myopathy, hypokalamic, 287

N
Naloxone (Narcan), 228
Narcan, *See* Naloxone
Narcissistic stage of pregnancy, 244
National Association for Perinatal Addiction
Research and Education (NAPARE),
164-165, 176
National Drug Abuse treatment referral
hotline, 176
Nausea, 298. *See also* Emesis gravidarum;
Hyperemesis gravidarum; Morning
sickness
behavioral interventions for, 356
Negative legacy, related to substance abuse,
176
Negative reinforcer, 351
Neglect, infanticide and, 16
Negligence, 22
professional, *See* Malpractice litigation
Neonatal complications of substance abuse,
170-172
Neonaticide. *See also* Infanticide
clinical findings, 189t
defined, 186-187
differential diagnosis, 189
maternal passivity in, 190
Neurobehavioral effects, of substance abuse,
in infants, 171-172
Neurologica diabolica, 214
Neurological signs, in hyperemesis
gravidarum, 287
Neurophysiology of pseudocyesis, 227-228
Neurosis
depressive, 119
hysterical, 206-209
Neurotic theory, related to emesis
gravidarum, 286
Neurotransmitters, 123
Newborn, *See* Infant
Nonmaleficence, 36, 37
Noradrenergic activity, depression and, 123,
125
Norepinephrine, 144
Nortriptyline hydrochloride, 130, 338
Nuclear families, 40
Nurses
attitude and reaction to abortion, 314-315
burn out, 315
Nutrition, changes, behavioral interventions
for, 354
Nystagmus, 321

O
Obsessive-compulsive disorders, 120-121
Obsessive ideas, in depression, 118
Obstetric complications
related to mental illness, 140
from substance abuse, 169-170
Obstetrical practice

changes in, 3
current problems in, 8
ethical dilemmas, 7. *See also* Ethical
issues
new reproductive technologies, 6-7
older pregnant woman, 5-6
prematurity, 5
prenatal care, 4-5
substance abuse, 7
legal issues, *See* Legal issues
Obstetrician. *See also* Physician;
Physician-patient relationship
attitude and reaction to induced abortion,
310-314, 316
training of, 319
Obstetrics, two-patient concept of, 32
Office environment, related to follow-up appointment after perinatal loss, 271-272
Older women
pregnancy in, 5-6
motivation for, 49
psychological adjustment to, 60
risk estimates for, 6
substance abuse in, 165, 166-167, 173
Operant and classical conditioning, 348, 350
aversion therapy, 352
reinforcement procedures and operant
interventions, 351
systematic desensitization, 351-352
Operant learning theory, 351
Operative complications, injuries related to,
malpractice and, 12, 13
Opiates, 165
in pseudocyesis, 228
Oral contraceptives, use, by adolescents, 59
Oral sex, 94, 297
Organic brain lesions, 337
Orgasm, 89
breast milk release during, 89
during late pregnancy, complications, 97
manual manipulation for, 95
during second trimester, 89, 90
Orgasmic phase dysfunction, 93t
therapeutic and prognostic factors in, 94t
Orientation, in delirium, 321
Ovulation, induction of, 248
in underweight women, 158, 158t
Ovum transfer, 39
Oxyphenomium bromide (Antrenyl), 292
Oxytocin (Pitocin), 99, 191
legal aspects of, 28

P
Pain
behavioral interventions for, 357
grief-related, 259
Panic disorders
diagnosis, 120
drug therapy for, 335, 336, 337-338
symptoms of, 73
Papilledema, 323
Pappenheim, B. *See* Anna O
Paranoid-delusional states, 218
Parent-child relationship, physician-patient
relationship and, 31-32